AMMA THERAPY

AMMA
THERAPY

A COMPLETE TEXTBOOK
OF ORIENTAL BODYWORK AND
MEDICAL PRINCIPLES

TINA SOHN
AND
ROBERT SOHN

Healing Arts Press
Rochester, Vermont

Healing Arts Press
One Park Street
Rochester, Vermont 05767
www.InnerTraditions.com

*Note to the reader: This book is intended as an informational guide.
The remedies, approaches, and techniques described herein are meant to supplement,
and not to be a substitute for, professional medical care or treatment.
They should not be used to treat a serious ailment without prior consultation
with a qualified health care professional.*

LIBRARY OF CONGRESS CATALOGING-IN-PUBLICATION DATA
Sohn, Tina.
Amma therapy : a complete textbook of oriental bodywork
and medical principles / Tina Sohn.
p. cm.
Includes index.
ISBN 0-89281-488-8
1. Massage. 2. Medicine, Chinese. I. Title
RA780.5.S64   1996
615.8'22—dc20   96-21032
CIP

Printed and bound in the United States

10 9 8 7 6 5 4 3 2

Text design and layout by Virginia L. Scott
This book was typeset in Life with Stone Serif and Copperplate as the display typefaces

Healing Arts Press is a division of Inner Traditions International

CONTENTS

PART ONE
THE PHILOSOPHY

PART TWO
THE PRINCIPLES

ACKNOWLEDGMENTS

We would like to express our sincere thanks to those who have contributed to the writing and production of this book.

Firstly, with deep gratitude we want to thank Faye Schenkman, diplomat in Chinese herbology and our senior student and therapist in Amma therapy and Oriental medicine for over twenty years, for being the major force in the proper expression of the principles and art of Amma therapy as presented in this book. Working side by side with us over the last two years, Faye was instrumental in organizing, coordinating, writing, and editing, putting in endless hours to insure that the true spirit of our teachings of Amma therapy, Oriental medicine, and the principles of wholistic health were accurately expressed in this text. Without her devotion, hard work, and initiative this book would not have been realized.

We would also like to acknowledge several individuals for their contributions to various chapters and sections in the book. Steven Schenkman, president of the New York College for Wholistic Health Education and Research and certified Amma therapist, contributed to the chapter on t'ai chi chuan, helped in organizing many of the aspects of the book from its inception through to its publication, and worked with us and his wife Faye on accurately detailing and recording the Amma therapy treatments. Dr. Sharon Borzone, D.C. and certified Amma therapist, assisted in detailing the channel diagrams and descriptions, creating a system for cataloging Tina Sohn points, and reviewing the galleys. Dr. Robert Borzone, D.C. and certified Amma therapist, contributed to the chapter on nutrition, developing with Dr. Sohn the contemporary sophisticated views of evolutionary medicine elucidated therein. Dr. Janice Stefanacci, Psy.D., contributed thoughtful insights to the chapter on ethics, an ever-important issue for bodywork professionals. Anneke Young, R.N. and certified Amma therapist, assisted in detailing the Amma therapy treatment assessments. Linda Saslow wrote the introduction on the history of Amma in America.

We extend our gratitude to Richard Rockwell for his original drawings, and to Marvin Mattelson, who drew additional illustrations for the basic Amma therapy treatment. Ruth Hallsworth, graphic designer, carefully remade the diagrams of the channels and helped to create the various charts in the book; Professor Wang Jin-Huai created the beautiful calligraphy on page 3.

Finally, we would like to thank Susan Davidson, project editor at Healing Arts Press, for her expertise in the editing of the manuscript and for her vision and support in making this into the first complete textbook of Oriental bodywork therapy.

Tina Sohn and Robert Sohn

FOREWORD

In looking back over how my path intersected with that of Dr. and Mrs. Sohn, I can only say that it was the most fortuitous event of my life. Sometimes in retrospect we can look over our lives and see a remarkable turn of events that results in something extraordinary occurring. So it was that I first met Robert Sohn in the summer of 1973. I had interrupted my doctoral studies in Chinese history at the University of Illinois to return to New York where my father was gravely ill, misdiagnosed with lung cancer—my first major interaction with the severe limitations of Western medicine. A relative who was a physician eventually correctly diagnosed my father's problem as pneumonia. Although he recovered from the pneumonia, my father had contracted hepatitis while in the hospital and was no longer able to work. His business failing, I could not return to school and so found employment teaching Chinese in two Brooklyn high schools. It was there that I became friends with another young teacher who in turn introduced me to her boyfriend, a karate student of Robert Sohn's. He told me Dr. Sohn was practicing acupuncture, which I had only casually read about in my studies, and to Dr. Sohn this man mentioned that he had a new friend who knew Chinese. Before I knew it I was translating acupuncture charts and texts from Chinese into English for Dr. Sohn; in those early years of the wholistic health movement there were very few books available in English on Oriental medicine. Becoming more fascinated as I read, I asked Dr. Sohn if he would treat me with acupuncture for some serious health problems that I had suffered with since childhood and had required years of ongoing medication. So began my excursion into the mysteries of acupuncture treatment and Chinese herbal formulas and the existence of energy, a concept I had never before considered.

Following a few acupuncture treatments and the implementation of some dietary changes, I was alleviated from major arthritic pain and severe allergies. I wanted to know more about energy as Dr. Sohn experienced it. By this time my relationship with Dr. Sohn was beginning to grow into that of student to teacher, and I was spending all of my spare time at his home with a growing group of students who were interested not only in karate and Oriental medicine but who had also come to hear Dr. Sohn teach about spiritual work. At his directive I began taking hatha yoga classes with his wife, Tina Sohn, to further work on my arthritic joints.

It was in my first yoga class that I was initially exposed to Mrs. Sohn's extraordinary sensitivity and powers. As she walked by me at the start of class she looked down at me and asked what was wrong. Before I could respond she took her finger and pressed an acupuncture point in my cheek. Miraculously the pain of a tooth extraction that had been lingering for weeks was gone. To this day I remember the initial experience of her finger seemingly melding into the point and touching the energy body to dissolve the pain. Mrs. Sohn had no prior knowledge of the extraction that had taken place weeks before, and there was no visible evidence of any swelling on my face. She said "That's better," and proceeded to walk to the head of the class; my eyes followed her as I sat in utter amazement, realizing that something extrasensory had just taken place, something on an energetic level. I knew I wanted to understand it. When I asked Dr. Sohn about my experience he told me about Amma therapy and Mrs. Sohn's royal background, about her early brush with death, and about her grandmother/teacher, a traditional Oriental physician in Korea who healed her granddaughter with Amma, acupuncture, and herbs. He explained his wife's extraordinary sensitivity, her empathic abilities, and her healing art.

When Dr. Sohn began expressing his vision for a wholistic health center as a means of revolutionizing health care in this country, I was so inspired by the idea that I wanted to be a part of it. When Dr. Sohn asked his students who would like to study Amma with his wife, I was quick to volunteer. So began seven years of daily training in this profound healing art. I married the man who introduced me to Dr. Sohn and who would later serve as the president of the New Center College for Wholistic Health Education and Research begun by Dr. and Mrs. Sohn.

I apprenticed with Tina Sohn for seven years before I was allowed to begin doing hands-on healing work with strangers. As a beginning therapist I was required to watch Mrs. Sohn, observing the treatment to learn what techniques and points needed to be used. As I watched Mrs. Sohn not only diagnose problems that Western medicine could not, but also treat the energy system that underlies the physical body, I experienced the suspension of time and space and the existence of higher dimensions. I saw Mrs. Sohn move energy, give the patient some of her own energy, cure ailments, and relieve pain and suffering. No matter how many times I observed her treat a patient, the experience was never less than awesome as she encompassed her patient's mindbody complex and honed in on what the patient needed to do to heal himself. I saw her treat a twelve-year-old child who had languished in a hospital for three months coughing up blood, her condition undiagnosed after every imaginable test turned up negative. After just a moment of laying her hands on the child's head, Mrs. Sohn declared that the child's sinuses were bleeding. The child's father leapt to his feet as he stated that the child's sinuses had never been checked, that all the tests had focused on body processes that basically take place below the neck, as the main concern was the child's cough. A few Amma treatments later and with the help of some herbs, the child was perfectly healthy again.

One woman came in with mysterious fevers, severe joint pain, and a long history of antibiotic use. She was looking for a diagnosis and some relief. She, like many patients, had a long history of medical tests that had all come back negative. As Mrs. Sohn was taking the patient's pulses she began to question her as to a possible history of high fever and deadly illness. At first the patient denied this and then suddenly recalled having suffered with malaria from a mosquito bite when she was a small child living in Europe. When Mrs. Sohn continued to question her regarding the onset of the current problem, the woman remembered being bitten in her garden by some bug that left a huge welt, one that lingered for days. It was soon after that experience that her symptoms began. Mrs. Sohn concluded that the bug bite had triggered a post-malarial response; she treated the patient and explained the process of detoxification. The patient complied with the treatments and recommendations and within four treatments was pain free.

Frequently when Mrs. Sohn would treat a patient with Amma therapy her intuitive sensitivity would immediately indicate to her whether the patient had been exposed to chemicals or if poor nutrition was at the root of his problem, and would often amaze patients by telling them exactly what they had been eating. Mrs. Sohn's sensitivity could cause her to become ill if she touched patients who

were on powerful medications, such as steroids or the drugs used in chemotherapy treatments. Unable to block the negative effects of these medications within her own body, she would absorb some of the drug into her system and begin manifesting their side-effects. While we always screened new patients to make sure Mrs. Sohn did not directly treat anyone who was on such powerful drugs, such patients would periodically make it to her table, as many of them had no idea what medications they were taking or when they were last taken. At those times Mrs. Sohn would be suddenly forced to leave the room ill and I would have to take over the treatment for her. Sometimes she would remain sick for days, and I would be left to ponder the mysteries of energy and sensitivity and her dedication to her art and her patients, for she always returned to treat again.

There were times when she would see upward of twenty patients in a day, treating and teaching wholistic lifestyle changes. Not all patients made those changes, but those who did found their health radically improved. In many cases the changes were lifesaving. At other times it was Mrs. Sohn who literally saved a patient's life. I remember quite vividly the time my husband had a raging fever for two days that did not respond to all my efforts with both Amma therapy treatments and herbs. Panic was starting to set in, but we were calmed by the knowledge that Mrs. Sohn was arriving that night from Florida. As soon as she walked in the door I asked Mrs. Sohn to see Steve. She went directly to him and began treating him with her wizard's fingers. After about twenty minutes of using her magical touch on points and channels, she moved an intestinal obstruction and the fever broke. Without Mrs. Sohn, my husband would have faced emergency surgery.

There was also the case of the young hairdresser with life-threatening asthma who came to see Mrs. Sohn desiring to breathe freely and to be rid of her inhalers and medications. Mrs. Sohn treated her, gave her strict dietary recommendations, and suggested quite strongly that she seek a new career, one in which she would not be exposed to chemical dyes and sprays. The young woman came for regular treatments, made radical dietary changes, and within months was breathing on her own, off all of her medications. She was so happy and impressed with her experience that eventually she began a new career as an Amma therapist.

A myriad of stories and case histories could be told, not only by myself but by other therapists who have worked closely with Dr. and Mrs. Sohn at the Wholistic Health Center. We as a group have borne witness to two remarkable lives, and to a vision that has blossomed as the New York College for Wholistic Health Education and Research. It has been our joy and privilege to be part of the teaching and healing that continues to spread among our many students and patients through the work of all our graduates.

Elucidating the principles of Amma therapy as taught and evolved by Mrs. Sohn by helping to put this book together has been a labor of love. Becoming a student of Dr. and Mrs. Sohn has inextricably altered my life in the direction of self-healing. After twenty years of practicing Amma therapy, observing Mrs. Sohn treat patients, learning Oriental medicine from Dr. Sohn, and working to

go beyond my own perceived limitations, there are days when I am treating when I find that intuition and sensitivity merge into higher levels of awareness. At those times I feel that Mrs. Sohn is in the room with me, instructing me and guiding my hands and fingers. Patients improve. I stand back in thankfulness and understand that I have been the recipient of a most wonderful gift.

Amma therapy is Mrs. Sohn's art and this is her book, a comprehensive text that explores Amma, a wholistic system of health care, as she has taught it. Advanced students can use the book not simply to learn the techniques but as part of their path to self-discovery. Beginning students should approach this book with respect for what has preceeded them and willingly put themselves under the authority of the teacher in order to learn what the teacher knows. Self-righteousness, an aversion to correction, or lack of willingness to accept a teaching in its totality has no place in the learning of Amma therapy. Beginners often approach profound arts with a full cup, thinking they "know better," and find that they must first empty that cup in order to learn.

Over twenty years ago I learned from Dr. and Mrs. Sohn that serious practitioners, no matter what their backgrounds, will find that there is always more to learn, more to know, more to understand. This book will help all healing arts students on their path.

Faye N. Schenkman
Dipl. Chinese Herbal Medicine
Dean of the School of Amma Therapy,
New York College for Wholistic
Health Education and Research

PREFACE:
THE ORIGINS OF
AMMA THERAPY IN AMERICA

Wholistic health care as we know it today had its origins in an ancient Chinese philosophy that regards man and the universe as one symbiotic and integrated whole. Developed over five thousand years ago, this philosophy began to be known in America in the 1970s as the fundamental underpinning of Oriental medicine. This was a time when yoga and other Eastern arts were being introduced into this country; outgrowths of the counterculture, they began to slowly enter the mainstream. The history of the wholistic health-care movement in America has been shaped by a small group of pioneers who, over the course of the last few decades, have revived these ancient bodymind-centered therapies or developed new techniques based on these therapies. At the forefront of this movement are Robert and Tina Sohn, whose vision was to articulate a wholistic approach to health and well-being that would positively impact the health care delivery system in America. This vision, sustained over many years, grew into a mission—to create a wholistic health-care facility that combined patient care with education and research. The personal histories of Tina and Robert Sohn provide insight into their paths of growth and development, and an appreciation for their impact on wholistic health in America.

At age three, Robert Sohn began asking questions that adults told him were unanswerable. His grandfather, an Orthodox Jew, was his first teacher, talking to Robert about a higher reality, a concept that few understood. After his grandfather died, Robert's questions were often dismissed with promises that he would understand when he reached maturity. His parents tried but ultimately could not answer the three fundamental questions that drove Robert Sohn, even at such an early age. Those questions were: What is the nature and purpose of reality insofar as I am an integral part of that reality? What is my nature and purpose in relation to that reality? and How shall I go about developing that nature and accomplishing that purpose?

His father looked for books that might help his son, and one day brought home a simple paperback on hatha yoga. It was a book that gave new direction to Robert Sohn's life. The book told him what he had been longing to hear—that through serious and long efforts at the development of the mind and body, one could learn the universal truth and experience that truth directly. Dr. Sohn practiced the exercises described in the book, which included exercises for physical strength and limberness, breathing techniques, and meditations. Throughout his childhood and teens, he continued to focus on the physical arts, practicing hatha yoga; gaining a fourth-degree black belt in tang soo do, a Korean karate system; and becoming a master instructor in t'ai chi chuan.

Robert Sohn studied philosophy in college. Following graduation he went to Korea as part of the United States Army, where he studied tang soo do, acupuncture, and herbal medicine. One of his teachers was Madame Ho Hyun, the grandmother of his future wife. Years of study and practice of the physical arts attuned Robert Sohn to subtle energies and taught him to channel the life force, or Qi, for many positive uses, from self-defense to healing to spiritual enlightenment.

Dr. Sohn used his knowledge of Eastern and Western philosophies, science, and the healing arts to serve as an active force in the development of the wholistic health movement. Over the years he has played a pivotal role in engineering the great shift in American consciousness toward natural, wholistic health care. As a master herbalist and acupuncturist, he has been influential in the promotion of acupuncture through legislative action in several states, particularly through the formation of the American Association of Acupuncture and Oriental Medicine (AAAOM), an organization for which he served as president for several years. Under Dr. Sohn's direction, the AAAOM, along with a core group of dedicated individuals who were also pioneers in the field of acupuncture, gave rise to the National Commission for Certification of Acupuncturists. The examination given by this organization is the basis of licensure in most states today. In 1986 Dr. Sohn was awarded the honor of Acupuncturist of the Year by the AAAOM for his outstanding service, dedication, and skills in the fields of acupuncture and Oriental medicine.

In keeping with his mission, Dr. Sohn founded two companies: Sunsource Health Products, Inc. and Mindbody, Inc. Through both companies Dr. Sohn has introduced millions of Americans to natural health technologies.

As his vision continued to grow, Dr. Sohn began to direct his energies in a new direction—toward planetary health and the environmental crisis that threatens our planet's ecosystem. He brought together noted scientists, engineers, and researchers to form another company, Sustainable Technologies, Inc., whose goal is to reform global energy practices and encourage environmental health.

Over the years Dr. Sohn has directed all of his knowledge and interests toward a single primary purpose: to help others understand the methods of spiritual development in order to promote individual growth. In essence, he has dedicated his life to serving as a teacher and spiritual leader. His mission to help others fulfill their true inner potential has taken him on a course from reforming personal health to reenvisioning planetary health. After all, inner potential can better be realized if one is in a balanced state of health, but what is the ultimate good of people enjoying better health if it is only a matter of time before the health of our planet fails? Dr. Sohn's vision reflects a deep understanding of the relationship between man, his environment, and the universe.

Tina Sohn was born into one of the eight hundred families who constitute the traditional ruling class of Korea. The royal Kim family was comprised of acupuncturists, artists, herbalists, philosophers, and masters of the martial arts. The women practiced the ancient healing arts while the men focused on the martial arts. Within the family, training in energy development and control began during childhood.

Along with the legacy of physical and spiritual training, Tina Sohn inherited a responsibility to the people she served. She began her training at the age of four, studying yogalike exercises and esoteric energy development. Her grandmother would execute a few Amma techniques on the child, then have her imitate these techniques to "help grandma feel better." Thus the basic skills of the Amma therapist were inculcated into the body and hands of the child with no need for intellectual intervention. To help with the necessary physical development Tina

Sohn trained as a long-distance ocean swimmer; by the time she was eleven years old she had attained the status of a champion endurance ocean swimmer. Her skill was so highly developed that she was invited by the Korean government to participate in the Olympic Games in the early 1950s. Her training was so stringent that it was not sufficient simply to win a seventeen-mile race in the Sea of Korea, but she was required by her coach/brother to win by several miles, and to accomplish this feat without straining. The significance of her success was not in the sport itself, but in the degree and intensity of training required to become a superior champion. Only by training in heat, cold, snow, and rain, when she was well and when she was ill, did Tina Sohn gain great strength and endurance.

When she was twelve years old, following the deaths of her eldest brother and her father within months of each other, Tina Sohn fell into a coma that lasted for thirty days. She awoke transformed—when she touched someone, she could actually feel that person's pain or illness. She "saw" her school teacher as a skeleton, and three months later he died of a consumptive disease. She felt pain in her kidneys while near a relative, and several weeks later he was hospitalized with severe kidney disease. Not yet understanding this ability to experience others' pain, illness, or distress, Tina Sohn believed that she was a demon who was causing these conditions in others. She tried to block the experiences, and for many years attempted to avoid contact and intimacy with other human beings. Only later did she realize her higher level of development and her ability to use her healing power to bring others to a state of wellness.

While still a teen, Mrs. Sohn was in an accident that shattered the bones of her right leg into nine pieces. After gangrene had set in, medical doctors in a Western-style hospital were ready to amputate the leg when her eighty-two-year-old grandmother removed her from the hospital. Over the next four years her grandmother worked the nerves in her leg, which the doctors claimed were dead, for sixteen hours a day, until she regained the use of the leg. To heal her granddaughter, the older woman used herbs, acupuncture, and Amma, the form of bodywork passed down for generations that Tina Sohn later evolved into a new healing art called Amma therapy.

At twenty-three, Tina Sohn met her future husband, Robert, who was then a soldier stationed in Korea and a student of martial arts. He was introduced to Tina's grandmother, from whom he began to learn acupuncture. During a sacred Buddhist ceremony Tina was told by a religious monk that she would marry Robert Sohn, and that he would become responsible for her training until she was thirty-five years old. After that time she would be released and would be responsible for her own growth.

Under the guidance of her husband and teacher, Mrs. Sohn pursued her destiny as a diagnostic sensitive and healer. She organized her diverse training into the development of Amma therapy, using it as a vehicle through which she manifested her inherent potential as a healer. Through her highly developed and disciplined skills as a therapist, she has been able to perceive an ailment and know how to heal it, often becoming the medium herself for healing. From years of self-study and internal psychological discipline and direction, this extraordinary healer with acute sensitivities and understanding learned to express her skills and to translate them into a series of diagnostic techniques that others could emulate.

When Tina Sohn came to America in 1964, she brought the healing art of Amma therapy with her. In 1976, Dr. and Mrs. Sohn founded the Institute for Self Development in Manhasset, New York—the first public expression of their teachings. For Dr. Sohn, the institute was the fulfillment of a fifteen-year-old dream—to provide an educational institution dedicated to the expansion of man's intellectual, emotional, and physical capabilities. Courses were offered in philosophy to promote intellectual development. For emotional development there were encounter groups, communication workshops, and counseling. Physical development was met by classes in hatha yoga, t'ai chi chuan, tang soo do karate, biofeedback training, nutrition, and health. Dr. Sohn introduced courses in the integrated healing arts, including Oriental medical principles and Amma therapy, which expanded from a twelve-week guide for self-learning into the basic curriculum at the New Center College. In total, the Institute for Self Development aimed to develop the three centers of the being—physical, intellectual, and emotional—in order that a student excel at whatever endeavors he or she would undertake.

As an outgrowth of the Institute for Self Development, the Wholistic Health Center opened one year later, providing health care that incorporated thousands of years of Oriental healing with modern knowledge and treatments of Western medicine. Patients were treated through natural, noninvasive therapies that were integrated for a truly wholistic approach to health care. Mrs. Sohn herself treated thousands of patients with Amma therapy, which became a registered service mark in 1990.

Dr. and Mrs. Sohn recognized that changing the face of health care must begin with wholistic education and training. That insight became their motivation to turn their attention to the evolution of a school and research center that would further develop and teach wholistic health practices and Oriental healing arts. They were inspired by patients who were requesting to learn the techniques that had helped to heal them, so that they could use these modalities to help others. Some of those first patients eventually became therapists and now teach Amma therapy.

In 1981 Dr. and Mrs. Sohn, along with the staff of the Wholistic Health Center, created the New Center for Wholistic Health Education and Research (now known as the New York College for Wholistic Health Education and Research). Located in Syosset, New York, the New York College serves as a regional health-care facility, a model for wholistic health care, a resource and innovator for other health facilites, and a school for future generations of wholistic practitioners.

The college's massage therapy program, its first educational program, started in 1981 and has since become nationally recognized. Students are trained in both European massage therapy and Amma therapy, and graduates qualify to sit for the New York State licensing examination to become licensed massage therapists. For students inter-

ested in more in-depth training, the program of advanced Amma therapy was created to allow for the propagation of this powerful healing art by exceptional students who demonstrated great sensitivity and kinesthetic awareness.

In 1992 the state of New York passed legislation licensing professionals to practice acupuncture, and the New York College's school for acupuncture was the first acupuncture program to be approved by the state's Department of Education. This was a milestone in the promotion of acupuncture through legislative action and a culmination of Robert Sohn's efforts over many years.

The college's programs in Oriental medicine and Chinese herbal medicine were both outgrowths of the school for acupuncture. The diploma program in Oriental medicine was a natural expansion of the acupuncture curriculum, while the diploma program in Chinese herbal medicine was the first three-year program of its kind in the United States to focus on Oriental medicine exclusive of acupuncture.

The program for wholistic nursing was created to meet a need for practicing registered nurses whose philosophy reflected wholistic principles and who were interested in caring for the bodies, minds, and spirits of their patients. The program, which includes the study of traditional Oriental medicine and Amma therapy, was designed to lead to the development of a wholistic nurse who is both an autonomous professional and an essential part of a health-care team.

All of the college's educational programs evolved over years of study and experimentation, and included a curriculum that integrated methodologies of the

East and the West for both preventive and curative medicine. In September of 1996, the Board of Regents of the New York State Department of Education awarded the New Center college status, making it the first New York college of wholistic medicine and the first educational institution in the United States to offer a college degree in therapuetic bodywork. As in the past, the emphasis at the New York College is on interactive education. Students study and train with a faculty whose members are intimately involved in many facets of the college. Most of the faculty actively treat at the Wholistic Health Center. Students benefit from their professional expertise in the classroom, as well as from assisting their instructors in the student clinics and observing the professional treatment of patients at the Wholistic Health Center.

The New York College clinic was started to provide both an opportunity for students to complete their training in a professionally supervised internship and for the community to benefit from therapeutic treatments in acupuncture, herbal medicine, European massage therapy and Amma therapy. By making these services affordable through the student clinic, the benefits of wholistic treatment modalities were extended to the general community.

As a resource for the community, the New York College has offered classes in t'ai chi and hatha yoga for both students and the public, with lectures on relevant health-care topics and workshops in varied subjects of interest to health-care professionals. The Wholistic Health Center, recognized as a pioneer in providing wholistic patient care, has integrated natural healing arts with patient education. Wholistic practitioners use comprehensive modalities such as Amma therapy, acupuncture, chiropractic, bio-feedback, Chinese herbal medicine, homeopathy, nutritional counseling, psychological counseling, remedial exercise programs, smoking cessation, and weight-management programs.

Since its inception the New York College has also emphasized the importance of research. The center formed several collaborative affiliations with nearby hospitals and universities to study the effects of different wholistic therapies on patients with various pathological conditions. By exploring new ways of combining ancient Oriental healing methods with current scientific advances or diagnosis and treatment, the New York College continues to function as an innovator in the field of wholistic health care.

Linda Saslow

PART ONE

THE PHILOSOPHY

1

WHAT IS AMMA THERAPY?

An introduction to Amma therapy must begin with a journey back in time to the origins of this ancient healing system, one that is rooted in the principles of traditional Chinese medicine (TCM). Whereas the use of therapeutic massage for healing is relatively new in the United States, therapeutic bodywork has been an integral part of the medical system in China for thousands of years.

In ancient Chinese, the word *am-ma* means "push–pull." The origin of Amma dates back approximately five thousand years to the period of the legendary Chinese Yellow Emperor, Hwang Ti. This mythical emperor, one of three legendary emperors of China, is credited with the authorship of China's oldest written medical text still extant, the great *Hwang Ti's Nei Jing* (known in English as *The Yellow Emperor's Classic of Internal Medicine*). While Hwang Ti's dynasty is recorded as 2697–2597 B.C.E., the first mention of this text is found in the annals of the Han dynasty, which existed from 206 B.C.E.–25 C.E. During this period China had a highly developed culture with a comparably evolved system of medicine, both rooted in a philosophy that included the earliest discussions of Yin and Yang and the Five Elements of the body as they related to organs and to the planets. Based on Taoist philosophy, the Chinese medical system expressed the belief that humans must live in harmony with the universe, known as the Tao or "the Way," and that they accomplished this through self-perfection, known as *teh*. Unlike American culture, the Chinese venerated their elders. From the Taoist monks the Chinese learned the art of living into a happy and joyful old age with health and vitality and an absence of disease.

Thus the doctrines of Chinese medicine developed through focusing not only on healing but on preventing illness as well, and the means employed toward these ends were therapeutic bodywork, acupuncture, herbalism, dietary therapy, exercise, meditation, and moderation in living. *Hwang Ti's Nei Jing* presented a wholistic picture of human bodies, the planets, and the universe, and provided the foundation of the entire medical system that is known in China today.

It is fair to suggest that, since oral tradition precedes written tradition, the ideas and concepts presented in the *Nei Jing,* if not the text itself, are of much older origin. Archaelogical excavations of oracle bones indicate that Chinese calligraphy dates back to at least 2,000 B.C.E. Early Chinese characters for massage recovered from stone etchings show a patient lying on a table with a hand working on the patient's abdomen, demonstrating that the use of massage therapy in the treatment of disease is thousands of years old. In *Hwang Ti's Nei Jing* we find one of the earliest written references to therapeutic bodywork. Chapter 13 discusses the different cures used by people of varying geographical locations in China, based on the four directions of the compass and the region

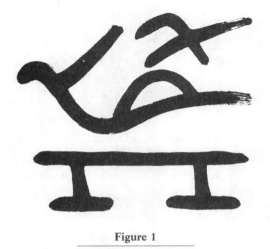

Figure 1

An ancient Chinese ideogram for massage

of the center. Each area was susceptible to different diseases and, as a result, different modalities were necessary for treatment. Of people living in the center, *Hwang Ti's Nei Jing* says:

> The people who inhabit the Center live on level, fertile ground and are able to obtain a varied diet without great exertion. Yet, they too are attacked by disease, mainly by complete paralysis, chills and fevers. The treatment prescribed for the people of the Center consists of massage, breathing exercises, and exercises of the extremities.

And chapter 27 of the *Nei Jing* says:

> One must first feel with the hand and trace the system of the body. One should interrupt the sufficiencies and distribute them evenly, [sic] one should apply binding and massage.

During the Han dynasty Chinese massage was known as *anmo.* Traditional physicians of this era were required to learn therapeutic bodywork as well as acupuncture and herbalism, because palpatory skills and sensitivity were essential for pulse diagnosis and channel and point location, as well as for diagnosis by touch. During the Tang dynasty (618–907 C.E.), therapeutic massage reached its peak. Recorded information from this period speaks of health professionals who used massage. These individuals were referred to as professors, healers of the highest respect. It was during the Tang dynasty that bodywork evolved to such a high level that a doctoral degree was offered at the Imperial

College of Medicine in Hsian, the capital of the Tang dynasty at the time. During this time physicians from Korea and Japan came to China to learn the healing arts, martial arts, and principles of Chinese medicine, and Buddhist monks trained in Chinese medicine brought these techniques to Korea and Japan. It was mandatory that anyone who wanted to become a doctor in Japan practice massage therapy. The Japanese called this practice *anma;* the Chinese principles of bodywork adapted by the Koreans were called by their ancient Chinese name, *amma*. Some evidence suggests that Jesuit priests who traveled to China and back again to Europe in the 1700s brought with them Chinese medical texts that contained information on bodywork techniques. It is suggested that this information formed the basis of what later became known as European or Swedish massage.

During the Sung dynasty (960–1279 C.E.) massage began to experience a decline, as touching became an inappropriate act among the nobility and the educated, and so massage fell into disfavor.* In succeeding dynasties the fortunes of bodywork rose and fell, ultimately declining with the growing Western military and missionary incursion into China. During the period of China's Republic (1911–1949), begun by Sun Yat-sen and continued by Chiang Kai Shek, traditional Chinese medicine came under increased scrutiny and skepticism. This came to a head in the 1920s when Chinese doctors who had studied

Western medicine abroad returned to China convinced of its superiority over traditional Chinese medicine. In the effort to thrust China into the twentieth century so that it could compete with the Western industrialized nations, anything of Western origin was seized upon as superior, including Western medicine. As Western medicine brought with it new techniques like surgery and the use of potent drugs, traditional Chinese medicine was overpowered by Western medicine and relegated to a secondary role among the middle and upper classes. But because the philosophy of traditional Chinese medicine was so much a part of Oriental tradition, the ancient healing arts survived among the masses, not simply in remote areas where it was not possible to obtain Western medicine, but even in the large cities where many continued to visit traditional physicians out of trust and belief in the traditional ways. In other Asian countries like Korea, the ideas of wholistic and preventive treatment were so profound that, even in the face of Western science, they could not be disregarded.

During China's civil war, the Communist soldiers who were forced up into the mountains by Chiang Kai Shek's troops were not privy to Western modalities and techniques and were forced to rely on traditional methods of medical care for their men. When the People's Republic of China was established in 1949, it was only natural that the medical modalities that had sustained Mao Tse Tung and his men be maintained as part of China's cultural heritage. It was also obvious to the Communist powers that the cadre of approximately seventy thousand Western-trained doctors was in no

---

* Therapeutic massage later came to be known as *tuina* during the Ming dynasty (1368–1644) and is still known by that name today.

way sufficient to offer medical treatment to a country of 650,000,000 people at that time. Traditional practitioners were called upon to help fill the void, and thus the "barefoot doctor" became a national fixture in the countryside and outlying regions of China.

Today medicine in China is a mix of both traditional Chinese therapies and Western medical techniques. Hospitals offering only traditional Chinese modalities exist side by side with those offering modern Western medicine. Therapeutic bodywork is considered a specialty and a doctoral discipline, with schools and hospitals devoted especially to its practice. The training involves five or six years of medical study with concentration in bodywork techniques.

It has been through the efforts of a small number of individuals that therapeutic massage has taken on a new life in the West. My years of training in Korea in amma techniques translated into a healing art that we know today as Amma therapy. Over the course of many years I evolved the technique to new levels and sensitivities. What emerged is a complex and highly refined system of bodywork therapy employing a wide variety of massage techniques and manipulations, and the application of pressure, friction, and touch to points and to channels on which the points are found. Rooted in the same fundamental medical principles as acupuncture and herbalism, Amma therapy focuses on the balance and movement of energy within the body. The techniques of Amma therapy aim to remove blockages and free the flow of energy in the body, thereby restoring, promoting, and maintaining optimum health.

Amma therapy is concerned with the balance and movement of life energy (Qi) in the human body. Whereas the acupuncturist will insert needles into these energy pathways to stimulate and move the energy and the herbalist will use appropriate herbal remedies to do the same, the Amma therapist relies primarily on the sensitivity and strength of the hands to manipulate and balance the life energy. Knowledgeable in related approaches, such as acupuncture, moxibustion (the application of heat to acupuncture points), skeletal manipulation, appropriate use of herbal medications, diet, and meditation, the Amma therapist is concerned with the flow and balance of energy in the pathways of Qi, commonly known as the channels, that form an energetic web throughout the body. The channels of Qi nourish and defend the body. As well, it is through these channels that harmful energies gain access to deeper regions of the body. The balanced and unobstructed flow of Qi through the channels is imperative for maintaining good health. Amma therapy utilizes all the techniques of the major forms of therapeutic massage. Deep pressure and point manipulation as used in shiatsu massage are applied in the administration of an Amma therapy treatment to attain the desired effects of energetic movement and release of muscular contraction. Foot reflex points are stimulated during the course of a treatment, a practice commonly known as foot reflexology. Stimulation of these points often has profound results on the deeper organs and tissues of the body. Deep fascial and connective tissue manipulation techniques similar to those used in Rolfing are part of the repertoire of the advanced therapist, as are the muscle stretching and pushing techniques commonly employed in European or Swedish massage. The master therapist is also well versed in the skeletal manipulations that form the basis of chiropractic. Amma therapy is therefore not simply a specific technique, but is rather a comprehensive healing art with a specific purpose and philosophy and a sophisticated mode of practice.

Amma therapy addresses all problems from this multisystem, multidirectional point of view. The process of assessment uses both Western and Eastern knowledge and techniques, combining traditional Oriental medical principles for assessing energy imbalances with a Western approach to organ dysfunction. A diagnosis is based on the Four Traditional Methods: looking, asking, touching, and smelling. This includes the assessment of every facet of the mind-body complex, including observation of the tongue; the taking of various pulses; palpation; and evaluation of diet, complexion, bowel movements, posture, emotions, vitality, personal likes and dislikes, smells, tastes, and sounds. Every sign and symptom reflects the internal state of the body and can be used in assessment, providing information about the psychological state of the patient as well as the prognosis of the disease or imbalance. Specific areas of the body are seen as a microcosm of the whole, revealing much about the entire organism. Once a comprehensive assessment is made and energy imbalances and organ dysfunctions diagnosed, the Amma therapist's hands and fingers can appropriately treat the body to remove blockages, free the flow of energy, and bring healing energy to problem areas.

In early civilizations, primitive people naturally sought to relieve pains by rubbing the body. The evolutionary position holds that Amma developed from early experimentation with rubbing that involved pushing and pulling the muscles of the body. However, the extreme sophistication of Amma makes such theories doubtful. This position is one that assumes evolution, while in the case of Amma and many other traditions of the Orient, devolution seems much more likely. Amma as practiced in modern China and Japan seems to be a devolved version of the original art in which the basic massage techniques are used exclusively, while the subtlety and power of Amma as recorded in the ancient texts has been lost. Given the profundity of Oriental medicine, beginning with the mapping of the energy patterns thousands of years ago, it seems clear that our ancestors were more sensitive to their subtle experiences than we are today; they were more aware of their bodies and could feel the flow of energy in their systems. While Oriental physicians of an earlier time generally never saw the inside of the human body, they were able to precisely delineate acupuncture points and knew the specific effects of these points on the physiology of the body. During that time they created charts describing the location of the pathways and their points, much of which has been confirmed by modern scientific research. The ancient texts of the "inner" or "soft" styles of the martial arts also indicate an awareness, sensitivity, and subtlety that is rarely found in practitioners of these physical arts today.

All arts—especially those that involve great attention to detail, extraordinary sensitivities, kinesthetic awareness, and control—are quite difficult to teach to others. The result is often a disintegration of the art, whereby the lower or more superficial forms of the original practices are taken on by the student. The intent of this book is to revitalize the practice of the ancient forms of Amma. As a tool for attaining these more subtle skills and sensitivities, this book will serve both as a text and reference for the serious student and Amma therapy practitioner, and as a detailed guide for knowledgeable bodywork therapists new to Oriental medicine. As sensitivity and awareness grow, so too will the effectiveness and beauty of the practice of Amma therapy. Due to the detailed and uncompromising way that Amma therapy has been taught at the New Center, it has begun to regain the respect it held in ancient years as a primary modality of healing, and in turn has helped elevate other forms of bodywork therapy to that same level.

At the Wholistic Health Center, trained practitioners have for over two decades used Amma therapy for both prevention and treatment of a wide range of disease conditions. Because Amma therapy works on both the Primary and Tendino-Muscle energy pathways of the body, it affects all the systems of the mindbody complex. It can therefore treat most illnesses. The decisions of what, when, and how to treat depends on a number of factors: the assessment of the therapist, the purpose of the patient's visit, and the severity of the symptoms and signs. Preventive Amma therapy treatments, along with proper diet and exercise, can discourage further pathological changes. In some cases Amma

therapy can reverse certain conditions; when a reversal of conditions is not possible, the therapist can at least alleviate the symptoms and pain.

The training of an Amma therapist emphasizes personal development. Great physical strength and endurance must be developed so that precise pressures can be applied without strain or fatigue. This physical strength must be accompanied by muscular control and kinesthetic awareness in order to provide the subtle differences in manipulative techniques that are necessary within the context of the treatment. All movements must be executed from the proper area of the hand without unnecessary strain on other muscle groups.

While the acupuncturist uses needles inserted into different points or loci in order to stimulate Qi flow, the Amma therapist uses the fingers toward the same general outcome. Achieving the proper effects of point application by the hand in Amma therapy requires sensitivity to pressure, angle, and force vectors, and a keen awareness of the use of the hands and fingers.

Sensitivity also plays a fundamental role in Amma therapy. The skill of the therapist in interpreting all the available data depends on the sensitivity and intuitive ability that develops from the continual application of knowledge with palpation. First, the practitioner must combine anatomical knowledge with the ability to palpate so that origins and insertions of muscles can be located, as can bony protuberances, sutures, and other anatomical landmarks. This sensitivity must also extend to the more evolved ability to locate with precision the superficial pathways of the channel system and points on these pathways. This requires a level of awareness and sensitivity that is tuned to the energy system. Amma therapy goes beyond the use of the fourteen major energy pathways (twelve Primary Channels and the Conception and Governing Vessels), also making use of the lesser known Tendino-Muscle Channels, the Connecting Channels, and the Cutaneous Regions. The Amma therapist must be prepared to feel extremely subtle changes in the skin as well as in the deep muscle layers. To help develop this sensitivity and ability to control the energy that flows within their own bodies, all Amma therapists at the New Center practice t'ai chi chuan.

Amma therapy can be a means for tremendous personal development for the practitioner, for ultimately the therapist develops the ability to use his or her own Qi to help heal others. For the Amma therapist, the highest level of accomplishment is becoming a healing sensitive—one who can experience a patient's pain, illness, and distress, and guide her hands and fingers to manipulate the appropriate points, channels, and tissues in order to bring the patient to a state of wellness. This ability to heal another is fundamentally unattainable unless a practitioner has brought herself to a state of health and vitality, a process that requires great self-awareness and inner control. The development of a true Amma therapist rests on the student's ability to develop control of her own inner emotional nature. When she is bound to her emotional experiences and to the pictures and ideas she has of herself, her ability to help another is severely limited. To break through the veils of fantasy and ultimately evolve into a capable Amma therapist, competent guidance in both physical and emotional directions is vital.

The exercises in this book have been used in the training of all Amma therapists at the New York College for Wholistic Health Education and Research. They represent the exercises that students have found most beneficial in preparing them for the rigors of practicing Amma therapy. The basic Amma therapy treatment used for general balancing and the more specialized treatments for specific conditions have been used successfully on thousands of patients at the Wholistic Health Center.

This book strives to codify and preserve an ancient healing art as it has evolved through the lineage of my family, and through my application and sensitivity.

THE DEVELOPMENT OF WHOLISTIC HEALTH CARE

A scientific approach to knowledge and understanding has characterized the dominant paradigm of reality in the twentieth century. The attempt to apply the methodology of the physical sciences to the biological and psychological sciences is called reductionism. Reductionists assume that by breaking things down into ever smaller pieces, greater understanding of that "thing" will emerge. While this approach obviously produces information, it results in a structural as opposed to a functional understanding of life. The application of this paradigm to medicine means that organs are removed, nerves are severed, and powerful pharmaceuticals are administered with little understanding of the consequences of such radical actions on the delicate biosystem of the living body. The prevailing viewpoint in the field of psychology is also structural. The mind is seen simply as the brain, with no existence separate from the structure of that organ. This materialist perspective disregards the dynamic, interactive quality of life processes, and therefore creates an artificial model of the human being.

Rapid technological development has brought with it a loss of the ancient wisdom of man's part in the ecosphere. In recent years we have been forced to reckon with the tragic effects of this loss. We now face a collective crisis in human health, evidenced by the appearance of new drug-resistant infectious organisms and the enormous rise in degenerative disease processes. At the same time, medical intervention has given more people the opportunity to live a longer life, a life that is often painful, crippling, and degrading. It is possible that historians will look back upon the relatively short history of reductionist-based medicine and see a great mistake—a folly as dangerous as the medieval practice of bloodletting.

To understand the evolution of reduction-based medicine, it is necessary to look back in time to the turn of the century. As civilized society began to move through the exciting and often painful birth process of the technological era, objective methods of investigation began to dominate scientific thought. This was not a sudden event, but was rather a logical result of many forces. The early work of Galileo and Descartes, as well as the work of physical scientists through the time of Newton, represented movement toward an intelligent attempt to systematically uncover mathematical relationships governing physical processes. The fields of medicine and biology demonstrated a long historical movement toward a more objective, systematic exploration of nature. Harvey, Darwin, Pasteur, and many others led the way toward seeking truths unencumbered by the dogma of religion. The refreshing winds of new discovery, unleashed by scientific method, carried the sciences toward seeking more objective methods in the search for knowledge.

At the same time the sciences were developing, the Christian church was fragmenting. Organized religion was weakening, and following centuries of directives and explanations given by religious leaders and based upon "God's will," a rebellion began to take place. This rebellion meant a negation of the spiritual and a concomitant deepening involvement with the material. The advent of the industrial and technological revolutions fueled the development of this materialist viewpoint. As never before, technology provided the means for exploration of the material world, and as the technology became available, physicists studied the nature of matter by attempting to break it down into its component parts by studying the properties of molecules, atoms, and subatomic particles. Physicists were studying inanimate matter (later discovered to be extremely animate) by reducing it to its most fundamental physical aspects. As technology evolved and physicists entered previously unexplored territories, great discoveries of atomic structure sped the advancement of technology.

Physics has always led the other sciences in the advancement of ideas related to the nature of the existence of the universe. As systematic methods of study were evolved by physicists, the other sciences sought to establish greater rigor in experimentation. With the rapid development of exploratory technologies, the biological sciences began to adapt a scientific method to the study of life. The method mimicked physics, and sought to use advancing technology to study life by breaking it down into smaller and smaller structural units. This approach gave primacy to biological structure, viewing function as a consequence of structure. While leading to enormous technological development and a greater understanding of biological mechanisms, it hardly offered greater comprehension of the nature of life. By looking at life microscopically, something was lost. By losing the awareness of the relationship between microcosmos and macrocosmos, scientists lost sight of the miracle of a living organism.

Like all great historical movements that were reactions to confined modes of thinking, the new surge toward materialism went to extremes. Scientific thought was directed toward what could be measured, and the new technology provided new rulers and scales with great rapidity. The trend in psychology then followed the biological and natural sciences. Classically considered a branch of philosophy, psychology, the study of the psyche, was suddenly considered a materialist study. Instead of adapting the use of scientific method to the classical study of psychology, it was suddenly declared a science and as a science it sought to provide objective measurement to human behavior. The approach of behaviorism aimed at studying smaller and smaller units of behavior in order to establish mathematical relationships by which one could measure and predict human action and response. Behaviorists felt that only observable phenomena were worthy of study. This approach soon became the dominant force of modern psychology, resulting in a concept of the human psyche that was measured by IQ scores, latency of response, and learning rates, but was grossly indifferent to the internal world of the mind.

Our health care delivery system reflects the reductionist bias in its orientation toward technological and mechanistic methods of caring for human beings. These extreme approaches have led to the nightmare of an extraordinarily complex, expensive, and specialized health care system. In the treatment of disease conditions, there is more emphasis placed on mechanistic manipulations available through surgery than on the importance of proper nutrition and exercise. The miracles of modern medicine have been accompanied by medical abuses that range from insensitivity and dehumanizing behaviors to the introduction of iatrogenic (physician- or drug-induced) diseases. Modern medicine has lost sight of health care methodologies that have endured, with good reason, for thousands of years. What is now considered medicine is just one of many approaches to treating disease and attaining wellness. In recent years, a rather ancient concept of the health/disease continuum has been resurrected and given the name *wholism*. The philosophy of wholism does not refute the potential value of reductionist thinking, but emphasizes the principle that the whole is greater than the sum of its parts. This important idea affirms the need to understand human health from a broad perspective. The human body is not a collection of organs, muscles, bones, and nerves, but represents something far more complex, integrating many systems that result in an ongoing dynamic process. Human beings have physical, emotional, intellectual, and spiritual lives that are intertwined and defy reductionist examination. Human beings do not exist in a vacuum but are part of the cosmos. The fact that each person exists within a physical, psychological, and spiritual environment is crucial to understanding the meaning of individual health. The word *heal* means "to make whole."

To understand health, one must have some understanding of the whole. This wider perspective (which includes reductionist information) is the basis of wholistic health care. Wholistic health shares a great deal with Chinese Taoist philosophy. The word Tao may be translated as "the Way of all things." Wholistic health care seeks to work in harmony with the Tao. That which opposes the Tao leads to disease. Comprehension of the Tao is not attainable by only studying at the level of the minutiae of cellular structure, but requires an ecological perspective of human health. Many intangibles are connected to the quality of life and the delicate balance of the human condition. As we acknowledge that our health is affected by factors that include human relationships, aspirations, and a rapidly changing society, old concepts of the boundaries between physical and psychological health must be radically altered.

A critical principle of wholistic health is that mind and body cannot be differentiated but instead must be seen as a single entity engaged in an ongoing dynamic called life. There cannot be a psychological problem that does not have a physical ramification, and the reverse also holds true. A constant dynamic exists between cognitive and physiological processes; this never-ending interaction between mind and body obliterates any clear distinction between the two. For example, heart attacks, with associated problems of hypertension and coronary artery disease, are highly connected to stress and one's psychological life. Countless studies have been done on the stress factors of modern life and the type A individual. Physicians today acknowledge the correlation between stress and heart disease, yet all too often they resort to their prescription pads for solutions. Such so-called solutions have made drugs like Valium among the most widely used

medications in the world. We recognize the negative effects of stress but at the same time we want quick and easy solutions. Consequently, we are the most drugged and drug-abusive society in history.

The concept of wholism, which expresses the unity of mind and body, hinges on a different approach to health care. It is impossible to treat a heart, arm, or lung as isolated from the dynamic of a living being. Since there is no division of mind and body, all diseases are of the mindbody, treatments are for the mindbody, and methods of maintaining health focus on the mindbody. In providing treatment, the wholistic practitioner seeks to follow a Taoist principle once eloquently expressed by Hippocrates: "First, do no harm." In *The Yellow Emperor's Classic of Internal Medicine* as translated from the Chinese, it is written:

The superior physician helps before the early budding of the disease. The inferior physician begins to help when the disease has already developed; he helps when destruction has already set in.

Taking a broad view of health, the wholistic practitioner recognizes that many cures are worse than the disease. With the advent of technology and potent pharmaceuticals, iatrogenic disease has become a major issue of modern health care. An examination of the ten top-selling prescription drugs includes a list of narcotics, diuretics, and anti-inflammatories that all have potentially dangerous side effects. A study done at Harvard University attempted to ascertain whether physicians prescribed drugs more based upon research papers or as a function of advertising by the pharmaceutical manufacturers. The study found that while physicians thought they were most influenced by research, their actual prescribing practices included drugs that were ineffective or had no value in treating the conditions for which they were prescribed. Although this information was available in well-documented research, the prescribing practices were a reflection of how the drugs were advertised. Hence, iatrogenic problems have become common. The view of a human being as a compartmentalized, structural phenomenon does not see the enormous potential damage of invasive methods on a carefully balanced biological system.

Wholistic health care tends to minimize these iatrogenic problems because it approaches human beings—the mindbody—with an almost religious awe. The recognition of the exceedingly complex nature of living things and the extraordinary web of interactive processes involved in health precludes the casual use of pharmaceuticals and invasive therapies. It requires a broader perspective of human health and a larger conception of time than the simplistic kill-the-symptom mode of healing. Wholism recognizes the profound power of health and healing to be inherent in the mindbody. Therefore, wholistic health practices seek to support and encourage healing whenever possible, rather than to force it. Such practices seek natural, safe, minimally invasive methods to help the mindbody heal itself.

Practitioners of wholistic health care tend to see themselves as agents or catalysts of the healing process, rather than as the source of healing. Much wholistic health practice is directed toward educa-

tion and the removal of sources of abuse to our health. However, when a patient is in an extremely critical, life-threatening situation, it may be necessary to use invasive and perhaps even dangerous procedures. Modern Western medicine excels in many procedures for acute and emergency health care as well as in its advanced diagnostic techniques. Wholism does not reject these methods, but values and integrates all approaches to health care.

A study of nonconventional medicine in the United States, published in the *New England Journal of Medicine* in 1993, found that nonconventional or alternative therapies have an enormous presence in the United States. According to the article:

> An estimated one in three persons in the U.S. adult population used unconventional therapy in 1990. The estimated number of visits made in 1990 to providers of unconventional therapy was greater than the number of visits to all primary care medical doctors nationwide, and the amount spent out of pocket on unconventional therapy was comparable to the amount spent out of pocket by Americans for all hospitalizations.*

"Unconventional therapy" was defined as sixteen interventions neither taught widely in United States' medical schools nor generally available in United States' hospitals. Among them were acupuncture,

---

* D. Eisenberg, M.D., et al., "Unconventional Medicine in the United States," *New England Journal of Medicine* 328(4):246–52 (1993).

chiropractic, and massage therapy. The majority of the respondents used non-conventional therapy for chronic, as opposed to life-threatening, medical conditions. Based on the results of the study, it was concluded that the use of nonconventional therapy in the United States was far higher than previously reported.

Wholistic approaches to health care emphasize changes in lifestyle, education, and overall patient responsibility. Patients must recognize that they are ultimately responsible for their own health and well-being based on their cooperative efforts with a professional. In seeking health, an individual must take an active role in the process: learning, making changes in daily habits, and eating and exercising properly. The potential of wholistic health care is actualized only when an individual moves from being a passive recipient to becoming an active participant in his or her own health and wellness development.

The wholistic practitioner has an additional responsibility beyond providing care and information. He must also serve as a model of the process. The relationship between patient and wholistic practitioner is not the "just do as I say, not as I do" relationship that is so often seen in allopathic health care. Obese, smoking, stressed out, and sedentary health professionals are living a lie. In ancient China, an acupuncturist did not treat patients when the acupuncturist was ill. A sickly physician was an impossibility. There is a great difference between being told about smoking, nutrition, and exercise by a practitioner who practices and understands what is expressed as opposed to being given a series of edicts by a practitioner who has no experience in their application.

Wholistic health care is health oriented. It seeks to avoid serious problems and prevent disease more than to quickly alleviate symptoms. This is in contrast to the disease orientation of the current Western medical model that focuses on the treatment of disease conditions rather than on the promotion of health. Although preventive medicine is part of the medical model, billions of dollars are spent each year on medical costs that are not for preventive measures. Insurance companies often reflect this bias, paying the costs for lung surgery but refusing payment for a program to help a person quit smoking. While the system is slowly changing, most people still see a doctor only when they are ill rather than working with a professional to develop their health to its maximum potential.

A wholistic approach is based on the theory that it is easier to maintain health, making minor adjustments in behavior as necessary, than to apply drastic intervention once the system has deteriorated to a serious condition. This is why the major "treatment" in wholistic health is education. Methods of treatment such as acupuncture, Amma therapy, herbalism, chiropractic, and biofeedback are necessary to help an individual return to health, but such therapies face an ongoing battle without a patient's commitment to making important changes in his or her lifestyle.

Perhaps the single most distinguishing characteristic of wholistic health is that it conceives of human beings in a way that is radically different from that of modern medicine. Unlike the reductionist viewpoint that sees the body in a materialistic way, the wholistic model views a human being as an energy system that controls and directs all physical functioning. The results of reductionist thinking have led to a medical system that is fragmented, where organs and systems are viewed in isolation from each other and structure is paramount. Thus, only repair or interference with structure is the basis of health care. A radically different and complementary concept of health care is the functional orientation that dominates the health care of the East. The energy model unifies and explains the other principles of wholistic health care, underscoring the need for a mindbody concept. Physical or psychological stresses often cause a disruption of the energy flow of the mindbody, resulting in disease. The disastrous effects of many medications and "simple" surgical procedures over time on the energy system are only beginning to be seen in the increasing number of iatrogenic problems. Many procedures, such as the indiscriminate use of steroids, simply mask symptoms while intensifying the problem and weakening the immune system. Wholistic health sees the energy system as underlying the physical system. For health to be maintained, the energy system, composed of opposing forces, must remain in a state of balance. Imbalance results in disease.

The implications of the human being as an energy system are profound, and must be explored in terms of human relationships, the effects of interactions between practitioner and patient, the quality of food and exercise, and ultimately the relationship between the individual and the cosmos. As material bodies we are individual beings, separate and distinct from one another. As energy fields, we are highly interactive and connected.

In summary, the delivery of wholistic health care reflects the following rational and pragmatic principles of health:

- A human being is a living energy system, not an arrangement of parts. Any disturbance in body, mind, or spirit reflects a disturbance in the whole system.
- Real health involves the whole person. Mind and body are integrated and inseparable.
- Wholistic health treats the whole person, not just symptoms and disease.
- Real health is not just the absence of disease, but a positive state of being.
- Real health is achieved by treating causes rather than symptoms, and by using natural and preventive approaches to health.
- In wholism, all approaches to health care are valued and integrated. Wherever possible, natural, low-risk methods that mobilize the individual's healing resources take precedence over drugs, surgery, and other hazardous therapies.
- Wholistic health recognizes the power of the body to heal the mind, as well as the power of the mind to heal the body.
- Each person has a responsibility for his or her own health and must be an active participant in his or her own healing.

The current theory of wholism was developed in reaction to the materialistic viewpoint of modern physics and its application of reductionism. With increasing technological development, modern physics has entered the world of subatomic or particle physics. Now the leading researchers in nuclear physics are articulating a very different view. The new physics claims that there is no material universe as it was previously understood. There is little more than the fabric of space itself, and the events that come in and out of existence from space itself. These events, which were first thought to be particles and are now considered to be wave packets, are clearly closer to our concept of energy than they are to our concept of matter. With this understanding one can better recognize the truth and wisdom of the ancient Chinese adage: "All that exists between Heaven and Earth is law and energy."

Physics is coming to the viewpoint that the universe is a highly interactive matrix of energies, each influencing one another in both direct and subtle ways. Einstein demonstrated the primacy of energy and the nonmaterial nature of reality. Bell's theorem suggests that the universe is completely interconnected, with events influencing each other without any restrictions on distance. Other theorists have offered similar notions of matter coming in and out of existence in a multidimensional matrix of reality. As physics has historically spearheaded the directions of study taken by the other sciences, it is possible that the reductionist-materialist-structuralist viewpoint has become outdated and that the new psychology, physiology, and medicine will be wholistic-energetic-functional. As we move in such a direction we will come to rediscover the truths that have existed for millennia, and, it is hoped, return to a place of greater rationality, humanism, and consciousness.

3

THE HOMEODYNAMIC MODEL

To the Amma therapy practitioner, identifying the causes and the patterns of disharmony of a patient's illness is of primary importance in developing a treatment plan. Without this knowledge, it is not possible to treat the patient effectively or guide her with appropriate recommendations that will prevent an exacerbation or recurrence of her condition and restore her energy system to harmony and balance.

The wholistic approach to health care is rooted in the Taoist philosophy of ancient China. The Chinese base their entire medical system on the idea of a polarity of forces that actively change throughout the day, season, and lifetime, but that maintain a certain balance. This philosophy regarded man as a microcosm of the universe and reflected on the relationship between man and his environment. In Taoist philosophy, the human being was considered to be an integral part of the universe, and universal forces were considered to be reflected in the human being. From this perspective it was imperative that man live in harmony with his environment—as an energy body comprised of the same universal energies, or Qi, surrounding him, he was highly connected and interactive with that environment. The ancient texts expressed this by saying "All that exists between Heaven and Earth is law and energy." Modern-day physicists have reached similar conclusions by their recognition that there is no material universe in the Newtonian sense; instead, the universe is a much more subtle and dynamic energetic process. Under normal conditions, the relationship between man and his environment is one of harmony and balance; when this balance is disturbed or disrupted, the source or origin of illness is born.

The corollary to these ideas in terms of physiology and its relationship to the external environment is found in the Western scientific concept of homeostasis. *Homeostasis*, or "steady state," refers to the bodily condition in which there is a balanced and harmonious functioning of all physiological activity. The human body is an exceedingly complex entity, activated in part by complicated biochemical, neurological, and mechanical processes that are all directed toward the maintenance of the delicate equilibrium that results in health. The continuum of energy moves from the finest energies, invisible to sophisticated scientific instruments, to the most dense, which manifest as organ, tissue, and bone. The body requires balance of its interactive functions on every level in order for health to be maintained. From a TCM perspective, this means that the energies moving through the body in complex pathways or channels, ebbing and flowing with specific times of the day and seasons, are actually regulating the functions of the organs and the body's complex physiological processes and helping to maintain the balance of Yin and Yang, Qi and Blood, and nutrient and protective energies.

This process is complex and extremely dynamic, with tides in the energy system causing constant changes of harmonious equilibrium. Rather than the term *homeostasis*, we use the term *homeodynamic* to emphasize the ongoing movement toward balance resulting from the activating and depressing functions of the various organ systems and the movement of energies throughout the system. This process is one of constant correction. A good analogy to the homeodynamic mechanism is the tightrope walker who must continually make subtle corrections as soon as any loss of balance begins to occur, lest he fall. Homeodynamic balance is the basis of function of the whole mindbody mechanism.

YIN AND YANG

In traditional Chinese medicine, the basic manifestations of the polar forces continually acting upon and within the human system are called Yin and Yang. The concept of antagonistic forces as being mutually supportive is not alien to Western medical thought. This concept can be recognized in the pairing of muscle groups into extensors and flexors, as well as in the complex chemical and neurological activities of the body, in that inhibition and stimulation are constantly at play to maintain the homeodynamic condition that is the organism's most stable state.

Yang is characterized as Heaven, Sun, Bright, External, Hollow, floating, and energetic, in relation to Yin, which is characterized as Earth, Moon, Dark, Internal, Solid, sinking, and material. Yet the energy of Heaven which is Yang moves down to become Yin and the energy of Earth which is Yin moves up to become Yang. The value of this concept of functional polarities is seen primarily in the differentiation of patterns that defines the basic diagnostic techniques of Oriental medicine. In relationship to the body process, Yang energies are considered to be activity and function, while Yin energies are considered to be the organs, structures, and vital substances of the body.

Oriental medical science further divides these two basic antagonistic/supportive forces of Yin and Yang into the Six Transitory Stages or Six Divisions of Yin and Yang and the Five Phases or Relative Motions (Energies), commonly called the Five Elements. In the Six Stages, the cycle of activity begins in the quiescence of the Great Yin, which then swells into the Absolute Yin. Absolute Yin, reaching the ultimate peak of Yin, turns rapidly into its opposite and becomes the Lesser Yang. The Lesser Yang grows into the Bright Yang. Then, swelling into the Great Yang, the ultimate peak of Yang turns rapidly into its opposite and becomes the Lesser Yin. In this way, Yin and Yang flow into, and thus transform into, each other. They are mutually supportive, yet they are in constant conflict. This flow of energies can best be shown in a modified representation of the classical Yin-Yang diagram (see figure 2).

The flow of Qi in the body shows clear patterns of ebb and flow, of increase and decrease, based on the Six Stages of Yin and Yang. The basic pattern of Qi flow in the organism begins at 3 A.M., as the Great Yin suddenly begins to rise, and peaks at 4 A.M., when its Qi drops off, rapidly passing into its opposite, the Bright Yang. As the Qi flows down from the upper torso it peaks in the Arm Bright Yang Colon Channel at 6 A.M., and then again in the Leg Bright Yang Stomach Channel at 8 A.M., where it returns to the Great Yin of the Leg, the pertaining organ of which is the spleen. The primary pathway of Qi continues through the remaining channels in a similar manner through the course of a full twenty-four hour cycle. This flow of energy from channel to channel is called the Nutrient Cycle; the times of the day when the

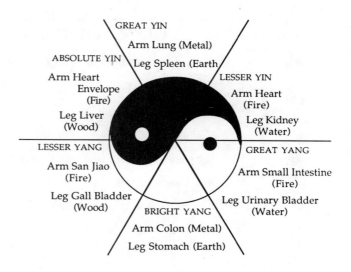

Figure 2

The Six Stages of the manifestation of Yin and Yang

energy is most active in a channel is known as the Cycle of Tides. These processes are summarized in the table on page 20, where '<' indicates increasing and '>' indicates decreasing from the peak.

THE PATTERN OF THE FIVE RELATIVE PHASES

The Five Relative Phases are commonly called the Five Elements. When Oriental medical concepts were first introduced to the West, the Five Elements theory elicited a negative response from many Western health professionals and others who knew that there were indeed more than ninety naturally occurring elements. But just as the ancient Greeks, in their philosophical search for the nature of the "underlying substance," used metaphors

THE NUTRIENT CYCLE AND CYCLE OF TIDES

CHANNEL AND PERTAINING ORGAN	PERIOD OF MAXIMUM ACTIVITY
Arm Great Yin Lung	3 A.M. < 4 A.M. > 5 A.M.
Arm Bright Yang Colon	5 A.M. < 6 A.M. > 7 A.M.
Leg Bright Yang Stomach	7 A.M. < 8 A.M. > 9 A.M.
Leg Great Yin Spleen	9 A.M. < 10 A.M. > 11 A.M.
Arm Lesser Yin Heart	11 A.M. < 12 P.M. > 1 P.M.
Arm Great Yang Small Intestine	1 P.M. < 2 P.M. > 3 P.M.
Leg Great Yang Urinary Bladder	3 P.M. < 4 P.M. > 5 P.M.
Leg Lesser Yin Kidney	5 P.M. < 6 P.M. > 7 P.M.
Arm Absolute Yin Heart Envelope	7 P.M. < 8 P.M. > 9 P.M.
Arm Lesser Yang San Jiao	9 P.M. < 10 P.M. > 11 P.M.
Leg Lesser Yang Gall Bladder	11 P.M. < 12 A.M. > 1 A.M.
Leg Absolute Yin Liver	1 A.M. < 2 A.M. > 3 A.M.

of major natural phenomena to describe the energies they were exploring, the East Indians and the Chinese used similar conceptualizations to express the relative forces at play in the universe in general, and used the same terms to describe similar forces at play in much more specific arenas, such as the human body. Thus the Five Relative Phases became the basis of much of the diagnostics of Chinese medicine.

The Five Phases, in most Yang to most Yin order, are: Fire, Water, Wood, Earth, Metal. The Five Phases correspond to organs, sense organs, tissues, colors, emotions, seasons, and climates, as well as other categories. The table on page 21 shows several of the important correspondences used in diagnostics. Clearly delineated in the medical literature, these correspondences formed the backbone of the diagnostic art of traditional Chinese medicine. Each major area

of concern was generally organized into a group of five aspects. In some cases there is a real correspondence, while others seem to be forced for philosophical continuity. Clinical experience is the best teacher of what is most true.

Although various combinations of the Five Elemental Phases are possible, two have great significance to the practitioner of Oriental medicine. Just as Yin and Yang are in a combined antagonistic/mutually supportive relationship, the Five Phases also show the same balanced stress in the Cycles of Creation and Control.

Figure 3 shows a graphic representation of the Cycles of Creation and Control. The outer circle shows the Creation Cycle, while the five-pointed star shows the Control Cycle. This pattern of relationship is based on the law of Mother/Son, in which Mother generates and nourishes Son, while the Mother of

FIVE ELEMENT CORRESPONDENCES

RELATIVE PHASE	YIN VISCERA	YANG BOWELS	SENSE ORGAN	TISSUE	COLOR	EMOTION	SEASON	CLIMATE
Fire	Heart	Small Intestine	Tongue	Blood Vessels	Red	Overexcitement (joy)	Summer	Heat
Earth	Spleen	Stomach	Mouth	Flesh	Yellow	Worry (excessive thinking)	Change of season*	Damp
Metal	Lung	Colon	Nose	Skin/Hair	Ash (white)	Sadness	Autumn	Dryness
Water	Kidney	Urinary Bladder	Ear	Bones	Black	Fear	Winter	Cold
Wood	Liver	Gall Bladder	Eye	Tendons	Green	Anger	Spring	Wind

* Earth corresponds to the transformation of one season into the next. This accounts for the large increase in Spleen and Lung syndromes in periods of seasonal transition.

the Mother controls the Son. Thus the Creation Cycle (the circle) shows that Fire is the Mother of Earth and therefore Earth is the Son of Fire; Earth is the Mother of Metal and therefore Metal is the Son of Earth, and so forth. The Control Cycle (the five-pointed star) shows that Fire, the Mother of the Mother of Metal, controls Metal; Earth, the Mother of the Mother of Water, controls Water, and so forth. Within the Creation Cycle, when the Mother is weak it does not feed the Son, weakening the Son in turn. Conversely, when the Son becomes excessive it can draw excessively on the Mother, injuring the Mother. In the Control Cycle, there can be either Overcontrol or an unnatural reversal (Insult), in which the controlled injures the controller. The complex relationships within the pattern of the Five Relative Phases constitute one of the most important diagnostic and treatment techniques of Chinese medicine.

Interpreting a common condition through the dynamics of the Five Phases shows the true wisdom of this traditional theory. If we think of the angry and stressful businessman who develops ulcers and finds it difficult to digest fatty foods, by studying figure 3 we can see how the Chinese functional model clearly explains this problem that only recently became slightly less opaque to the structurally oriented physician. Note the controlling function of the Wood Gall Bladder and Liver over the Earth Stomach and Spleen. Excess Anger is an overactivation of Liver Wood, which results in an overcontrol of Earth by

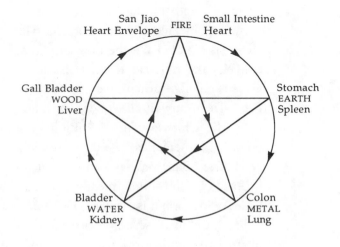

Figure 3

The Creation Cycle and the Control Cycle

Wood. This overcontrol injures the Spleen, (disturbing the whole digestive process) and further causes the Stomach to act inefficiently and eat its own lining, thus causing an ulcer. The excess of the Gall Bladder makes its digestive function highly inefficient, and the resulting condition is as indicated above. The Amma therapist must treat the Liver and Gall Bladder to calm and correct their functions, while treating the Stomach and Spleen to support and assist the Liver and Gall Bladder. Stress management and dietary recommendations would also be appropriate.

Traditional Amma therapy is based upon these concepts of Yin and Yang, the Six Transitory Stages, the Five Elements, and the Cycles of Creation and Control. Differential diagnosis is attained by studying these interrelationships. The same principles guide the course of Amma therapy treatments, directed toward the establishment and maintenance of the vital homeodynamic balance in the body through the treatment of the Tendino-Muscle Channels and the superficial pathways of the Primary (Organ) Channels, and through the activation of specific points along these channels. The channels conduct Qi, the bioenergy that enlivens the physical form. (Chapter 6 gives detailed information on these channels.) The term *point* is a poor translation from the Chinese. The definition of a point in mathematics is "a dimensionless geometric object having location but no property." The actual meaning of the Chinese ideograph is "cavern" or "hole," indicating that these points are not simply invisible dots positioned on the body but are actual openings into the energy pathways. Stimulation of these "points"

(as we know them) can move the Qi and Blood of the immediate area. Such stimulation also carries the potential to treat large areas or regions of body, as, for example, in treatment of the Lower Burner. Stimulation along the channels can affect the organ that is related to that channel and, through internal connections, affect other organs and channels as well.

A person is considered to be in a state of health when energy of the proper quality is moving through the system in a balanced, harmonious way. Health is defined as a state of vitality, well-being, and vigor. Overall, health is a state of ease. It is when the system ceases to be in a state of balance that "dis-ease" begins to manifest, reflected first in minor signs and symptoms and eventually in more serious ailments. The homeodynamic model of health is a paradigm that seeks to show what happens when this delicate balance is disrupted. It expresses exactly what the various sources of imbalance are, as well as the different means for restoring harmony.

It is important to note that the bioenergy system will naturally tend toward homeodynamic balance and will seek to maintain that balance when a source of interference presents itself. From the wholistic perspective, there is no dichotomy between the mind and body. It is the complete, harmonious functioning of the mindbody that defines health. In this way we see the truth of the Taoist principle that the mindbody is a microcosm of the ecosphere, with complex relationships providing a check-and-balance system to maintain internal and external harmony. We have seen demonstrations of this truth in our modern world, where the destruction of rain forests on one side of the world can affect the atmosphere, producing far-ranging consequences that often have disastrous effects.

The homeodynamic model represents a functionally based interactive prototype where an effect on one aspect of the model often has extensive effects in other areas, demonstrating the unity of the mindbody complex. For example, an apparent structural problem catalyzing sciatica can also interfere with energy associated with the Bladder Channel, and subsequently produce energy blockages that will affect the genitourinary system. Conversely, an organ dysfunction can catalyze energy disturbances in its corresponding channel, inducing pain and discomfort along the pathway of that channel. Constipation, for example, can result in shoulder pain, since the Colon Channel moves through the area of the trapezius. It is therefore important that energetic blockages and areas of stasis be corrected, and, when possible, the sources of such imbalance be corrected as well.

THE INTERNAL SOURCES OF DISEASE

Many different factors can disrupt the balance of the homeodynamic system. These factors were carefully delineated thousands of years ago in ancient Chinese medical texts and are still as relevant today, for as long as man must interact with his environment, he must strive for balance with it. Traditional Chinese med-

icine categorized the various sources of disruption into internal and external sources. While useful for the purposes of assessing the patient, it must be understood that these categories are not mutually exclusive. It is most common that many sources of imbalance interact to produce any disease condition. In fact, since the etiology of disease is so interactive and complex, it is sometimes difficult to differentiate the sources of disharmony of the energy system.

The section that follows is an examination of the internal sources of disease.

CONSTITUTION

The term *constitution* is used to describe the physical, emotional, and mental inheritance that we receive from our parents. In one sense, it is our genetic makeup, specifically determined at the moment of conception and dependent on the overall health of our parents, particularly upon their health at the moment conception takes place. At the moment of conception there is a fusion of the Pre-Heaven Essence, the Jing, from the mother and father, that manifests in our material world as sperm and ova. The constitution is also contingent on the health of the mother during pregnancy. If the mother smokes, drinks, or takes drugs (including medications), or suffers emotional stress during pregnancy, the constitution of the developing child can be adversely affected.

The Jing from both parents fuses and is then stored in the child's Kidney as the life force that will be responsible for the baby's growth, development, and ultimate reproduction, and will determine

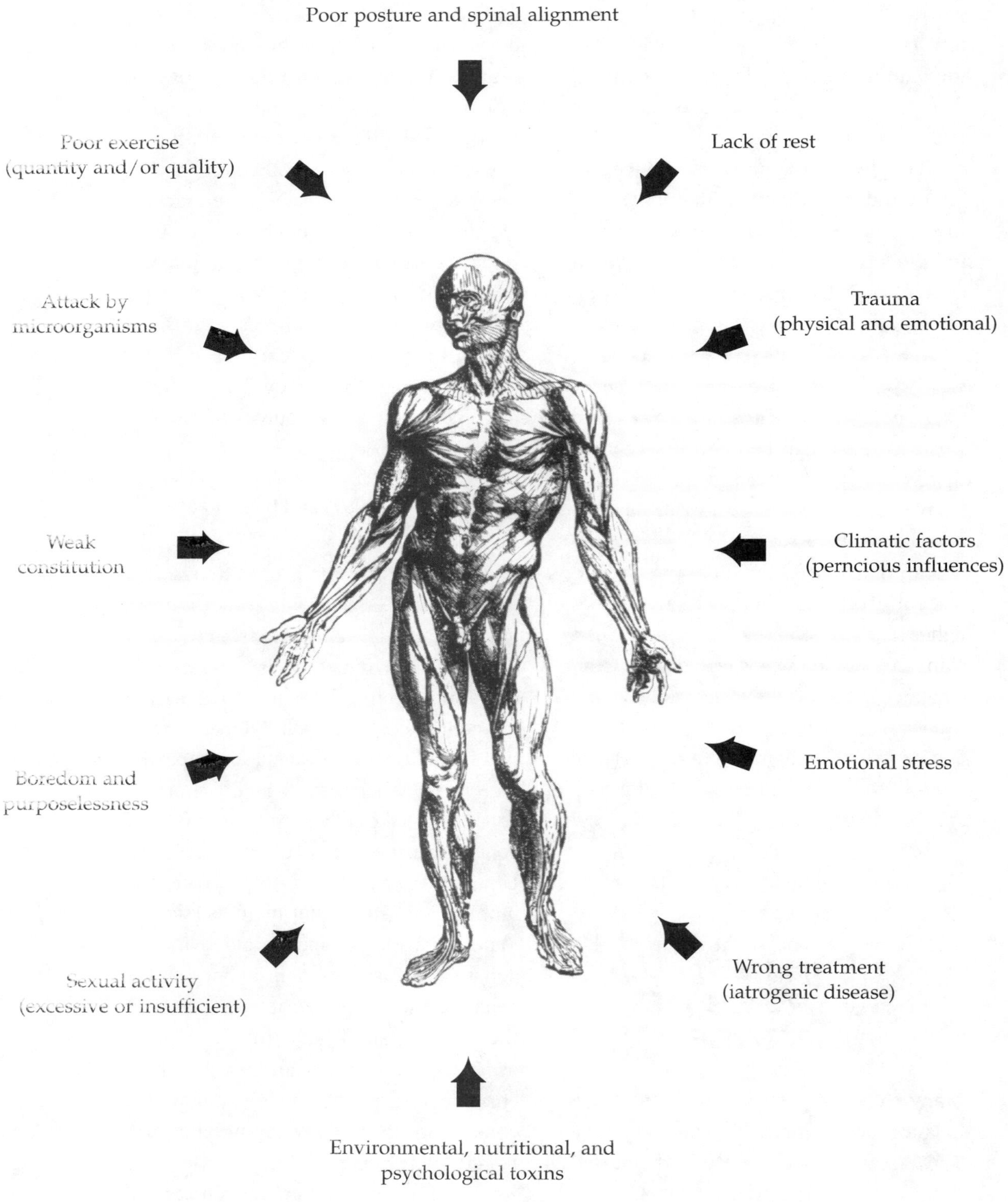

Poor posture and spinal alignment

Poor exercise
(quantity and/or quality)

Lack of rest

Attack by
microorganisms

Trauma
(physical and emotional)

Weak
constitution

Climatic factors
(pernicious influences)

Boredom and
purposelessness

Emotional stress

Sexual activity
(excessive or insufficient)

Wrong treatment
(iatrogenic disease)

Environmental, nutritional, and
psychological toxins

Figure 4

The sources of imbalance in the homeodynamic model

the length of the lifespan and the health of the individual during that time. To a large extent, what is inherited is fixed and cannot be changed. Some people are born with very strong constitutions while others are born with weak ones. However, to a certain extent the constitution can be improved, although it is much more difficult to build the Jing than it is to deplete it through alcohol, drug abuse, excessive sexual activities, and a stressful lifestyle. Preventive measures, proper energetic treatment, healthy nutrition, a balanced emotional life, and proper exercise can benefit the constitution and improve upon our inheritance.

For thousands of years the focus of Chinese medicine was mainly on the conservation and building of the Kidney Essence, and its transformation into higher energies. The driving force behind Chinese medicine was the Taoist monks, the Immortals of the Mountains, who quested after longevity and immortality through herbal elixirs, breathing exercises, and special forms of the martial arts, such as t'ai chi chuan. These inner schools of the martial arts were designed to build up the Jing and the vital energies of the body. The result of these efforts has been a wealth of knowledge and practices concerning the strengthening of the constitution.

It is important for the Amma therapist to get a sense of the patient's constitution from the assessment through the Four Traditional Methods, which includes gathering information from the medical history, pulses, tongue color, palpation, and inquiry regarding lifestyle and dietary habits. (The traditional methods of diagnosis are described in chapter 8.) Studies of inherited weaknesses, organ dysfunc-

tions, and congenital defects have resulted in the creation of several systems of somatotypology, that is, the categorizing of human beings according to their constitutional propensities toward certain diseases.

While such categorizing suggests exclusivity, most every person is actually a combination of types, having a unique pattern of innate strengths and weaknesses. For thousands of years traditional Chinese medicine has recognized the patient's physical appearance as representative of specific energies based on the theory of Five Elements. Hippocrates also recognized varieties of types and temperaments and their influence on disease. In the 1700s, physiognomy—the study of facial features to deduce temperament and character—was popular in France but later fell into disfavor. During the 1930s and 1940s in the United States, Dr. William Sheldon studied the most deep-seated similarities and differences between human beings, in order to differentiate between heredity or the constitutional patterns of the individual personality and the effects of environment. He believed this would help provide solutions to many social problems as well as further efforts to treat disease. It is interesting to note that a landmark study of somatotypes by Dr. Sheldon was maligned by many of his colleagues because catagorizing people was unfashionable in a democracy, where everyone is supposedly created equal. However, later studies on typology by Carl Jung, H. J. Eysenck, and R. B. Cattell supported Sheldon's theories.

It is helpful for the therapist to be aware of these studies of somatotypes, because they give him more information with which to assess potential sources of health problems. Clearly not everyone is born equal with regard to physical, emotional, and intellectual constitution. By having a good concept of the patient's constitution, the therapist will be better able to gauge the degree to which he can help the patient and the expectations for improvement, and can make specific recommendations on what the patient can do to strengthen his constitution.

EMOTIONS

Amma therapy recognizes that optimum health is achieved through the treatment of the physical body, the bioenergy, and the emotions that reflect and are bound into the neuromuscular system. At the core of treatment is the fundamental principle that everything is comprised of Qi, the only distinction between matter and energy being density. Emotions are considered a form of energy that play an integral role in the development of health or illness. In fact, TCM has traditionally viewed the emotions as one of the primary causes of disease. This is in direct contrast to the reductionist viewpoint of Western medicine, which has fragmented the human being and separated the psyche from the physical body. Western medicine has traditionally viewed the emotions as secondary factors to the cause of disease. A person suffering from ulcers sees a gastroenterologist and receives medication for his pain, but the stress that may be the cause of his problem is not addressed. In contrast, Oriental medicine recognizes the innate connection between the mind, the body, and the emotions.

Emotions become a causative factor in relation to disease when they are persistent and extended over a long period of time, when they are excessive and intense, and when they are not expressed but repressed. Because the mind, body, and emotions form a gestalt within the human being, emotions are not only a source of disease but can also be a result of illness. For example, anger harbored over a long period of time can injure the Liver; on the other hand, liver disease can be the source of angry outbursts and depression. Explaining these connections to the patient often relieves the patient's anxieties and fears as he comes to understand that his emotions are related to his physical problems and his physical problems are connected to his emotions. This helps the therapist guide the patient accordingly and, where appropriate, to recommend psychological counseling.

Traditional Chinese medicine acknowledges seven emotions. These are not meant to be narrow labels but rather broad and often overlapping categories. Each of the major organs is affected by and connected with a particular emotion that affects the Qi in a particular way. The seven emotions are:

+ Anger, which affects the Liver
+ Melancholy, which affects the Lungs and the Heart
+ Joy or Overexcitement, which affects the Heart
+ Fear, which affects the Kidneys
+ Worry and Excessive Thinking, which affects the Spleen and the Lungs
+ Shock, which affects the Kidneys and the Heart

Many of these emotions will turn to Heat

and Fire if they become intense and prolonged, because emotions lead to stagnation of Qi, and stagnation accumulating over a long period of time will give rise to Heat. To better understand the impact of these emotions on human physiology, it is helpful to examine them in greater detail.

Anger is an umbrella term for a host of negative emotions, including frustration, irritability, rancor, acrimony, resentment, deep-seated hatred, antagonism, hostility, and enmity. When these emotions become long-standing, they cause Liver Qi Stagnation or Liver Blood Stagnation, resulting in the rising of Liver Yang or Liver Fire. The resultant symptoms often affect the head and manifest as headaches, tinnitus, visual disturbances, and dizziness. Anger can also have a negative impact on digestion, as stagnating Liver Qi can invade the Middle Burner and disrupt the normal flow of Stomach and Spleen energies. Anger that is intense and chronic will often transform into depression. The classic example of this connection is the alcoholic whose emotions swing from angry outbursts to depression while his liver deteriorates from abuse. The more he drinks, the more dysfunctional his liver becomes, and consequently the more emotional he becomes; the more emotional he becomes, the more he depletes his Liver energies, and consequently the more diseased his liver becomes. In this way the diseased organ and the emotions become intricately intertwined in a negative spiraling cycle of illness.

Melancholy, grief, or sadness weaken both the Lung and the Heart, together known as the Upper Burner. This dissipates Qi, leading to Lung Qi and Heart Qi Deficiency, which manifest in such symptoms as fatigue, weak voice, depression, crying, shortness of breath, frequent sighing, and anxiety. Since the Lung is responsible for the descending and dispersing of Qi, Blood, and Fluids, the effects of Lung Qi Deficiency can be widespread throughout the system.

It is hard to imagine the emotion of Joy as being a source of disease, but it is more easily understood when we define an imbalance of Joy as a state of overexcitement that can negatively affect the Heart. Too much excitement or overstimulation is injurious to the Heart. We see this in people who crave excitement and live on the edge. Symptoms of Overexcitement include insomnia, restlessness, palpitations, and easy excitability. Overexcitement can also be a form of shock. For example, a person who is given a surprise party may experience a state of anxiety and suspension of Qi in his chest, which can have a negative impact on the Heart.

Fear causes Qi to descend and depletes the Qi of the Kidney. Fear can be a chronic, ongoing state of anxiety, dread, and fright, or it can be a sudden terror. Soldiers in battle who suffer incontinence when faced with potential death exemplify Qi descending from fright. Fear is also a frequent cause of enuresis in children. Fear is commonly experienced in later years as one's Kidney Essence wanes. Fear can also affect the Heart, as it can create a Kidney Yin Deficiency and a rising of Apparent Yang to the Heart, resulting in palpitations, insomnia, and night sweating.

Worry and Excessive Thinking entangle or knot the Qi, causing a stagnation of Qi that effects both the Spleen and the Lung. What is meant by Excessive Thinking is not a positive state of deep thinking but rather a state of excessive cerebrating, ruminating, or fretting. This includes thinking too much about past events, worrying about the future, and otherwise obsessing over things in one's life. It also includes excessive mental work, as with the student cramming for exams or the computer operator who sits for long hours entering data until his mind becomes foggy and unclear. Both Worry and Excessive Thinking can affect the Lung and cause shortness of breath, hunching of the shoulders, and a dry cough. In affecting the Spleen they can cause loss of appetite, fatigue, abdominal pain, and bloating, as the digestion becomes sluggish.

Shock suspends Qi and will affect the Heart and the Kidney. Anyone who has heard of the death of a loved one has felt that suspension of Qi at the news; this sensation results from a sudden dissipation of the Heart Qi, which can lead to palpitations, shortness of breath, and insomnia. Shock can also harm the Kidney because the Kidney will automatically seek to replace the suddenly depleted Heart Qi with Kidney Essence. This can result in Kidney Yin Deficiency symptoms, such as night sweating and dizziness.

It is important to note that, under normal conditions, emotions are not a cause of disease. Since energy is inherently neutral, the same emotional energies that can be misdirected toward illness can also be harnessed for positive growth and development. Each emotion has its positive side, an aspect that can be utilized for making a productive and wholesome emotional life. For example, the Yang energy of the Liver, with its tendency to rise, is a very powerful energy that, when brought under control and directed, can be used for making positive decisions and changes in one's life. The Liver's partner is the Gall Bladder, which gives courage to the decision-making process and works in concert with the Heart and Small Intestine. This courage comes from the positive directing of the Liver's energies, which are supposed to be free flowing and smooth.

The same energy that produces Worry and Excessive Thinking, which affect the Spleen, can be transformed into a powerful capacity for memory and the ability to concentrate and contemplate. The positive complement of Fear is willpower and the ability not only to have a strong memory but to be resolute and determined, focused and energetic in the accomplishing of one's goals. Properly harnessed, Kidney Qi is reflected in having specific aims in life and going after those aims with gusto and drive, not being easily discouraged by adverse conditions. Instead of depleting energy from the Heart, that same energy can be used to strengthen the Shen or Spirit of the Heart and improve mental functioning. The energies of the Lung can be used for strengthening breathing, which in turn helps to calm the mind.

The relationship between breathing exercises and meditation was recognized long ago by the Taoist monks of China as well as by Buddhists and practitioners of other esoteric philosophies. By focusing on breathing the mind is quieted, allowing the individual to reach higher levels of consciousness within himself. The best way of relating to one's emotions is not through disregarding them or repressing them but by acknowledging and facing them, and redirecting those energies for internal growth and development.

Emotional states are now being looked at by Western medicine with a new eye toward their relationship to disease. An accumulating body of research links psychological stress with emotions and disease. A study on the interrelationship between the mind, body, and emotions in cancer was done at the School of Radiation Therapy Technology, University Hospital and Clinics at Madison, Wisconsin, in 1990. The results of the study concluded that there is an interrelationship between the mind, body, and emotions in the fight against cancer. "Stress seems to play a key role in the generation and continuation of cancer and there appears to be cancer-prone personality patterns associated with the propagation of increased stress levels."[*] The new field of psychoneuroimmunology has recognized dramatic links between emotional states and the immune system, demonstrating that stress is associated with immunosuppression. This finding has resulted in the unprecedented sharing of information between the fields of psychiatry, immunology, the neurosciences, and endocrinology. As well, a significant body of research links emotional stress with cardiovascular and respiratory problems, which is easily understood in terms of the fight-or-flight mechanism in animal physiology. An article appearing in the July 1994 issue of the *Journal of Cardiovascular Nursing* stated that "the current biologic, unidimensional, reductionist, technologic approach to the treatment of heart disease must be expanded to include the psycho-social-spiritual dimension."[†]

Energy-balancing therapies, such as acupuncture or Amma therapy, can result in dramatic changes in emotional states, but serious emotional work is also necessary for real, permanent change. Many extreme disease conditions, including cancer, have been linked to general emotional states.[††] Continuing research in these areas gives further scientific confirmation to the truth of the homeodynamic model.

MUSCULOSKELETAL MISALIGNMENT

Musculoskeletal problems can manifest as poor posture, skeletal misalignment, or muscular tension, all of which can block the free flow of energy in the system and can result in various health problems. One of the fundamental concepts of the practice of t'ai chi chuan is the deliberate effort to maintain proper posture and detailed alignment of the limbs, down to the hands and fingers. Proper postural alignment allows energy to flow through the system, while misalignments result in Qi stagnation that bring a wide range of disease conditions.

Postural problems can result in muscles

---

[*] R. Morrison, "Interrelationship of the Mind, Body, and Emotions in the Cancer Fight," *Radiologic Technology* 62:28–31 (1990).

[†] B. M. Dossey and C. E. Guzzetta, "Implications for Bio-Psycho-Social-Spiritual Concerns in Cardiovascular Nursing" *Journal of Cardiovascular Nursing*, 8:72–88 (1994).

[††] S. M. Levy, "Biobehavioral Interventions in Behavioral Medicine," *Cancer* 50:1928–35 (1982).

being tense or in spasm, causing energy stagnation and blockages that then have a reverberating effect on the channels that pass through those muscles and their related organs. Chiropractic is founded around this concept, and is quite effective when used in conjunction with Amma therapy. Practices such as hatha yoga and t'ai chi chuan can be extremely helpful in maintaining musculoskeletal alignment. Most ancient wholistic therapies such as Amma and acupuncture include a number of techniques to establish realignment of the spine and promote energy flow through the system.

EXCESSIVE SEXUAL ACTIVITY OR INSUFFICIENT SEXUAL ACTIVITY

According to traditional Chinese medicine, the Kidney Essence manifests as sperm in men and as ova in women. During ejaculation for men and orgasm for women, some Kidney Essence is depleted, though under normal conditions this Kidney Essence is regenerated and is therefore not the source of disease. However, excessive sexual activity in which the body does not have the time or the proper energies to recoup what has been lost leads to Kidney Essence being depleted faster than it can be restored, ultimately causing Kidney Yin Deficiency. Logic dictates that this loss occurs more frequently in men, since through ejaculation sperm is releasd from the body, whereas in a woman's orgasm there is no such loss, although there will be some depletion. The fact that women retain more of their Kidney Essence probably accounts in part for the reason why women generally live longer than men. Taoist monks practiced special nonejaculatory sexual techniques to conserve and build their Kidney Essence. These techniques, also practiced in India as advanced techniques of Tantra yoga, were used as a way to build spiritual energies.

What constitutes normal versus excessive sexual activity is a difficult question to answer, as it is dependent on the health of a person's constitution, the quality of the Kidney Essence, and the overall strength of the Kidney. Sexual excess, however, is marked by lower back pain, fatigue, and genitourinary problems. It should be noted that women who have successive childbirths in a short period of time will also deplete their Kidney Essence, which can result in menstrual difficulties.

Lack of sexual activity is also a cause of illness, for the sexual organs need to be exercised in the same way that muscles need to be utilized to retain their strength and tonicity. Lack of exercise can lead to atrophy and to an accumulation of sexual energies, that, if denied their normal outlet, can be turned inward and become the source of disease.

Every Organ possesses both Yin and Yang energies. Yin energies refer to the vital energies and substances of the body, such as Qi, Blood, and Fluids, while Yang energies denote the activities or functions of the Organs, such as the sexual function of the Kidney. A strong and healthy Kidney will be reflected in healthy sexual desire. If there is frigidity, lack of desire, or an inability to attain orgasm or to enjoy sex, it is generally due to Kidney Yang Deficiency. However, if the Kidney Yin is Deficient, this can cause a flaring of Apparent Yang, resulting in excessive sexual desire. Both of these conditions can be successfully treated through Amma therapy, acupuncture, and herbal therapies. As stated earlier, the converse can also hold true. An unhealthy and unhappy sexual relationship or a relationship lacking in love and tenderness will lead to stress and anxieties. These emotions can deplete the Kidney Essence and encourage disease.

THE EXTERNAL SOURCES OF DISEASE

An examination of the internal sources of disease leads to discussion of the external sources of imbalance. The Oriental medical perspective postulates a broad definition of the concept of a pathogen. In Western medicine, the definition of a pathogen is limited to a microorganism or substance capable of producing a disease. The homeodynamic perspective recognizes a more expansive definition, one that includes negative energetic forces, climatic excesses, and environmental toxins and poisons as forms of pathogens. Anything that has the potential to be the source of disease, including microorganisms, is considered from the homeodynamic perspective to be a pathogen. The ancient Chinese forefathers of Oriental medicine did not have microscopes, and did little invasive work on the human body. However, by observing the changes in clinical signs and symptoms, they became acutely aware of how environmental changes could affect human health and disrupt the balance of Yin and Yang energies, Blood and Qi, and the flow of energies in the Organs and channels. Five thousand years of clinical evidence attests to the profundity of their observations, analyses, and treatment strategies.

THE SIX PERNICIOUS INFLUENCES

The Six Pernicious Influences, also referred to as the Six Excesses, Six Evils, or Six Devils, are the six climatic conditions of Wind, Cold, Fire, Dampness, Dryness, and Summer Heat. Normally the Protective Qi (Wei Qi) will shield the body from exogenous pathogenic factors as it circulates through the skin and the Tendino-Muscle Channels. The body has an inherent defense mechanism called Upright Qi or Zheng Qi that resists disease as the body seeks to maintain homeodynamic balance.* Climatic forces become a source of disease when the balance between the body and the outside environment is disturbed. This can occur when the weather becomes very unseasonable for the particular time of year or when the mindbody's protective energies weaken in relation to the climate. This weakening of the body's defenses does not necessarily indicate a constitutional weakness. A person can be generally quite healthy and still be invaded by climatic pathogens, if the pathogen is stronger than the body's defenses at the time of the attack. This demonstrates how environmental conditions carry a particular energetic influence, and emphasizes the interactive nature

---

* Zheng Qi is a general term encompassing the various Qi energies that protect the body from exogenous forces. Wei Qi is one type of Zheng Qi.

between man and his environment.

Exogenous pathogens are often seasonal. Summer Heat invasions occur in the summertime and Cold invasions are more dominant in the winter. However, the creation of artificial environments by air-conditioning and central heating allows for the manifestation of pathogens at any time of the year. People who work in occupations in which they are continuously exposed to certain pathogens, like butchers who have to go in and out of refrigeration units or marine biologists who spend much time in the water, are more susceptible to illnesses caused by exposure to those influences.

In addition to the Six environmental Excesses, the Chinese also postulated a seventh pathogen called Pestilential Qi, a term that refers to epidemic pathogenic factors that have the ability to enter the body through the nose and mouth. This type of Qi was thought to be contagious and quite poisonous, and was considered to be the cause of epidemic diseases centuries before the discovery of the microscope and microorganisms. Even in these situations, the resistance of the body's Protective Qi in relation to the pathogen was a primary factor in who fell ill and who did not as, even in the worst epidemics, some people always managed to survive. Current scientific research has shown remarkable parallels between bacterial and viral infections and the Six Pernicious Influences. Oriental methods of treatment for these pathogens have shown to be effective, and hold promise in the treatment of modern-day scourges such as autoimmune and immunodeficiency diseases.

Exogenous pathogens enter the body through the skin or through any orifice in the body, including the nose, mouth, and Lower Burner outlets, which include the anus, urethra, and external genitals. One of the major areas of penetration is in the back of the neck, where the Yang channels, which are the more superficial channels, converge. When a pathogenic factor lodges in the exterior portions of the body (the skin, muscles, or flesh, or in the superficial pathways of the Organ Channels,) it is considered an Exterior pattern, and is much easier to treat than when the pathogen penetrates into the deeper recesses of the body and into the organs themselves. Once that occurs, the resulting condition is considered to be an Interior pattern, even if it began with an exogenous invasion. If a person has a pre-existing propensity toward illness in a particular organ, he may be more easily affected by a particular pathogen's entry, since each organ is negatively influenced by one of the pathogenic factors.

Each of the six pathogens causes specific and unique types of clinical manifestations. For example, Cold causes muscle contractions and pain; Dampness is characterized as heavy and sticky and results in fluid accumulation and discharges; Dryness dries up the fluids of the body; Wind causes a rapid onset of symptoms, and the symptoms and signs move from place to place in the body; and Heat produces symptoms of thirst, fever, scanty urine, and constipation. Once they have penetrated into the body, many of these pathogens can alter their nature, most of them eventually turning to Heat.

Some diseases are the result of internally created pathogenic factors that have nothing to do with the exogenous factors but, because they mimic the manifestations of the external pathogens, they are given the same names. For example, internal Wind, mimicking the movement of wind in nature, causes tremors and convulsions, while internal Fire, in the form of Liver Fire Rising, can cause headaches, tinnitus, and vertigo. Treatments to rectify these imbalances are geared toward dispelling Wind, cooling Heat, moistening Dryness, draining Fire, transforming Dampness, and warming Cold.

MICROORGANISMS

In traditional Chinese medicine, any sort of infectious process, whether viral, bacterial, fungal, or parasitic in origin, is considered to result from the influence of microorganisms. The ability of the mindbody to resist disease is a direct function of its general state of health and its constitutional strength. Clearly, the more balanced the system, the greater its potential to resist disease mechanisms due to the harmonious functioning of the biological and psychological systems of the mindbody. Many people believe that infectious problems are caused by an invasion of the system by bacteria, viruses, and other such microbes. However, there are many kinds of microorganisms in regular contact or living within the ecosphere of the human body. More often than the presence of the microorganism, it is the disruption of balance that is the source of infectious disease. Usually the mindbody, when in a state of homeodynamic balance, integrates and tolerates the presence of such organisms in the system in the same way that the body adjusts to the influence of climatic factors. When a system is tending toward imbalance, microorganisms,

which tend to manifest in excessive numbers, can move the system quickly into a state of disease.

Infectious problems can also be simply a matter of poor hygiene. Attention to cleanliness is a simple yet powerful method of preventive medicine that is too often forgotten, since the focus of our culture is on external appearances, not internal cleanliness. As stated earlier, traditional Chinese methods of treatment have been found to be effective in the treatment of many infectious diseases.

ENVIRONMENTAL TOXINS

Exposure to pesticides or noxious chemicals, air and water pollution, noise pollution, or persistent stressful living or working conditions are other significant external factors that can lead to disharmony. People living in modern societies ingest, breathe, or touch toxic substances every day. Usually the mindbody is capable of ridding itself of such pollutants. However, excessive intake or extremely toxic substances can result in serious disruptions of the energy system. Petrochemicals, radiation, and asbestos are realities of a "civilized" society, as are food additives and artificial colorings, flavorings, and preservatives. Individuals have varying sensitivities to such substances. Contact with or ingestion of poisons is a central issue when evaluating a patient's pattern of disharmony.

NUTRITION

Improper nutrition is an obvious source of systemic imbalance. Foods filled with preservatives, stabilizers, colorings, hormones, antibiotics, and other substances that are not food demand more energy expenditure from the body as it endeavors to detoxify itself. Certain foods, such as highly refined carbohydrates, sugar, artificial sweeteners, and dairy products, put great stresses on the mindbody and can be responsible for disrupting the functioning of the internal organs, particularly the Stomach, Spleen, and Liver. When artificially manipulated, some foods become carcinogenic. Other foods become mucus forming, adversely effect metabolism, or are simply devoid of any nutritional value.

The effects of poor diet can manifest after many years or very quickly. Energetic treatments directed toward rebalancing the system are most effective when they are accompanied by intelligent dietary changes. The mindbody is capable of dealing with a great deal of abuse, but will eventually deteriorate when that abuse becomes chronic. Thousands of years ago, man did not have to ingest food that was tainted with chemicals. Modern practices in food raising, preparation, and storage pose problems that did not exist for our ancestors. Technological "advances" in food processing and preparation have resulted in changes in the energetic quality of foods in ways that are detrimental to our health. There is a clear energetic difference between foods baked by microwave and those prepared by conventional heating methods. A study reported in the renowned British medical journal the *Lancet* stated that microwave cooking transforms food in such a way as to cause "structural, functional, and immunological changes" in the body.* Unfortunately, the effects of such changes may not be understood until many generations later.

Poor nutrition not only includes eating nonnutritional foods; it also includes improper eating habits and eating an insufficient quantity of food. While we often think of malnutrition as a Third World problem, malnutrition also exists in modern society in less obvious ways. Current-day diseases of anorexia and bulimia can lead to malnutrition. As well, strange diets undertaken for the purpose of losing weight often cause weakening of the Spleen and Stomach. Senior citizens frequently are forced into malnutrition due to living on fixed incomes, or simply because they lack the ability or motivation to cook for themselves. Malnutrition will cause Blood and Qi Deficiencies and weaken the digestive organs. Overeating, a more common problem in our society and an increasing problem among our youth, will also weaken the Stomach and Spleen and lead to digestive problems. Modern-day habits of eating too fast, eating under stress, and eating on the run cause interference with digestion and can lead to long-term, chronic conditions.

MEDICATION

It is important to note that over-the-counter and prescription medicines are forms of poison and toxicity that can also severely affect the homeodynamic balance of energy. Medication should be used with extreme caution, because its

---

* G. Lubec et al., Amino Acid Isomerisation and Microwave Exposure (letter), *Lancet* 2(8676):1392–93 (1989).

prescription does not include an awareness of the homeodynamic balance but only seeks symptomatic relief. One of the great double-edged swords of our society has been the rapid growth of the pharmaceutical industry since the 1930s. The development of antibiotics initially saved many lives, however the overuse of antibiotics has led to a new phenomenon wherein one strain of bacteria can pass its immunity to particular drugs on to totally unrelated strains of microorganisms. As a result, antibiotics that would normally have treated those strains also become ineffective. The consequences of this situation are evidenced by untreatable strains of tuberculosis and other previously treatable diseases. As more and more strains of resistant organisms develop, the long-range effects of the overuse of antibiotics are still to be known.

The enthusiasm for the pill-ingesting approach to health care has also resulted in tremendous abuse and excess in both the prescribing and consuming of medications. A cursory look through the *Physician's Desk Reference* demonstrates the enormous number of side effects and contraindications for virtually every pharmaceutical. It is fundamentally problematic that many physicians and patients fail to recognize the fact that medications, while sometimes valuable and useful, are too often applied for symptomatic relief without consideration of the sources of the problem or the effects of those drugs on the whole mind-body system.

The rebirth of herbal medicine is one response to this problem. The herbal aspect of Oriental medicine approaches the mindbody from a wholistic perspective, which mitigates side effects.* As a rule, botanical preparations are less toxic than their synthetic counterparts and offer less risk to the user. One of the other advantages of herbs, as compared to drugs, is that they contain numerous active ingredients instead of one isolated ingredient. The constituents of herbs both within a single herb and within an entire formula are said to act synergistically to produce the desired actions and lessen side effects. In Chinese medicine, herbs are generally given for short-term use. The exception is tonics, many of which have been shown by modern scientific research to have adaptogenic abilities. An adaptogen increases resistance to negative influences through a wide range of physical, chemical, and biochemical processes, and usually produces a harmonizing action regardless of the direction of the pathologic state. An example is the tonic herb ginseng, which has been shown to have antistress and harmonizing qualities.

Many homeopathic physicians believe that the current use of medications to suppress acute symptoms can result in an increase of chronic diseases, such as arthritis or cancer, later in a person's life. It is possible that physicians may look back one hundred years from now and wonder how we could have been so cavalier in our overuse of drugs.

ACCIDENT

▼

Accident refers to any sudden trauma to the mindbody; this category includes

---

* Herbalism is one aspect of Oriental medicine, along with bodywork and acupuncture.

physical trauma; psychological trauma; and serious shocks to the mindbody system, such as the death of a loved one, divorce, or a change in careers. Any such trauma results in disruption of the energy system, causing stagnation of Qi and Blood and requiring that energy be directed toward the healing of the injury. Very often the system will simply return to balance as the injury heals, but in the case of severe injury, injury to vital organs, or injuries that directly disrupt the channel, some intervention is necessary. This could take the form of helping the injury to heal by promoting circulation, lymphatic drainage, and care for the wound, or by actually reestablishing the proper flow of energy.

Injury in the area of specific energy channels or acupuncture points can result in disruptive consequences that are either seen as separate, unconnected symptoms or produce problems months or years later. For example, a knee injury from years past may be the reason a person develops arthritis in that same knee after exposure to exogenous Cold that invades the area and comes to rest there. An injury to the index finger, which relates to the Colon Channel, can often result in constipation or diarrhea. Scar tissue along energy channels can also be extremely disruptive until the course of energy is restored or rerouted by acupuncture or Amma therapy. This is a consideration unknown to most surgeons, yet it often provides an explanation for unusual postoperative difficulties.

It is important to recognize that even apparently minor traumas can have far-reaching consequences. This recognition requires a shift in perception on the part of the health practitioner, since it requires seeing the patient in a time perspective, linking past events and other aspects of the health history to help understand the patient in his or her present situation. Disease conditions are rarely specific or simple in their etiology. Even apparently simple explanations, such as "I fell and hurt my knee," should be considered in larger terms. Does the patient have a history of falling accidents? Is there a propensity toward injury of a particular joint or side of the body? Is there a history of inner ear problems affecting equilibrium? The larger the perspective of the therapist, the greater the understanding of the patient's pattern of disharmony. On the other hand, it is equally important to recognize simple problems as such, and not to create pathologies that are not really there. Only through careful assessment and experience can such evaluations be made.

EXERCISE—TOO MUCH, TOO LITTLE, OR THE WRONG KIND

Our society is often one of extremes when it comes to exercise, exemplified by the disparate images of the jock and the couch potato. Proper quantity and quality of exercise is essential for good health, as is proper rest. A general lack of exercise results in weakness and atrophy of muscles, skeletal misalignment, poor circulation of Qi and Blood, and poor metabolism. Exercise is also the fundamental means of stimulating the lymphatic system and detoxifying the body via perspiration. Exercise reduces cholesterol levels and stimulates an increase in bone density, which reduces the risk of osteoporosis. Emotional well-being is also connected to proper exercise. Homeodynamic imbalance is a direct result of a lack of exercise.

The role of exercise in health care is becoming increasingly important in our sedentary society. Unfortunately, modern exercise systems are often as mechanistic as the reductionist health model. The idea of simply moving parts of the body or increasing cardiac and respiratory rates has become the popular conception of exercise. These approaches do not conceive of the homeodynamic model and miss the overall view of health. Excessive exertion that does not evenly exercise the whole body can cause stagnation of Qi. For example, jogging causes problems with the ankles and knees, and tennis causes problems with the elbows and wrists. Excessive exercise is harmful to young girls if engaged in during puberty, and can be the source of many genitourinary problems later in life.

For the most part, insufficient attention is paid by most people to quality of exercise. Exercise systems such as hatha yoga, t'ai chi chuan, and other martial arts are based upon establishing a balanced and unimpeded flow of energy in the mindbody. Such systems can be important partners to valuable mechanistic approaches, such as weight lifting, because they encompass a larger view of health. They are not directed toward a cosmetic approach to health or confined to a narrow view aimed at developing one aspect of the body, such as the cardiovascular system focused upon in aerobic conditioning. They are instead directed toward establishing homeodynamic balance. Certain types of movement that encourage excessive muscular, skeletal,

or cardiovascular stresses and are not carefully executed tend to result in imbalance, injury, and potential illness.

Generally, some exercise is better than none at all, and some exercises are better than others. When embarking on an exercise program, careful study and preparation are extremely important. The chosen exercises should be balanced in regard to purpose, needs, and the state of one's health. A program that includes some form of martial arts, t'ai chi chuan, or hatha yoga, in combination with weight lifting for maintaining muscular strength and tonicity and bone density, is the best system for maintaining overall well-being. Balance is always the key. A balanced lifestyle is the key to good health.

EXCESS WORK

There are basically two kinds of work: physical and mental. Because the Spleen rules the muscles and flesh, excess physical work can exhaust Spleen Qi. Overusing one part of the body can cause stagnation of Qi in that area—imagine, for example, the aching shoulder and arm of a waiter or waitress. An inordinate amount of standing or lifting will weaken the lower back and, in turn, weaken the Kidney. Excess mental work is often performed by people working in sedentary occupations, who usually also work under a great deal of stress. The continued concentration required of the bookkeeper or the individual sitting in front of a computer doing data entry can also weaken the Spleen. This, combined with poor and irregular eating habits, results in Spleen Qi Deficiencies and Stomach Yin Deficiencies.

Since a balanced lifestyle is essential for health, a proper balance must exist between work, recreation, and rest. When we engage in our work under normal conditions, we are using up a certain amount of Post-Heaven Qi, which is formed by the Stomach and Spleen. The Post-Heaven Qi is restored by the food and drink we take in, and by appropriate diet and rest. However, when a person works for long periods of time without sufficient rest to restore what has been lost, the body begins to deplete its Qi faster than it can be replenished. When that happens, the body begins to draw upon its Jing, the source of all energies. This leads to Yin Deficiency conditions that in turn result in more chronic and degenerative disease conditions and a shorter life span. Once again, the conditions brought on by excess work point to the need for regular energetic treatments such as Amma therapy or acupuncture, the use of appropriate herbal tonics, and the importance of energy-building exercises.

IATROGENIC SOURCES OF DISEASE

▼

The term *iatrogenic disease* refers to diseases that are induced by a doctor's actions. Iatrogenic conditions can result from incorrect treatment, as in treating a patient for a heart condition when he in fact has pneumonia, or they can result from side effects produced by medications or radical and invasive treatments, such as in the patient who receives thirty radiation treatments for his cancer only to die of cirrhosis of the liver induced by the radiation or in the patient who winds up with diabetes from years of high blood pressure medication. Unfortunately, iatrogenic disease is a growing phenomenon in our society, creating a new field in which reductionist physicians can now specialize. At the Wholistic Health Center, practitioners are confronted daily with patients suffering from the side effects of medications or from surgeries and tests that have caused new illnesses. One of the most gratifying features of Amma therapy is the absence of iatrogenic effects since Amma therapy is completely noninvasive and relies on the treatment of the energy body. The potential for iatrogenic effects does exist with herbs, however, since herbs have Organ and channel affinities. For example, if a patient suffering with a cold condition was prescribed cold herbs instead of warming herbs, his condition would worsen. It is for this reason that patients and students should never take herbs without consulting a qualified practitioner.

These categories of the sources of imbalance are not mutually exclusive; many of them are clearly interconnected and influence each other. The wholistic approach to health is essentially homeodynamic therapy—all efforts are directed toward helping the mindbody return to harmonious balance. The focus is to support and stimulate health and prevent illness rather than to simply treat a disease. While Amma therapists must often work to alleviate symptoms, they never lose sight of their aim, which is the prevention of disease and the maintenance of health. The various forms of homeodynamic interference clearly suggest that the Amma therapist should not work in a vacuum, but in concert with other wholistic practitioners to help restore homeodynamic balance. For example, chiropractic and exercise in conjunction with Amma therapy have proven invaluable for the treatment of musculoskeletal problems. Emotional stress can be reduced through psychological counseling, biofeedback, and exercise. Acupuncture is often alternated with Amma therapy treatments to treat a wide range of chronic problems.

The homeodynamic model offers a much broader approach to the disease process and a multimodality approach to treatment, where wholistic practitioners who share the same principles approach health problems as a team, working together for the health of the patient. The Amma therapist is a vital and integral part of the wholistic team. The success of the Wholistic Health Center, which employs the team approach to health care, attests to the efficacy of this method.

NUTRITION: EVOLUTION, THEORY, AND PRACTICE

Receiving proper nutrition is more than the sum of the processes of ingesting, assimilating, and utilizing nutrients. Our nutritional requirements are a reflection of the evolutionary processes that shaped our ancestors, and attending to those requirements by eating healthy food is one of the last connections we have to the natural world around us. Modern man has lost touch with and insulated himself from natural processes by creating a world of concrete and asphalt in which he is bombarded by electromagnetic fields and microwaves, lives in climate-controlled and artificially lighted rooms, breathes noxious fumes, and ingests refined, processed, and chemically altered foods. This trend toward "civilization" has eliminated the possibility of natural selection in our society. The homeodynamic mechanisms that determined the survival of our ancestors have become subordinate to the attempts of modern man to maintain his personal homeostasis by unnaturally controlling his health and environment. In his will to survive he has undermined the processes of natural selection, jeopardized his survival, and compromised his evolutionary potential.

The genetic makeup of each organism is constantly being honed and reshaped to fit the environments that organism encounters. A high degree of genetic diversity, healthy reproductive functioning, and random mutations from generation to generation makes more certain the survival of a species by allowing organisms to accommodate changes in their environment. Man has similar adaptive abilities, and any change that improves our chances of reproducing is beneficial to our drive to survive, which is the fundamental purpose of our genetic code.

Diseases are dynamic evolutionary processes in intimate relationship with environmental and ecological factors. Genetic tendencies are only manifested in an environment that allows their expression; by controlling our environment we can, to some degree, control the expression of our genetic code. In addition to our genetic material, we inherit certain social mores, customs, lifestyles, and eating habits from our parents. By living and eating in the same way as did our parents, we become subject to the development of similar states of dis-ease; however, by creating a healthier environment—that is, by changing our living and eating habits—the genetic propensity for an illness might be delayed or diverted by virtue of the fact that we are altering our internal environment.

Our genetic programming and our dietary habits work synergistically to fuel and regulate the adaptive mechanisms that influence our health. The most common causes of disease in childhood are trauma and diet. While both can produce problems in later life, it is diet that can more directly influence the child's adaptive abilities, and it is diet that is more easily controlled. Diet is the primary factor in fueling the growth and development of the child. When the reproductive capabilities of the child are realized, the adaptive mechanisms that optimize survival of the genetic code are fully operational, and the influence of diet is secondary to the evolutionary drive of the genes. The adaptive efforts of the child are focused on survival from day to day whereas in the sexually mature individual the focus is on the generation of offspring and the transmission of the genetic code through time. During our adult life, from puberty until the loss of our reproductive functions, the genetic drive to maintain life protects us by producing the adaptive changes to secure our survival that occurred in the generations preceding ours. Once our reproductive life span is eclipsed, diet and genetic programming no longer work synergistically to regulate adaptation and maintain health, and the likelihood of dying or developing senescent diseases increases dramatically.

Along with exercise, mental stimulation, and emotional stability, diet is an important factor for maintaining and protecting our health and influencing our survival as we age. Today osteoporosis develops quickly in postmenopausal women, and heart disease, our primary killer, is common in men over fifty years of age. Dietary intervention is extremely important for arresting and even reversing these disease processes. In our later years when the genetic program has aborted, diet and supplementation become significant factors in regard to our survival.

NUTRITIONAL REQUIREMENTS OF THE BODY

If we consider the body as an aggregate of physical and chemical parts that are organized and given form by an energy field, we can look past the conventional view of food as chemical substances and consider a more wholistic view, one that considers the properties, effects, tastes, colors, textures, and growing patterns of foods as reflections of their energetic qualities. Let's take as an example the differences in the qualities of a hot red pepper and a cucumber. The pepper is a hot, spicy, stimulating food that is a diaphoretic; the cucumber is a cool, sweet, moistening food that is a diuretic. Their effects and uses are different, and are predicated upon their energetic qualities. Cabbage and broccoli are both cruciferous vegetables that have antitumor properties, and both are green vegetables high in vitamin C. However, cabbage is a warming, sweet-flavored, moistening food that improves digestion, is high in iodine, and is good for certain thyroid conditions, while broccoli is a cooling, bitter-flavored, diuretic food that can disrupt the body's ability to use iodine and should therefore be avoided by people with hypothyroid conditions. If we considered only the vitamin, mineral, and fiber content of these foods, they would appear to be similar in nature; however, when their individual energetic qualities are taken into account, they are vastly different and have distinct uses and applications in the treatment of illness through diet.

A nutrient is any substance that affects the nutritive or metabolic processes of the body by either directly supplying or stimulating the production of some needed substance or energy in the body. In order to nurture the life of an organism, a food must supply some form of active energy. The quality and quantity of that energy will be determined by the nature of the food, how natural and unprocessed it is, how it is grown or harvested, and how it is prepared. For example, a fresh apple will produce a normal blood sugar curve as it is metabolized and assimilated by the body. Applesauce, with its reduced fiber content, will produce an increased fall in blood sugar values, indicating a greater

secretion of insulin by the pancreas. Concentrated apple juice, which is sweeter and has no fiber, produces an even more precipitous drop in blood sugar levels, requiring more work for the body to return to homeodynamic balance. This minimal processing of a natural food changes its qualities and results in physiological changes in the body.

Whole, natural, unprocessed foods will supply the most complete and easily assimilated nourishment. Similarly, refined, chemically processed, fragmented foods will be incomplete in their properties and insufficient or detrimental to the nourishment of the body. This difference can easily be seen by comparing fresh to frozen or canned vegetables or drinking fresh wheatgrass juice versus taking a wheatgrass supplement. The energy of freshly prepared foods is much greater than the energy of processed, prepackaged foods.

In order to consider what to eat and what not to eat, it is necessary to first consider the body's requirements. The desire for certain categories of foods, which is based on the need to survive, has changed over time as the availability of nutrients has changed and the genetic need has made these foods difficult to eat in moderation. For example, in agriculturally based societies of the past, the primary nutrients were vegetable-based proteins and carbohydrates. The occasional consumption of fatty meats or salty foods led to some type of advantage for survival that was naturally selected and produced a genetic craving for these rare dietary substances. As a result, these foods are still required components of the modern diet and are difficult cravings to overcome. However, fats and salt are now readily available in our diets and our cravings for them have led to excessive consumption and resultant illnesses. Our modern craving for refined sugar had similar beginnings as a favorable trait. In his book *Sugar Blues,* William Dufty describes the transition from the medicinal use of sugar in ancient times to its overuse and abuse in the modern diet. What may have once been a favorable trait has become an illness-producing habit that is difficult to overcome.

AIR

In addition to the proper balance of nutrients, the body is also fueled by the air we breathe. In the broadest sense, air is our most vital nutrient. We can only live without air for four to six minutes. Air brings oxygen, nitrogen, and other elements into the body. Of these, oxygen is the most important because of its function in the oxidative processes and biochemical reactions of the body. The final process of cellular respiration by the mitochondria of the cells is the splitting of the oxygen molecule and its coupling with hydrogen ions. Without oxygen, energy production is impaired and cellular respiration stops. Breathing exercises can help us to improve the intake and utilization of the vital nourishment that is in the air, thereby increasing cellular respiration. Proper intake of clean, unpolluted air is vital to good health. The incidence of asthma and other respiratory diseases continue to increase as the quality of our air continues to worsen.

According to traditional Chinese medicine, proper breathing allows the Lung to extract vital energy from the air. Da Qi, or the Qi of Air, is an essential component in the production of Nutrient Qi, which takes place in the chest. Nutrient Qi nourishes the entire body and is produced and distributed through proper breathing. Deep abdominal breathing, which allows the diaphragm to descend completely, will not only ensure the proper development of Da Qi but will also facilitate the circulation of blood, lymph, and Qi, increase gastrointestinal motility, massage the abdominal viscera, and conserve water (half of the daily loss of water is through the lungs and skin). This will result in increased physical strength (which is under the control of the Lung) and emotional calm, and an overall increase in energy.

WATER

Clean water is vital to every cell of the body. In *Job's Body,* by Deane Juhan, a human being is described as a connective tissue container invented by water so that water can walk around. He goes on to describe how the ground substance of the connective tissue, the most abundant tissue of the body, acts as a fluid crystal that fluctuates between a watery sol state and a viscous gel state. A constant supply of water is necessary to maintain the fluid sol state of this and all other tissues of the body. The body is approximately 70 percent water, and it is the medium in which all intracellular and extracellular transformations and reactions occur. As the need to metabolize waste increases, so does our need for clean water. An accumulation of wastes or mineral salts is likely if adequate quantities of water are not consumed; in fact, 75 percent of all kidney stones are caused by dehydration.

Adequate water consumption is considered to be 40 to 48 ounces per day.

Water quality has become a major global problem. The output of most water-treatment plants in the United States today is not satisfactory from a health standpoint, and it is necessary for people living in most locales to use spring water, or distilled or otherwise purified water, to avoid the residual chemicals present in municipal water systems and their carcinogenic and other negative effects. Mineral supplementation will alleviate any deficiencies that may result from drinking distilled or purified water.

In TCM, the Stomach is responsible for digestion; the Stomach needs adequate fluid in order to extract the refined essence from ingested food and drink. The Stomach uses body fluids and ingested fluids to perform its digestive function, and also ensures that body fluids are formed from the ingested food. When fluids are abundant, digestion will be good and the production of Nutrient Qi will be normal. When fluids are deficient, digestion will be poor and Nutrient Qi will be lacking, affecting one's overall health and vitality. The stomach normally secretes two liters of fluid per day, which is equal to the secretion of the entire small intestine. This fluid is essential for lubricating the digestive tract and liquefying the digested foods. Dehydration, a condition not uncommon to the elderly, can lead to constipation. Hypochlorhydria, a condition of diminished acid secretion, is another common digestive problem of the elderly that may be associated with dehydration. Clean water in adequate quantities is essential to the proper functioning of the Stomach and the production of Nutrient Qi.

In considering the Yin and Yang qualities of our food, we can say that the essence or energy of a food or the caloric fuel it provides is its Yang aspect, while the stored or structural components derived from the food are its Yin aspect. Generally speaking, the macronutrients that are the source of caloric fuel for the body are the Yang aspect of the diet, and the vitamins and minerals that constitute the noncaloric, regulating factors for our metabolic processes are the Yin aspect of the diet. Both constituents must be balanced, and both are mutually dependent on their counterpart for their proper functioning. Carbohydrates have both Yang and Yin qualities. The energizing, tonifying quality they possess is Yang compared to the stored (glycogen) and structural (glycoproteins of cartilage) forms, which are Yin. Proteins provide energy and create enzymes and hormones, which are metabolically active molecules with Yang characteristics. Proteins are also the basis for all the structural elements and connective tissues of the body, which are Yin in comparison. Fats contain more energy than any other food and form cholesterol and hormones, giving them a Yang quality. Lipids are important components of cell membranes and are stored in adipose tissues, both structure and storage being characteristically Yin qualities.

CARBOHYDRATES

▼

Carbohydrates are the primary energy source of the body. They consist of sugar units (saccharides), which are the fundamental fuel of the cells. The group of foods called carbohydrates consist of starches, natural or refined sugars, and celluloses (fiber). Starches, such as grains, vegetables, and beans, are complex or whole carbohydrates. These foods are the fundamental elements of a balanced, healthy diet. According to TCM, the sweet taste that complex carbohydrates provide has a tonifying and harmonizing effect on the body. The sweet taste that we associate with refined sugars found in soda, candy, ice cream, and the other confections we consume is so extreme that it cannot be balanced and therefore has no place in one's diet according to Chinese medicine.

PROTEINS

Proteins make up the basic structure of every living cell and are an essential life-giving and life-sustaining ingredient of the diet. Animal protein is more concentrated and has a warm or hot quality, which means it provides energy for the system. It is anabolic and promotes growth, making it important for building or strengthening during conditions of Deficiency. Vegetable protein is less concentrated, which means larger amounts are needed. It has a cool or cold quality which tends to draw from the system by breaking down and stimulating elimination. It is catabolic and therefore useful during conditions of Excess. A balanced diet will contain a variety of both vegetable and animal proteins.

FATS

Fats, an essential element of the diet, are necessary for the synthesis of hormones, cholesterol, and cell membranes, and for the transport of fat-soluble vitamins. From a TCM viewpoint, fats build tissues, enhance fluid metabolism, and direct nutrients into the nervous system. They also provide energy and warmth, which produce the feeling of satiety that is associated with fatty meals. In cold climates, a diet high in fat is superior to a carbohydrate diet for supplying deep, internal heat.

VITAMINS

The word *vitamin* is a general term for a number of essential organic compounds needed in small amounts for the normal metabolic functioning of the body. Vitamins are generally subdivided into two groups: the fat-soluble vitamins (A, D, E, and K) and the water-soluble vitamins (the B complex and C.) Each vitamin has specific functions in the body and is essential for proper metabolism, growth, and development. Although vitamins supply no calories to the diet, they are high-energy substances that catalyze various transformational processes in the body. Vitamins ingested in whole foods will be complete sources of this vital energy. However, due to the poor quality of commercially produced foods, our vitamin needs may not be met. Organically raised produce and grains are better sources, but the quality of the soil they are raised in is still questionable and will have an important impact on the vitamin and mineral content of these foods. It seems that supplementation is a viable alternative. Whole-plant or food supplements are preferred; for example, fresh wheatgrass juice will provide more

B vitamins, enzymes, minerals, and chlorophyll than a chlorophyll supplement or B-vitamin tablet. However, for reasons of practicality, a natural vitamin complex may be preferred. A high-quality supplement will contain no added preservatives, colorings, sugars, salt, or yeast, and will be produced from a natural source.

MINERALS

Like vitamins, minerals are only needed in small amounts, and are vital to the normal functioning of the body. Minerals are important regulators of hormones, enzymes, and muscle and nerve function, making them important components in the homeodynamic mechanisms of the body. All minerals in the body are in a delicate, dynamic balance; if a deficiency of one mineral exists, then others will also be out of balance. In nature, the elemental chemicals that our bodies require for survival are in inorganic forms that cannot be absorbed or metabolized. They are therefore transformed into organic, ingestible forms by land and sea plants. These chelated minerals are found in vegetables, seaweeds, grains, and some fruits. Eating a wide variety of organic vegetables, including seaweeds, and taking a high-quality supplement will ensure the proper intake of all required minerals.

FIBER

Fiber is the structural part of plants that cannot be broken down by human digestive enzymes. Fiber is found in the cell walls of all vegetables, fruits, and legumes. Water-soluble fibers, gums, mucilages, pectin, and some hemicelluloses, all found in fruits, oats, barley, and legumes, act to delay stomach-emptying and intestinal-transit time, and lower blood cholesterol levels. Water-insoluble fibers, cellulose, lignin, and some hemicelluloses, all found in vegetables, wheat, and cereals, act to accelerate intestinal transit time and increase fecal weight. Fiber encourages healthful bacterial growth in the colon, which aids in the assimilation of nutrients and the formation of cancer-resistant bowel acids. Refined and processed foods are low-fiber foods and tend to cause digestive problems, such as constipation. Improper colon function will lead to toxic buildup and liver congestion, which will produce changes in fat metabolism (increased cholesterol). The most balanced approach to fiber intake is to eat a variety of different types of fiber in the form of whole foods.

MILK AND DAIRY PRODUCTS

Breast milk is a maternally secreted fluid, a short-term nutrient for newborns. Nursing is an instinct provided by nature for only the very youngest of mammals. The mother of any mammal will provide her milk for a short period of time immediately after birth, and when the time comes for weaning, the young offspring is introduced to the proper food for that species. Man is the only species that drinks milk as an adult, and he drinks the milk of a different species!

According to traditional Chinese medicine, the excess consumption of dairy products produces a condition of

Dampness or Phlegm in the body by impairing the transportation and transformation function of the Spleen, much like sugar does. The mucus-forming properties of these foods is a manifestation of the Dampness they produce. This Dampness congests the body and leads to the development of abdominal distention, bowel problems, edema, cysts, tumors, yeast infections, urinary tract infections, upper respiratory infections, and allergies.

Here are several suggested alternatives to cow's milk.

- Soy milk is available in health food stores and some major supermarkets, or it can be made by blending 2 cups of ice cold water with 8 tablespoons of soy powder. Add vanilla, sorghum, barley malt, maple syrup, carob, or another sweetener to taste, then blend well.
- Rice milk and amasake, a brown rice kefir-like drink, can be found in health food stores. Rice milk and amasake are generally sweeter than soy milk. Like soy milk they include vegetable oils, but often have about half the fat of soy milk.
- Sunflower milk is another alternative to cow's milk. You can make sunflower milk by blending ¹/₂ cup raw sunflower seeds and 1 cup of ice cold water for 30–90 seconds, until smooth. Pour in additional cold water to fill the blender, and add a sweetener to taste. Blend to mix.
- Nut milk can be made by following directions for sunflower milk, substituting nuts or nut butter for sunflower seeds.

SUGARS

According to traditional Chinese medicine, the sweet flavor is Yang in nature and has warming, energizing, and ascending qualities that help tonify the body. Sweet foods build the Yin of the body—the tissues and fluids—thereby strengthening weakness and deficiency in general. The sweet taste that tonifies and harmonizes is different from the sweet flavor to which Westerners are accustomed. Sweet whole foods like fruits, grains, beans, and vegetables are complex carbohydrates that are balanced and provide a constant and enduring energy. When sugar is refined and concentrated in juices, white flour products, soft drinks, and candy, the natural balance of the food is upset and the energy becomes very dispersing. These foods then lose their tonifying and harmonizing qualities and produce imbalances in the energy system that lead to disease. The sweet taste enters the Spleen (pancreas) and Stomach, which are the root of Post-Heaven Qi, the source of vitality. These Organs are responsible for transporting and transforming the essences of foods and fluids into Qi and Blood to nourish the entire body. Excess consumption of sweet foods will impair the transporting and transforming functions of the Spleen and lead to Dampness, which will manifest as a heaviness, tiredness, and a congested condition that is associated with edema, obesity, hypoglycemia, diabetes, yeast infections, arthritis, menstrual problems, poor concentration, and emotional upset.

DIET AND WHOLISTIC THERAPY

In response to an ever-changing environment, man is constantly transforming in order to maintain balance. He must follow the natural changes that occur around him and adapt to the unnatural changes that he has produced through the creation of an artificial environment. By creating this environment he has stopped the process of natural selection as he is, rightly so, valuing the life of man for its own sake and is no longer allowing the natural selection process to operate. However, he has thereby lost the advantage his predecessors had gained through their adaptation by natural selection. What remains are uncontrolled cravings and maladaptive changes that are supported by his ingestion of unnatural, chemically altered foods. In order to maintain balance, a small portion— approximately 5 percent—of our diet needs to be "junk" food. This is in keeping with the homeopathic principle that "like cures like." Ingesting a small amount of a noxious substance will assist the body in resisting its harmful affects. By ingesting small amounts of chemically altered foods we can keep our systems honed for developing resistance toward these substances.

Wholistic treatment focuses on every aspect of the patient. Diet is an important part of the wholistic practice of Amma therapy. The foods a patient eats reflect his history and influence his present and future condition. Cravings for fat, salt, and sugar must be recognized and put into proper perspective when dealing with a patient and counseling him about diet. The genetic cravings for these foods should be considered when trying to adjust the diet, however they should not be used as a justification to indulge in cravings. A patient's diet should evolve as his needs change. Eating a variety of healthy foods will allow this process to proceed smoothly and harmoniously. Balance is the keystone of health, and diet can promote this balance or produce imbalance, depending on how healthy or unhealthy our food choices are.

Finally, it is important to recognize that a truly wholistic healing art such as Amma therapy not only looks at the present state of the patient but also considers the evolution of the patient's condition from past to present and into the future. The whole lifetime of the patient is thus incorporated into the treatment, and the recommendations evolve with each patient as his condition and health consciousness evolves. The superior Amma therapist is in harmony with the Tao, the constant contraction and expansion of the Universe, the constant flux of nature. The therapist's art evolves in concert with the changes around her and she rides the crest of the wave of change instead of merely being carried by its force. The Amma therapist tries to bring her patients to that same place of responsibility and control.

HIGHLY RECOMMENDED FOODS, AND THOSE TO AVOID

Making the transition to a more healthful lifestyle begins with basic dietary changes. Recommendations from the

U.S. government's report prepared by the Senate Select Committee on Nutrition and Human Needs include these suggestions:

+ Increase complex carbohydrates by consuming more fresh fruits, vegetables, whole grains, and legume products.
+ Decrease refined carbohydrates and processed sugars to no more than 15 percent of total food intake.
+ Decrease fat consumption from the present 40 percent to 25–30 percent of total intake by eating lean meats, less beef, and a greater proportion of poultry, fish, and vegetable protein. Trim fat from animal foods; do not eat the skin of poultry; be aware that most hamburgers are 50 percent fat; eliminate dairy intake; and eat little or no fried foods. Limit animal protein intake to no more than four ounces per day.
+ Change the balance of total fat intake to a majority of unsaturated fats. Try to effect a 2:1 ratio of unsaturated to saturated fats.
+ Limit sodium intake by decreasing total salt intake (content in all foods eaten) to one teaspoon per day.
+ Increase fiber intake significantly (fruits, vegetables, grains, beans, nuts, and seeds).

The following general dietary recommendations are based on the information that I have shared with Amma therapists and students for the many years that the Wholistic Health Center has been helping patients. Proper diet is a fundamental way to prevent illness and restore and maintain health. A general diet is offered

here to help begin the transition to a more healthful lifestyle. This diet limits, but does not eliminate, salt, refined sugar, and saturated fat intake. In addition, this diet will limit one's exposure to preservatives, colorings, and other chemicals that are added to our foods.

The recommendations made below should be implemented slowly to allow the body to adapt and better tolerate the change to a healthful lifestyle. For example, if you eat a lot of dairy products and sugar-laden foods and drink a lot of coffee, it would be wise to completely eliminate the dairy products first and then cut down on sugar and coffee consumption. Instead of six cups of coffee per day, reduce your consumption to three, and then to one and one-half cups. A slow transition is necessary to allow your metabolism to change and the detoxifying and eliminating pathways to be activated.

In eating a sensible diet, the following foods should be avoided:

+ Refined simple sugars: White, raw, brown, turbinado, or yellow sugar; honey; corn syrup; corn sweeteners, dextrose, and fructose. Dried fruit, raw honey, and maple syrup should be limited when a blood sugar imbalance exists. (Honey and maple syrup are highly allergenic, highly concentrated sugars that are excessively sweet.) Avoid all artificial sweeteners.
  Alternatives: Fresh fruit, malt barley, rice syrup, blackstrap or sorghum molasses, and carob—all in moderation.
+ Refined starches: White flour; bleached, enriched wheat flour;

degerminated corn meal; corn starch; white rice; rye bread; and white flour products (cakes; cookies; pastries; pizza; and most breads, bagels, rolls, and crackers.) These foods are essentially refined sugars and will produce the same negative effects as the refined simple sugars listed above.

Alternatives: Whole wheat and whole grain breads and pastas; artichoke pasta; brown rice and whole grains, such as barley, kasha, rye, oats, millet, quinoa, amaranth; potatoes.

✦ Chemical Additives: All additives, preservatives, artificial coloring agents, stabilizers, softeners, emulsifiers, artificial flavorings and sweeteners. These substances place an additional burden on the liver, which has to metabolize and neutralize these chemicals. Many of these chemicals are used to retard or stop bacterial growth and will have negative effects on the healthy flora of the gastrointestinal tract, producing a number of different digestive problems.

Alternatives: Whole, fresh, unprocessed foods.

✦ Beverages such as coffee, tea, cocoa, soft drinks, and alcohol should be limited. The various chemical substances found in these beverages will have adverse effects on the body, and thus should be moderated. The ingestion of alcohol or caffeine-containing beverages may produce temporary relaxation or stimulation, but ultimately the liver will be burdened with the job of detoxifying these substances. Coffee consumption should be limited to no more than two cups per day.

Alternatives: Cereal beverages (Roma, Pero, Cafix, Postum, Bambu); fresh fruit or vegetable juices; distilled or spring water, and seltzer. (Do not substitute club soda for seltzer. Club soda contains sodium.)

✦ Salt: Including additives such as MSG, HVP, sodium propionate, sodium bicarbonate, sodium metabisulfate, and most canned foods. Salt consumption is associated with water retention, which leads to edema and hypertension and will weaken the Kidney.

Alternatives: Eat "low-sodium" or "low-salt" products. Use natural sea salt in moderate amounts in food preparation.

✦ Dairy products: Milk, cream, ice cream, sour cream, cheese, yogurt. Limited use of butter is acceptable and preferred over the use of margarine. These foods are the most common allergens and are mucus forming. The dampness that they produce by weakening the Spleen congests the system and leads to many chronic problems.

Alternatives: Soy milk, rice milk, or diluted apple juice (for cereals).

✦ Nightshade family foods (may aggravate arthritis and other degenerative conditions): White potatoes, tomatoes, eggplant, paprika, garden peppers. These foods disrupt the acid-alkaline balance of the body and can upset calcium metabolism, leading to arthritic problems.

Alternatives: Russet or sweet potatoes, yams, whole grains, turnips, and Jerusalem artichokes.

+ Shellfish: Should not be eaten on a frequent basis. As filter feeders, shellfish collect and concentrate the pollutants and chemicals from the water into their flesh. Consumption of these foods should be limited to one or two servings per year. The high iodine content of these foods can disturb the hormone balance in sensitive women. These foods also stimulate the production of fluids and should be avoided by those suffering with genitourinary problems and all women with menstrual problems.

Alternatives: Small whole fish, such as trout, flounder, snapper, and sardines. Farm-grown fish are preferred over ocean fish because of the high contents of mercury and other heavy metals found in large saltwater fish, such as tuna, salmon, and swordfish.

+ High-fat foods: Ice cream, whole milk, sour cream, cream cheese, hard cheese, heavy butter sauces, red meat, pork, duck, oil, nuts, and seeds. Excess fat is a contributing factor in all chronic degenerative diseases, including atherosclerosis, heart disease, and cancer. These foods are severely limited or eliminated in a health-promoting diet.

Alternatives: Organic lean meat, chicken, turkey, farm-grown fish.

+ Meats: Beef, pork, and veal that have been treated with chemicals such as nitrites, nitrates, and other preservatives. Organ meats are often loaded with waste products of the animal's metabolism. Commercially prepared meats contain hormone and antibiotic drug residues which have to be metabolized by the liver and cause serious imbalances to the internal environment of the body.

Alternatives: Organic or natural meats, fowl, and eggs; fresh farm-grown fish, fresh small ocean fish.

+ Delicatessen foods: All chemically processed cold cuts and pickled or marinated foods (olives, tomatoes, peppers, salads, pickles). Prepared salads like cole slaw and potato salad are often high in fat and sugar. Because of their high salt, fat, and sugar contents, deli foods should be avoided. This trio of offending substances accounts for most of the diet-related problems seen today.

Alternatives: Homemade salads with low-salt, low-fat dressings; fresh turkey or chicken breast; fresh roast beef.

While specific medical conditions require further dietary changes, these recommendations are for general health and well being. Taking control of your eating habits contributes to a healthier, more vital life.

The following natural, unrefined foods are recommended:

+ Fresh organic vegetables: steamed or stir-fried and raw salads.
+ Fresh organic fruits in season.
+ Fresh organic poultry.
+ Fresh farm-grown fish.

✦ Organic beef (limit to one 4-ounce serving per week). Eat no pork, veal, liver, duck, or shellfish.

✦ Whole grains: Brown, basmati, or wild rice; wheat, bulghur, rye, millet, oats, barley, quinoa, amaranth; whole-grain bread, pasta, muffins.

✦ Beans, peas, and lentils (limit to two servings per week—these are highly allergenic).

✦ Raw, unsalted nuts and seeds: Almonds, cashews, pumpkin, sunflower. Eat no peanuts—this food is highly allergenic and difficult to digest. Moldy peanuts produce a chemical that is a known carcinogen. Also eat no walnuts—these nuts are very fatty and the skin of the nut is difficult to break down and can congest the Kidney.

✦ Beverages: Distilled or spring water, lemon and water, vegetable juice, diluted natural fruit juice, low-salt seltzer. Coffee (limit to two cups per day). Drink coffee substitutes such as Roma, Pero, Cafix, Bambu, Postum.

✦ Salad dressing: Vegetable oil and vinegar, lemon, garlic with vegetable oil.

✦ Spices and Seasonings: Garlic, ginger, parsley, cayenne pepper. (Garlic and ginger should not be used together because their beneficial properties will be canceled out.) Eat no black or white pepper, as they irritate the stomach.

✦ Vegetable oils: Sunflower, safflower, canola. Eat no peanut or sesame oil—both of these oils are highly allergenic.

✦ Eggs: Limit to four to six per week. This includes all eggs in cooked and baked foods.

Some specific foods that can aggravate certain conditions should be limited in their consumption. As part of this transitional diet, the following guidelines should be followed:

✦ Fried foods limited to once per month.

✦ Tomato sauces (Italian food) limited to once per month.

✦ Dessert once per week.

✦ Animal protein (meat, fish, fowl) limit to three servings per week.

✦ Yogurt (4 oz.) once per week.

✦ Tuna fish once per month.

The following is a sample menu that can be used as a helpful guideline.

Upon rising:
Drink a glass of water with the juice of one-half fresh lemon added to it.

Breakfast:
1 cup of coffee or grain beverage (Postum, Cafix, Bambu) or herbal tea.

Choice of:
a. Two Nutri-Grain waffles with natural unsweetened jelly or natural maple syrup.
b. Hot, whole-grain cereal (Quaker oats, cream of rye, oat bran, and so forth).
c. Cold, whole-grain cereal with rice milk (Nutri-Grain, shredded wheat, puffed rice, and so forth).
d. Whole-grain muffin with natural unsweetened jelly.
e. Whole-grain pancakes with natural unsweetened jelly or natural maple syrup.

f. Two eggs with whole grain toast.

Lunch: Choose between any two of the following.

a. Salad with sprouts and unlimited steamed vegetables. Salad can contain any of the following: Bibb or romaine lettuce, sprouts (any variety), endive, carrots, radishes, radicchio, arugula, cucumber, beets, cabbage, chickory, mushrooms, hard-boiled egg, turkey, chicken, chickpeas, brown rice, pasta.

b. Homemade soup.

c. Sandwich on whole-grain bread, pita, or roll: turkey, chicken, egg, fish, nut butter (almond, cashew).

d. Russet potato, sweet potato, or yam, boiled or baked with vegetables.

Dinner:

Salad with sprouts and unlimited steamed vegetables.

Choice of protein:

a. Beans (limit to two servings per week).

b. Fish.

c. Chicken or turkey.

d. Beef (limit to one 4-ounce serving per week).

Choice of complex carbohydrates:

a. Whole grain (brown rice, kasha, millet, barley, oat, rye).

b. Whole-grain toast, whole-wheat pita, or whole-grain English muffin.

c. Pasta (whole wheat, De Boles artichoke, spinach) with vegetables (no cheese).

d. Russet potato, sweet potato, or yam, boiled or baked.

e. Homemade soup with any ingredients listed above.

Snacks:

Two snacks can be consumed daily.

a. Fresh vegetable juice or fruit juice.

b. 3 ounces nuts or seeds (no peanuts, walnuts).

c. Two rice cakes with 1 tablespoon natural, raw nut butter (cashew, peanut, or almond) and/or jelly.

d. 1 cup plain air-popped popcorn (no salt or butter).

e. One serving of fresh fruit.

f. Fresh raw vegetables.

Good nutritional health begins with a diet of whole, natural foods, and is enhanced by natural vitamins and minerals. The body most easily absorbs and most effectively uses natural supplements. Prepared properly, natural supplements are in the right form and ratio for optimal activity. All products should be hypoallergenic and free of additives, preservatives, coloring agents, sugar, starch, and yeast.

No listing of daily vitamin and mineral requirements can take into consideration individual lifestyle and environmental factors. To ensure that the body's basic nutritional needs are met, a general supplementation program should include:

✦ Multiple vitamin/mineral: One per day, taken with a meal.

✦ Vitamin C (with bioflavonoids): 1000 mg. with each meal.

✦ Vitamin B complex: One per day, taken with a meal.

✦ Multiple minerals: One per day, taken at bedtime.

PART TWO

THE PRINCIPLES

CHAPTER

5

THE FUNDAMENTALS

The purpose of the following discussion on the basic principles of Chinese medical theory is to introduce the apparently exotic basis of this medical science. The subsequent chapters of this section will detail Oriental anatomy and physiology and diagnostic techniques, and will attempt to explain the diagnostic- and treatment-pattern concepts so that they can become the basis of a realistic evaluation of the patient. Part IV gives further diagnostic information, particularly related to syndromes and Western disease patterns, along with the appropriate Amma therapy treatments. In this chapter we wish to acquaint the first-time student of Chinese medicine with the proper philosophical basis for understanding the purpose and nature of the art of Amma therapy.

Oriental medicine recognizes the existence of twelve Organ/Function complexes, each of which encompass a set of tissues, pertaining organs (from which the name of the Organ/Function complex is derived), sense organs, and physiological and psychological functions. It also recognizes a number of less important organs that are only regarded in the context of their dysfunctions. The six Yin Viscera are the Lung, Spleen, Heart, Kidney, Heart Envelope, and Liver. The six Yang Bowels are the Colon, Stomach, Small Intestine, Urinary Bladder, Three Burning Spaces, and Gall Bladder. The minor Organs, such as the Brain and the Uterus, do not enter into the primary and secondary energy cycles, and are therefore given limited consideration. The Uterus is considered significant not only for its function of housing the fetus, but also because it is the place of origin of certain Extraordinary Vessels. The sense organs are connected to the orbs of influence of the Bowels and Viscera.* Other important tissue groups are also related

---

* Following Dr. Manfred Porket, I will at times refer to the Organ/Function complex as the orb of influence, or simply the orb.

to the control or influence of certain Organ/Function complexes.

As we discuss the Organs it will become apparent that we are not discussing the Western physical structures. The structures are indeed noted and are even outlined in the charts of the channel pathways in chapter 6. However, it is the function that is the focus of our interest. The surgical removal of an organ structure does not remove the function, although it definitely hinders that function. Oriental medical tradition speaks of each Organ in the singular. The reason for this is easily understood in the case of the Lung, when one considers the Lung to be the central bronchus and its branches, rather than the two masses of air sacs. The difficulty in reconciling this practice with the anatomical fact of two distinct kidneys reminds us again that the reference is not the simple physical organ or organs, but the Organ/Function complex with the same name.

It is necessary for the student of Oriental therapies to reorient his or her thinking process so that the functional elements—as opposed to the structural elements—of the diagnosis become the primary basis for treatment. To facilitate this reorientation we have chosen to capitalize words that would not ordinarily be capitalized, in order to remind the reader of the extraordinary usages being implied. This practice, common to English writings on Oriental medicine, compels the reader to distinguish the functional and energetic meanings of words in traditional Chinese medical tradition from the concrete meanings of the same terms in Western tradition. In the following chapters you will notice that more than one phrase or term may be used to describe the same concept. This results from the fact that the Chinese medical concepts are more inclusive in meaning than their English counterparts, and therefore often require additional terms to indicate alternative uses of the same complex concept. This tendency toward using more than one term to describe the same concept also results from the rather poetic and sometimes forced patterning present in the old Oriental medical texts.

Oriental diagnosis and therapy is concerned with the dynamic balance of the interactive forces of each human being's individual cosmos. Structure may be considered to the extent that it is beyond doubt that a structural defect is the basis of a patient's disease condition. The following brief story from my experience with acupuncture illustrates the functional concern of Chinese medicine as opposed to the allopathic physician's structural concern.

Many years ago a young woman of twenty-five who had been totally deaf in her right ear since the age of four as a result of childhood otitis media asked to be treated with acupuncture, since she had read that deafness was being cured in China by acupuncture. After twenty treatments the hearing in her deaf right ear was totally restored. She could cover the left ear and hear perfectly, even when conversations were whispered. She could talk on the telephone with the phone held against her previously deaf ear, and she could no longer sleep through storms and sirens even if her "deaf" ear was exposed and the other ear was buried in a pillow. Her life, vis-à-vis her hearing, became absolutely normal. She went to an ear specialist who was amazed at the results and asked to do a test on the right auditory nerve. The examination showed that the nerve was dead and could not be conducting the sounds that she heard. The allopathic physician then announced solemnly *that the acupuncture had not worked* and that the young woman was *still deaf in the right ear*. His concern lay with the functionless structure, while my concern, and that of my patient who contended that she was no longer deaf, was with function—even an apparently structureless function that constituted her ability to hear again.

As is clear from this story, the traditional Chinese physician has a view of the problem that is more akin to that of the patient's. When the patient has pain, the Amma therapist should seek the cause of the pain in the imbalance of Yin and Yang and, if there are indeed structural disturbances, be aware that although the repair of structure may relieve the problem, it also may not. Though apparently irreparable by traditional Western means, the structural disturbance may be easily resolved by traditional Oriental means. As well, many functional repairs can be made in spite of a structural disturbance, as is so clearly illustrated in the deaf woman's functional recovery.

FUNCTIONAL VERSUS STRUCTURAL VIEWPOINTS

The interesting and important difference between the views of the Western and the Oriental health practitioner—the dichotomy between the significance given to form and the significance given to function—has deep and primary implications. This distinction defines the entry point and primary direction of the whole of the theoretical and practical processes of each health care system. While the Western practitioner is very conscious of form, his Oriental counterpart is primarily concerned with function. This difference is most markedly obvious in the study of the Oriental concept of the Organs.

The study of physiology, which is a significant part of the Western structural orientation, is replaced in Chinese medicine with the study of the Zhang Xiang Xue Shou, which can be literally translated as "the theory of the phenomena of Internal Organs." Here *phenomena* means "visible external expressions," indicating that the physical entity is of little consequence in the considerations of the Chinese medical practitioner. His concern lies not with the organ as a physical entity but with its functions in the body, whereby functions are regarded as generalized phenomena and not specific mechanically defined processes. This is a radically different focus from Western anatomy and physiology, whose students investigate the structures of the major body systems and the organs of the body. The osseous, nervous, cardiovascular, lymphatic, genitourinary, endothileal-reticular, gastrointestinal, integumentary, and pulmonary systems, as well as the sense organs and other structures, are studied in minute detail, and their functions tied directly to their individual structures and to structural relationships. Thus, function is defined in terms of structure.

While Western anatomy and physiology are concerned with the physical body in its most concrete form, Oriental healing arts have deeper concerns related to the underlying and sustaining body of energy that enlivens the physical form. Thus our concern is not with the structure and structurally related functions of the physical body, but with this energy and with functionally related structures. Most of traditional Chinese medical theory and its underlying principles are based not on anatomy but on observation of the functional activities observable by an external observer, on pathophysiology, and on the therapeutic results obtained through many years of observation and experimentation. Had we Westerners discovered this aspect of Chinese medicine early on, we might have found another nomenclature to express functional groupings instead of affixing the name of the pertaining organ to the channel. The Chinese tended to refer to the channels by their Six Divisions nomenclature. The Six Divisions naming provides more information about the channel, indicating not only its pertaining organ but also the Six Stage phase with which it is associated and the limb through which it flows.

As an example, Western anatomical understanding of the spleen is highly evolved, going into the most minute detail regarding tissue structure and its differentiation, organ innervation and vascularization, and specific details as to its size, shape, placement, support, position in relation to other organs, attachments, and every other imaginable physical detail, yet there is little knowledge (and not a great deal of conjecture) as to the function of the spleen. This organ is removed when there is internal bleeding. Of course, the spleen can be injured beyond repair, but the concept of why it ought to be repaired is missing. The pancreas is known in the same minute detail as the spleen, and its function is recognized to some degree, however the ability to repair that function is not considered. It is instead considered as necessary to supplement the secretions of the pancreas as soon as blood sugar balance becomes consistently impaired.

Oriental medical science, on the other hand, gives virtually no description of the spleen or the pancreas. Some simple drawings that have been made by curious physicians show the spleen as a roundish organ in the left hypochondriac region with a long tail reaching almost to the liver. This tail is obviously the pancreas, since there is no knowledge of the pancreas as a separate organ; indeed, in TCM the functions of the pancreas are considered to be part of the Spleen. The Spleen is specified as the controller of the digestive function. It harbors Yi, or the aspect of the human soul involved with reflection and intention. The Spleen communicates with the Lung (they share the same type of energy differentiation), and enters into disease syndromes involving many other Organs. It couples with the Stomach, and together they constitute the Middle Warmer wherein the process of digestion is accomplished. Its energy is the Great Yin (see figure 2, page 19), and it is therefore the very beginning of the cycle of life, which commences with the ingestion of air into the Lung and the ingestion of food into the Stomach. Since the Spleen is the controller of the total digestive function, it regulates, balances, and nourishes but does not directly digest the food.

This clear distinction between the

two medical systems shows that they indeed can be complementary and not antagonistic, as many in both communities seem to feel. Chinese medicine is clearly better suited to the prevention and treatment of chronic and functional disorders, while Western medicine succeeds at emergency therapy and the repairing of structure. Dr. Manfred Porket takes great pains to elucidate this truth in the introduction to his book *The Essentials of Chinese Diagnostics,* wherein he describes the complementary nature of the Chinese synthetic as opposed to the Western analytic approach. I highly recommend reading that introduction to gain a more thorough understanding of this important issue.

BASIC CONCEPTS UNDERLYING THE CHINESE MEDICAL MODEL

Before discussing the basic concepts we will briefly introduce the Chinese Organs called Zang and Fu Organs. These are translated as Solid (Zang) and Hollow (Fu) Organs; Organs of constant activity and Organs of intermittent activity; Organs that create and distribute Qi, Fluids, and Blood and Organs that deal with the digestion and elimination of nutrient substances. (We shall sometimes refer to the Organ/Function complex and sometimes to the Organ with the name capitalized. These are both understood to mean the orb of influence of the Organ/Function complex.) The Fu Organs, or the Bowels—the Stomach, Large Intestine, Small Intestine, San Jiao,

and Bladder—are the five Organs generated by the energy of Heaven, and their energies bear a resemblance to the energy of Heaven. Thus, they drain off things without storing them up, they receive muddy energies (impure fluids) from the five viscera, and they excrete waste products. The sixth Fu Organ, the Gall Bladder, neither receives muddy energies nor excretes waste products. It has special qualities which will be discussed later. The Zang Organs, or the Viscera—the Lung, Spleen, Heart, Kidney, Liver, and Hsin Pao Lao (Heart Envelope)—are generated by the energy of Earth. They store up Yin energy without draining it off, and for that reason they can be filled to capacity but cannot be oversupplied. Conversely, the Fu Organs, including the Gall Bladder, are such that they transmit Yang things without storing them up, and for that reason they may be oversupplied but cannot be filled to capacity.

The Bowels are Yang and the Viscera are Yin relative to their functions and anatomical descriptions. The Zang Organs (the Viscera) are responsible for the manufacture and storage of essential substances (Vital Essence and pure fluids). They are also responsible for the mental and emotional functions. The Fu Organs (the Bowels, including the Bladder and Gall Bladder) are responsible for the reception and transmission of the gross substances from which the Qi of Food and Vital Fluids are made, as well as the temporary storage and final discharge of the waste products. The Fu Organs generally more closely parallel the Western organ concepts.

The Odd and Constant Organs, also named the Extraordinary Organs, are the Brain, Marrow, Bone, Blood Vessels, Gall

Bladder, and Womb (Uterus). They are neither Viscera nor Bowels. They are said to be stored in Yin, implying that these Organs and their functions are deeper than the Viscera. They are like the Viscera in that they store things up without draining them off, but like the Bowels they are hollow. The Gall Bladder is a middle Bowel for storing clear energy (pure fluid, or Gall), and is in tune with the Liver and assists the Heart's function of decision making. The Gall Bladder is therefore considered an Odd and Constant Organ, although it also functions as a Bowel in the cycle of the Five Relative Phases (see page 19).

QI, BLOOD, AND FLUIDS

One of the most fundamental tenets in the Chinese medical model is the concept of Qi (pronounced *chee*) which, although commonly translated as "energy," has not been understood by the Western practitioner in a real and dynamic sense. Most people in the New Age and new medicine movements who speak of energy are speaking of an abstract idea, not something with which they have a direct experiential relationship. Qi in its many manifestations is a real and concrete experience for those who seek to realize its presence. In its simplest conceptual form, the state of one's Qi is expressed in the phrase "I have a lot of energy today," and in its counterpart, "I feel really low on energy. I can't seem to think straight (get anything right, finish my work, etc.)." For the practitioner of Amma therapy and other Oriental medical arts, Qi

has a wide variety of manifestations, and it is the differing expressions of a patient's Qi that the Amma therapist seeks to evaluate and assess in making a diagnosis and creating an appropriate treatment protocol.

Yin and Yang are the great dichotomies of Qi. The Six Stages or Six Divisions of Yin and Yang are one description of the forms that Qi takes; another is the Five Relative Phases. However, these descriptions are general, abstract concepts; Qi becomes more specific when we begin to look at the Organ complex and the creation and transformation of various forms of the active Qi of the body.

Before birth the fetus is sustained by the Qi of the mother. A very precious substance is created and passed on to the child in the procreation and birth processes. This is the Prenatal Qi, also called the Qi of Prior Heaven. Prenatal Qi can be conceived of as the hereditary constitutional potential of the body. In its kinetic aspect, it is known to circulate in the channels and to enter into all transforming processes. It is then called Yuan Qi, or the Active Essence of the Kidney. This substance is stored in the Kidney and carried by the Leg Lesser Yin Channel, as well as in the San Jiao and eight Extraordinary Vessels. (These channels are discussed in detail in the following chapter.) The Yuan Qi motivates or activates the flow of Qi in the channels; it is also the energy that acts as the catalyst for all the processes of energy creation through digestion and energy usage and generation in the organs.

After birth the infant breathes and ingests not only oxygen as it is known in the Western world, but also Da Qi or the

Qi of Air. As the child eats and drinks its food, the Stomach and Spleen extract the Gu Qi, or the Qi of Grain, which is transmitted by the Spleen to the Lung. There the Qi of Air and the Qi of Grain combine with the influence of Prenatal Qi to form the Nutrient Qi that flows in the channels.

In addition to the work of transforming and transporting Qi, the digestive function is concerned with the creation of two additional substances. Along with the extraction of Gu Qi, the Spleen begins the process of extracting pure fluids from the food substance. These fluids are circulated and a number of different substances, including serous fluid, saliva, sweat, synovial fluids, and so forth, are created. Some of the pure fluid is combined with Qi to produce Blood, which only in part refers to the substance of blood as we in the West know it. In the Chinese view, one rarefied form of Blood flows in the channels with the Qi (as, of course, Qi flows with the more material aspect of blood in the blood vessels). Blood is a complex substance that changes as it moves through the system and partakes of both material and energetic qualities. Blood is the Yin of the Heart while Fire is the Yang of the Heart, and Blood could be regarded as the most Yin or palpable part of the Qi. Many of the disease syndromes or patterns are considered to be conditions of the Qi or Blood. The relationship between these two is not unlike the relationships between the Yin/Yang pairs of the channels, to be discussed in the following chapter.

In addition to its other functions, the Spleen produces a great deal of Nutritive Qi in the regular internal energy cycle that creates Blood. It is primarily the Heart that is responsible for using the Fluids and the Qi that is generated by the Spleen, Lung, and Kidney. The Spleen is called the Source of Blood, because it is the Viscera responsible for the initial production of Qi and Fluids. The Blood is more energy than matter, except that its most Yin part takes the form of a literal fluid as it flows in the blood vessels. Much of the Blood flows in the channels with the Nutrient Qi, and is much more energetic than material.

The Marrow is another product of the energetic functions of the body that is named like a substance of Western medicine but is not a direct counterpart. Formed by the Kidney, Marrow is a special binding substance that produces bone marrow and the bones, and fills the spinal cord and brain. The Brain is thus called the Sea of Marrow; it has a physiological connection to the Kidney. The Oriental medicine classics of the twelfth century and beyond claim that Marrow assists in the production of Blood.

Many of the ideas implicit in the Oriental medical model are alien to usual Western patterns of thought or ways of looking at the world. We in the West tend toward detailed analysis of structure, and have achieved amazing feats of mechanical accomplishment relative to maintenance and repair of the human body. The Chinese view is basically outside the consideration of details; it is instead based upon observation of interactions, variations, similarities, and patterns of phenomena. The Chinese view therefore leads to an entirely different approach regarding the diagnosis and treatment of disease. Everything in the universe—all phenomena—is divided into Yin and Yang and subdivided several times, some with reference to the Five Phase Cycle and the Six Divisions of Yin and Yang. As can be seen in figure 2 (see page 19) the Qi of the channels is divided into Yin and Yang according to the Six Divisions. The Yin channels include the Lung and Spleen (Great Yin), the Heart and Kidney (Lesser Yin), and the Heart Envelope and Liver (Absolute Yin). The Yang channels include the Colon and Stomach (Bright Yang), the Small Intestine and Bladder (Great Yang), and the San Jiao and Gall Bladder (Lesser Yang).

Besides the Primary Channels, their connecting Vessels (the Jing Luo), and the manifestations or the orb of influence of the Organs, the Chinese recognized the existence of the actual physical entities of the Zang, Fu, and Odd and Constant Organs. However, the physical organs were not of much concern, as their functions were generalized into the manifestation of the Organs, and there was no need to be concerned with the minutiae of detailed processes expressed by general energetic transformations.

To a large extent, Oriental medical diagnosis is concerned with establishing the condition of various factors relative to both the material substratum and the active energy of the body, and the underlying disturbances that lead to perceived conditions of imbalance. Treatment is designed to reestablish harmony. The vital energies and substances that are examined include:

Qi—The generalized concept of the Organ and its function.

Yang—The activity of the Organ, such as the Stomach ripens food and moves the dregs down to the Small Intestine; or, the Spleen produces and moves Gu Qi to the Lung.

Yin—The essence of the Organ that underlies the processes; the material substratum of the energetic events.

Pure Fluids—Produced by the Yin Organs, the Pure Fluids are divided into thin fluids (such as tears and sweat) and thick fluids (such as synovial fluid and cerebrospinal fluid).

Blood—A product of the Qi of Grain (produced by the Spleen) and Pure Fluids, and flowing as the thick red liquid of Western blood, Blood also includes a continuum of refined energy qualities that flow throughout the body, including within the channels of Qi.

The conditions of these substances and energies as recognized through symptoms reported by the patient and signs observed by the health practitioner point toward specific sources of dysfunction brought on by constitution, pathogens, or lifestyle, and indicate the Organ/Function complex in which the dysfunction is manifest. The level of the condition is also evaluated in determining prognosis. These evaluations are both energetic, as in the Four Level Differentiation of Syndromes and Six Level Differentiation of Syndromes, and related to the division of the torso into three portions, as in the Three Burning Spaces Differentiation of Syndromes.

QI

It should be understood that Qi manifests as a wide variety of "substances" that have differing and necessary functions. Fluids also exhibit a variety of states. The various forms of Qi include:

Jing Qi—This form of Qi is comprised of the Vital Essences that combine to form the fetus. These are Yin Jing and Yang Jing, and specifically the female ovum and the male sperm. When looked upon as the Essence of Life, Jing is Yin while Qi is Yang. Jing is the Acquired Essence that, along with the Original Essence (see Prenatal Qi, below), is stored in the Kidneys as the Essence of the Organs.

Prenatal Qi or Qi of Prior Heaven *(Xian Tian Qi,* pronounced *syan tyan chee)*—Passed on to the fetus in the procreation and birth processes, this substance can be conceived of as the hereditary constitutional potential of the body not simply as defined by Western medical science, but including the substance that underlies the true health and dynamic potential of the organism. The Prenatal Qi, (also called the Kidney Essence), remains in the Kidney and is slowly depleted in the natural order of life. Its active component, Yuan Qi, begins to function at the moment of birth and is the activating factor of all processes in the organism.

Yuan Qi—The kinetic aspect of Prenatal Qi, Yuan Qi is known to circulate in the channels and to enter into all transforming processes. It is therefore called the Active Essence of the Kidney. This substance is stored in the Kidney and is carried by the Leg Lesser Yin Channel as well as in the eight Extraordinary Vessels. It also circulates in the Triple Burner, from which it enters the Primary Channels to surface at the Organ points (Source or Yuan points). Yuan Qi is the energy that motivates or activates the flow of Qi in the channels. This energy also acts as the catalyst for all the processes of energy creation through digestion, as well as the cycle of energy usage and generation in the Organs.

Postnatal, Post-Heaven, or Acquired Qi *(Hou Tian Qi)*—During inspiration, the Lung, under the stimulus of Yuan Qi, extracts the Qi of Air from the inhaled substance, and combines it with the Qi of Grain to form Acquired Qi.

Nutrient or Nourishing Qi *(Ying Qi)*—Once True Qi (see further down this list) is activated by the Yuan Qi, the Nutrient Qi is formed and can move through the channels and the Organ complex. This aspect of Qi, which nurtures the gross anatomical structures and flows in the blood vessels with the Blood as well as in the channels, is called Ying Qi.

Channel Qi *(Jing Luo Qi)*—Nutrient Qi that flows in the channels.

Pectoral or Ancestral Qi *(Zong Qi,* pronounced *dzung chee)*—Not ancestral as in the sense of prenatal, this form of Qi is rather the first manifestation of Acquired Qi and the forerunner of all other Qi transformations in the body. It is the energy in the chest that is used by the Lung for respiration and activation of the voice, and by the Heart for the movement of the Blood into the vessels. This energy is often blocked by emotional factors that affect the Heart and Lung functions.

Qi of Air *(Da Qi)*—When the lung inspires, the Lung extracts the material oxygen and other finer substances from the inspired Air. This Qi of Air and the Qi of Grain are used in conjunction with the Prenatal Qi to form the total Qi content of the organism.

Qi of Grain *(Gu Qi)*—This Qi is extracted from the ripened and rotted foodstuff by the action of the Stomach under direction of the Spleen. The Spleen then transmits the Gu Qi to the Lung for the production of Zhen or True Qi.

True Qi *(Zhen Qi, pronounced jen chee)*—Resulting from the transformation of the Ancestral Qi under the catalytic action of Yuan Qi, the True Qi is in a form that can be used for the various needs of the organism. Because True Qi is transformed into Nutrient Qi and Protective Qi, it is easy to suggest that all the subsequent names for Qi may indicate specific actions rather than variations in the form of the True Qi.

Organ Qi *(Zang-Fu Qi, pronounced dzang fu chee)*—The Qi present in the Yin Viscera and the Yang Bowels that nourishes the Organs and maintains their functions.

Center or Middle Jiao Qi *(Zhong Qi, pronounced jung chee)*—The Qi of the Spleen and Stomach that transforms Postnatal Qi.

Protective or Defensive Qi *(Wei Qi)*—As the Qi flows through the Organ cycle (discussed in chapter 7), each Organ uses what is necessary for its functions and adds to the general flow. As well, some of the Organs generate Defensive Qi, which flows in the Tendino-Muscle Channels and in the Cutaneous Regions. It is believed that the Defensive Qi may flow in the Divergent Channels as well. (These channels are thoroughly described in chapter 6.) This energy is the most superficial energy of the system and is responsible for the protection of the body from external pathogens. If the Wei Qi is highly developed, the skin will resist even insect bites. Wei Qi is also responsible for opening and closing the pores under the direction of the Lung, so that the fluid metabolism and temperature remain in balance.

Correct or Upright Qi *(Zheng Qi, pronounced jeng chee)*—A term used to describe the Protective Qi that defends the body from invasion by pernicious influences.

Vital Essence—The substratum of all the active Qi of the body is the Yin aspect or Vital Essence that constitutes the products of the Viscera, the Essence of the Viscera, the stored Qi of Prior Heaven, and Acquired Qi. Any substance or energy necessary for the processes of the body is called Vital Essence or Vital Substance.

FLUIDS

The various fluids include:

Serous fluid—This fluid is produced by the Kidney and also by serous tissue throughout the body. The fact that serous fluid production is under the control of the Kidney but is not confined to the organ of the same name clearly illustrates the nature of the Organ/Function complex, in that the orb of influence is necessarily differentiated from the anatomical structure.

Tears—This fluid that lubricates the eyes is produced by the Liver, which is inclusive of the eyes.

Sweat—This fluid is a function of the Heart and Blood Vessels.

Saliva—This fluid, produced by the Spleen, is responsible for all digestion.

Mucus—This fluid is created by the Lung. The orb of influence of the Lung includes the mucous membranes throughout the body.

Synovial fluid—This fluid lubricates the joints and sinews under control of the Liver.

Turbid Damp—During the extraction process when the Qi of Grain and fluids are extracted from food in the Stomach, a small amount of fluid residue called Turbid Damp is created. Under the impetus of Kidney Yang, Turbid Damp is carried to the tongue, where it acts as a fine diagnostic indicator by creating the coating on the tongue.

We can see that Chinese medicine views the human being not simply as a conglomeration of structural organs functioning together, but as a complex interaction of mind, body, and emotions resulting from the interplay and transformation of specific vital energies and substances, ranging in a continuum from the most dense, such as bone and body fluids, to the finest, immaterial energies, such as Jing. However, the foundation of the human existence, as it is for the basis of the universe, is always Qi. Qi is as much material as it is energetic.

In the following chapters we will explore the pathways of Qi and their interconnections and relationships. We will then examine in detail the Organ/Function complexes or orbs of influence of the Bowels and Viscera.

THE ANATOMY OF ENERGY

As a result of the original and limited translations of Chinese medical texts, early Western students of Oriental medicine named each main channel after the major pertaining organ of that channel. The common abbreviation for each Primary Channel therefore tended to be an abbreviation of the pertaining organ name. (Due to the imposition of Western medical viewpoints onto the Oriental medical model, a few of the channels have a number of different names connected to them, a situation that has led to a certain degree of confusion as Oriental medicine has become more widely taught in the West.) This limited terminology has led to a misunderstanding of the whole channel system. The Chinese in fact named each Primary Channel for its location (arm or leg), its energetic quality (one of the six differentiations of the Yin/Yang polarity), and its pertaining organ or function (Lung, Heart, Three Heaters, and so forth). (Figure 2 on page 19 shows these relationships.) In most cases this was a rather simple and straightforward delineation. However, in regard to the two rather odd function-oriented channels—the Heart Envelope and the Triple Heater—the question of nomenclature was complicated by Western assumptions about the information available to the ancient Chinese doctors.

In this chapter we will explore the anatomy of the pathways of Qi in the body. The list on page 68 will familiarize you with the names and abbreviations of the Primary Organ Channels. We will then discuss the names of the two function-related channels before moving on to detailed descriptions of the individual channels.

PRIMARY ORGAN CHANNEL NAMES AND ABBREVIATIONS

The Arm Great Yin Lung Channel is abbreviated Lu (Utilizing the first and second letters of the term Lung to establish the abbreviation)

The Leg Great Yin Spleen Channel—Sp

The Arm Lesser Yin Heart Channel—Ht

The Leg Lesser Yin Kidney Channel—Ki

The Arm Bright Yang colon Channel—Co or LI (for Large Intestine) Co is preferable, to avoid confusion with the "Li" of the Liver.

The Leg Bright Yang Stomach Channel—St

The Arm Great Yang Small Intestine Channel—SI

The Leg Great Yang Urinary Bladder Channel—UB or Bl

The Leg Lesser Yang Gall Bladder Channel—GB

The Leg Absolute Yin Liver Channel—Li or Liv

The Arm Absolute Yin Channel is the first of the two difficult-to-comprehend channels of Qi. In Chinese, the name of the so-called pertaining organ is Hsin Pao Lao (Xin Bao Lao), which translates literally as "the Envelope of the Heart." Early translators assumed that the Chinese medical practitioners were referring to the pericardium, the membrane which does indeed surround the heart. Western science is quite aware of the existence of the peritoneum, the membrane that surrounds and holds the organs in the abdominal cavity. The membrane surrounding a bone is called periosteum, and the membrane surrounding the heart is specified as the pericardium ("around the heart"). Thus the original name chosen for this channel was the Pericardium Channel. With time and study it became clear that Chinese medical science was not concerned with, and probably not aware of, the existence of the pericardium or any other of the peritoneal membranes; they were regarded as part of the organ and given no individual significance.

As time passed, it was repeatedly observed that the primary effect of treatment on this odd channel produced effects on sexual function as well as on vascular circulation, and so the channel was often called the Circulation-Sex Channel. With the increased recognition of the channel's effects on the circulatory system, it became clear that that which enveloped the Heart was indeed the circulatory system, and that the sphere of influence of the channel extended deeply into the circulatory function, which accounted for the channel's effects on sexual function. Somehow, the term "Heart Constrictor" began to be used, as well as the more logical term "Envelope of the Heart." Subsequently, Dr. Reinhold Voll showed that the points of the channel located on the hand were capable of very specific and direct influence on the major aspects of the vascular function, including the arteries and the veins.

We are now left with the following list of abbreviated names that are all used to describe this channel: P, HC, CX, EH, HE, and Cir. These refer, respectively, to

Pericardium, Heart Constrictor, Circulation-Sex, Envelope of the Heart, Heart Envelope, and finally, Circulation.

The second channel that has caused difficulties in naming is the Arm Lesser Yang Channel. In traditional Chinese medicine, the pertaining organ (or function) is called San Jiao or Three Burning Spaces (or Three Cauldrons, since there is a basis in Taoist philosophy for this name). In Chinese medical thought, the body is divided into Upper, Middle, and Lower Heaters. (In this respect, the words *heater, warmer,* and *burning space* are used interchangeably.) The Upper Burner consists of the Lung and Heart, the Middle Burner of the Stomach and Spleen, and the Lower Burner of the Colon, Bladder, Kidney, Liver, and Small Intestine. (The Liver is also considered to be part of the Middle Burner by virtue of its location.) This leads to the basic view of the function of the Arm Lesser Yang Channel as the controller of the three processes of assimilation, digestion, and elimination, respectively.

The Chinese medical view of the function of the Spleen is primarily that of the controller of the digestive function. Thus, digestion takes place in the Stomach (the Middle Burner), where tradition says that the Qi of Grain is separated from the substance of food, under the control of the Spleen. From here the Qi of Grain passes into the Lung (the Upper Burner), where it mingles with the Qi of Air to become the Nutrient Qi of the body. Under the control of the Heart, it is then distributed throughout the organism. Thus, the Upper Warmer controls assimilation. Finally, the impure solids pass into the Colon (the Lower Burner), and the impure Fluids into the Kidney and Bladder for elimination. There is no ques-

tion about the clinical use of the Arm Lesser Yang Channel for the purpose of treating conditions related to digestion, assimilation, and elimination.

Recognizing the Taoist spiritual influence in the channel names Three Cauldrons and Three Burning Spaces, a number of acupuncturists began to explore the validity of using the channel to effect the Shen, or Spirit, and consequently found great clinical value in treating emotional distress and emotional accompaniments to disease conditions through this channel. As Dr. Reinhold Voll and his colleagues in Germany began to explore this channel, much detail about the direct effect of certain hand points of the Arm Lesser Yang Channel became clear, and points were discovered that had powerful and direct influences on specific endocrine glands. As a result of the work by Dr. Voll and his colleagues, acupuncturists and advanced Amma therapists are able to treat dysfunctions related to the endocrine glands with a new level of accomplishment.

Thus, the orb of the Arm Lesser Yang Channel is recognized as influencing three major areas; the processes of digestion, assimilation, and elimination; emotional factors; and the functions of the endocrine glands. The abbreviated names for this channel are: TH, TW, SJ, and End, which refer respectively, to Three Heaters, Triple Warmer, San Jiao, and Endocrine Channel.

THE PATHWAYS OF QI

Most books and charts that intend to teach the concepts of Oriental manipulative therapy show the superficial branches of the principal Organ pathways of Qi. These do indeed have great significance for the acupuncturist, who uses the loci (points) on the superficial branches of these main channels to assist in diagnosis and as the primary points of treatment, as well as to the advanced Amma therapist, who also uses them for evaluation and treatment purposes. Rarely discussed, however, are the deep internal pathways of the channels and the particular type of channels that are generally used for treatment by the Amma therapist, primarily the Tendino-Muscle Channels. This has resulted in a serious misunderstanding of the true nature of the art of Oriental manipulative therapy.

I would like to digress here for one moment to discuss the nomenclature of the pathways. For a very long time there was a paucity of English translations of Chinese medical literature available to the acupuncturist, and a complete absence of literature on traditional Oriental manipulative therapy available to the would-be therapist, save for a few very basic books outlining the art of shiatsu from Japan. This resulted in the mistaken idea that the twelve bilateral meridians ("imaginary lines") and the two midline vessels ("closed containers") constituted the defined scope of the system, and were used by acupuncturists and manipulative therapists alike. This has resulted in the creation and use of the word *acupressure* (*acu* = needle), a misnomer based on the assumption that the manipulative therapist treated the same "imaginary lines" as the acupuncturist.

A far more conceptually correct term for the pathways of Qi is *channel* rather than *meridian* or *vessel*. In fact, the pathways of Qi are neither imaginary lines on the surface of the body or closed vessels containing some fluid energy (as are blood vessels, for example). The term *channel* implies a pathway that can increase and decrease, ebb and flow, stagnate and rush, or diminish and overflow. This is, indeed, a more proper understanding of the bioenergetic system, which is the basis of Amma therapy and related Oriental medical arts.

The bioenergy enlivens the physical form. According to the Bharta Dharma (the philosophy of India), the mind uses a dual system to interact with the world. This system is composed of the *manomaya kosha* (the body of food) and the *pranamaya kosha* (the body of energy), and these two taken together are called the living physical body. The channels of Qi constitute that bioenergy or pranamaya kosha, which is without doubt a complex and active system. It has been described in great detail in Chinese literature with the same kind of scientific study and precision as any Western anatomy, insofar as such was possible with the primitive measuring instruments of ancient China.

In the early 1990s the government of China began sponsoring extensive research into the nature of the channels. This topic is being actively pursued, and numerous validations of traditional views have resulted. Studies at the University of Toronto, the New York College for Wholistic Health Education and Research, UCLA, other American institutions, and numerous institutions abroad have also begun to corroborate the Chinese view of the polar bioenergy. Modern allopathic physicians can have no quarrel with the basic concept of bioenergy, as they recognize the bioelectrical activity of the nervous system, the signals in the heart and elsewhere, and the greater and lesser areas of bioelectric potential both on the surface and within the body. The major difference between the results of Eastern and Western research lies in the application of observation and theory to the bioenergy, in order to discover and understand the nature of the patterns of the flow of Qi and its relation to disease and health. Historically this has not been accomplished in the Western world to the extent that it has been in the East; only in the last sixty years has any serious study been undertaken in the West on the nature and significance of bioenergy. Of course, the works of Wilhelm Reich, Baron Von Richenbacker, and magnetic healers, which were often ridiculed by the simplistic and narrow scientific establishment of the times, should not be overlooked for the depth of their understanding and effort in the face of a hostile environment.

The system called Jing Luo, the channels and collaterals, consists of the complex of energy pathways that enliven every area of the body. Just as the neurological and vascular systems, when isolated from the rest of the body, show the shape and size of the whole, the bioenergy system also could stand alone as a body of energy showing the shape and size of the whole. The system itself is quite involved. Twelve major internal pathways—the Primary Channels or Organ Channels—wind and unite through the total organism, passing in and out of the major organs and extending into the superficial regions of the body. These superficial branches are the channels upon which the acupuncturist locates his points and inserts needles to a depth of between one-eighth and four inches, in order to make contact with the Qi of the Primary Channels. Lying within the deeper regions of the body, and extending the range of effect of the Organ Channels, are the twelve Divergent Channels. These are branches that diverge from the Primary Channels; they allow energies to reach areas where the primary pathway does not flow. All Divergent Channels send energies deep into the body and ultimately to the head. The longitudinal Luo or Connecting Channels, and the transverse Luo Channels, which are short branches between coupled Primary Channels, act as reservoirs of channel Qi and further extend the distribution of Qi. Connecting and regulating the six Yin and the six Yang channels, as well as binding all the channels at the transverse midline of the body, are the Extraordinary Vessels. The Extraordinary Vessels number eight in total. Enlivening and feeding the muscles and tendons are the Tendino-Muscle Channels. These channels form a more superficial network at the level of the muscles, with some deeper branches connecting internally to the spine, the ribs, and the tongue. Finally, the twelve Cutaneous Regions lying at the surface of the body are the superficial residences of the Qi of the channels.

Most of the channels and their branches disperse into broad webs of energy, not unlike the capillaries of the vascular system. Just as the neurological and vascular systems act both as channels for dispersing disease deeper into the body and as carriers for the healing substances introduced from the outside or generated from within the body, so do the channels of Qi act to defend, protect, and nourish the whole, while still allowing perverse energy access to the deeper regions of the body.

Figures 5 through 16 show the superficial and internal pathways of the Primary Channels. Because the Tendino-Muscle Channels, the channels with which the Amma therapist primarily works, follow the path of the channel with which they are allied, the superficial pathways are of great value for reference in studying the Tendino-Muscle Channels. Note also the direction of the flow of Qi. Yang Qi flows down from Heaven and Yin Qi flows up from the Earth. (In the Chinese anatomical position, the arms are always raised.) This sometimes seems contradictory to superficial observation, and has even led to confusion among some advocates of macrobiotics. Yin is heavy and internal; Yang is light and external. Yin is the interior; Yang is the surface. These truths about the qualities of Yin and Yang often interfere with the understanding of energy and its movements and qualities. If one keeps in mind the poetic concept that Yin is Earth and Yang is Heaven, and further, the concept of the transmutation of Qi into its bipolar quality, as indicated in the basic symbol of Yin/Yang, it will become apparent that Yang flows down from its source in Heaven, and in that downward flow is converted into its polar quality to take on various Yin forms on Earth. The Yin of the Earth flows up toward Heaven, and, undergoing like transformation, feeds the Qi of Heaven and nourishes the Yang.

Figures 17 and 18 show the two midline channels, the Conception Vessel and the Governing Vessel, which are the only two of the eight Extraordinary Vessels to be studied in detail in this text. These channels are significant in that they have branches to many other channels—the Conception Vessel to the Yin channels and the Governing Vessel to the Yang channels—as well as to the channels of German electroacupuncture (Electroacupuncture According to Voll). The Conception Vessel controls the genitourinary area; it is necessary for this channel Qi to be flowing for conception to take place. Control points for the functions of the Three Warmers are also found on this channel. The Governing Vessel includes control points for each of the Viscera, Bowels, and several other functions.

Figures 19 to 30 are detailed illustrations of the Tendino-Muscle Channels, including several branches not generally indicated in the academic literature and some modifications to the traditional academic view of the exact pathways. These corrections are the result of my decades of training, study, and practice. It is quite possible that the pathways are somewhat modified as a result of time; the corrections may also reflect differences in the population of patients, as the classic texts are based on the study and treatment of an ancient Chinese population, while my work is based on the study and treatment of modern Koreans and modern Americans.

Some modern books on Oriental medical arts present the thesis that the Tendino-Muscle Channels refer to the network of tendons and muscles that coat the underlying viscera, nerves, and bones. Although the Nutrient Qi of the muscular system as well as the Defensive Qi on the surface is delivered by the Tendino-Muscle Channels, it is not accurate to identify the channel system with the physical form of the muscles. More than one Tendino-Muscle Channel is often found to feed the same muscle, and the channels are found to be far more thin than the muscles through which they move, as, for example, the branches of the Bladder Tendino-Muscle Channel over the gluteal region. They are, however, the major channels of Defensive Qi and are responsible for the protection of the body energetically, as the muscles are structurally.

Figures 31 to 33 show the six (or as some would prefer, the twelve) Cutaneous Regions, the areas on the surface of the body, from the superficial aspect of the Tendino-Muscle Channels through to the superficial aspects of the dermis, that reflect the six basic differentiations of the primary Yin/Yang polarities. The twelve Cutaneous Regions correspond to the Arm aspects and the Leg aspects of the six forms of energy.

POINTS USED IN APPLICATION OF PRESSURE IN AMMA THERAPY

The manipulation of acupuncture points found on the superficial branches is not the basis of Amma therapy. The hallmark of Amma therapy is the full-body manipulation of the Cutaneous Regions, the Tendino-Muscle Channels, and the superficial aspects of the twelve primary Organ Channels and the Governing and Conception Vessels. Manipulation of these channels promotes the stimulation and circulation of Qi, Blood, and Fluids, leading to beneficial and often profound effects on the channel system and Organs. However, Amma therapists will often utilize acupuncture points, as well as traditional extra points generally found off the channels and a class of points known as Ah Shui points, a word that translates roughly as "ouch!" Ah Shui points are

used in the treatment of such conditions as sciatica, tendonitis, and muscular pulls and strains. The location and tenderness of these points often indicate the nature of a disease, and they can therefore be used for both diagnostic purposes and treatment. The acupuncturist palpates for tender spots on the Tendino-Muscle Channels and needles these points (if they are not directly over an artery or nerve) with amazing and rapid results. Midlevel and advanced Amma therapists also palpate for these points, and apply finger pressure instead of needling the point.

It may be noted here that the system of trigger point therapy, which was originally applied to musculoskeletal problems, in some cases parallels both superficial channel points and Ah Shui points. Trigger point therapy is not, however, parallel to Amma therapy conceptually, nor are the majority of the points used contiguous with those used by Amma therapists. It is not surprising that many loci on the body will be within the scope of practical application of a number of different systems.

TINA SOHN (TS) POINTS

A special category of points frequently used by advanced Amma therapists is Tina Sohn (TS) points. These are extra points discovered during my many years of intensive practice. These points, tested repeatedly on thousands of patients by me and by senior Amma therapists, have proven extremely effective. Some of these points are extra points located on the channels; others are located off the channels. These extra points have very specific local and distal actions, and can treat

Organ and channel dysfunction. Twenty-six TS points appear within the treatment protocols described in part IV of this book. These points are a small sampling of the many that will be elucidated in future volumes on Amma therapy.

This discussion and the channel descriptions that follow should be sufficient for the beginning therapist to initiate an exploration of the nature of the channel system, and to learn firsthand that stimulation of the superficial aspects of the body can have profound effects deep within the organism. While the channel descriptions name the location of many points along a given pathway, the points that are labeled on the illustrations are major points pertaining to each channel. These can be used as guideposts to help the student gain an experiential knowledge of the pathway. In the illustrations, black lines indicate superficial channels and white lines indicate deep channels. Triangles represent Intersecting points with other channels (Intersecting, Organ, and Luo points are defined in chapter 14.) The reader can consult other texts on Oriental medicine (see Suggested Reading) for a visual description of all points along a given pathway.

A tsun is an acupuncture unit of measurement (AUM). There are two methods of measurement; both are described on page 253.

A SUMMARY OF THE FLOW PATTERNS OF THE QI

As the pathways of Qi are complex and rather numerous, it should be helpful to summarize the most important flow patterns.

QI CYCLES IN THE CHANNELS

The Nutrient Cycle	Begins in the Lung and flows as follows: Lu Co St Sp Ht SI Bl Ki HE SJ GB Liv.
The Yin/Yang Pairs	Each coupled set of inner/outer channels has an independent flow through the mediation of the lateral Luo Channels. Each pair is of the same Five Phase quality: Lu/Co; St/Sp; Ht/SI; Bl/Ki; HE/SJ; GB/Liv.
The Arm/Leg Pairs	Because the channels are paired in the flow of each of the Six Stages of Yin and Yang, there are strong influences between the arm and leg branches of each of the six energy types: Lu/Sp; Co/St; Ht/Ki; SI/Bl; HE/Liv; SJ/GB.
The Tendino-Muscle Channels	It is often said by acupuncturists that these channels carry only Defensive Qi. If this were so, there would be no method for distribution of Nutrient Qi to the superficial regions. It is probable that the Defensive Qi flows primarily in these channels for twenty-five cycles during the day and in closer proximity with the inner pathways at night for twenty-five cycles.
The Midline Channels	Although little mention has been made of this rather significant pair of the eight Extraordinary Channels, it is necessary to mention that they have many connections to other channels—the Governing Vessel Channel to the Yang and the Conception Vessel Channel to the Yin—and that there is a distinct circulation between the two, which is the subject of much study in esoteric and modern scientific circles.

QI CYCLES IN THE VISCERA

The Creation Cycle	Follows the outer Five Element pattern: Ht Sp Lu Ki Liv.
The Control Cycle	Follows the inner Five Element pattern: Ht Lu Liv Sp Ki.

THE TWELVE PRIMARY ORGAN CHANNELS

ARM GREAT YIN (TAI YIN) LUNG METAL CHANNEL
▼

This channel begins in the Middle Burner, DEEP to CV12. It descends to loop around the transverse colon. It then ascends, passing the cardiac orifice of the stomach, where the stomach and the esophagus meet. The channel passes through the diaphragm to CV17, then enters into the lungs. It moves up toward the throat and then crosses the upper thorax. The channel surfaces (SUPERFICIAL) below the acromial extremity of the clavicle, 1 tsun lateral to the mammillary line, 6 tsun lateral to the Conception Vessel. It ascends to Lu2 and then descends the anterolateral arm, following a pathway that falls between the long and short heads of the biceps brachii. Lu5 lies lateral to the biceps tendon at the cubital crease. The channel continues in its descent, passing between the brachioradialis and the pronator teres to the anterior aspect of the styloid process of the radius where Lu7 is found, 1.5 tsun proximal to the wrist. It crosses the wrist fold to Lu9 (the Organ point), continuing between the opponens pollicis and the abductor pollicis brevis to the thumb, where it ends at Lu11, 0.1 tsun proximal to the lower corner of the nail root on the radial side of the thumb.

A DEEP branch splits from Lu7 and crosses over the dorsum of the hand to the radial aspect of the nail bed of the index finger to connect with Co1.

TRANSVERSE LUO: Lu7 to Co4

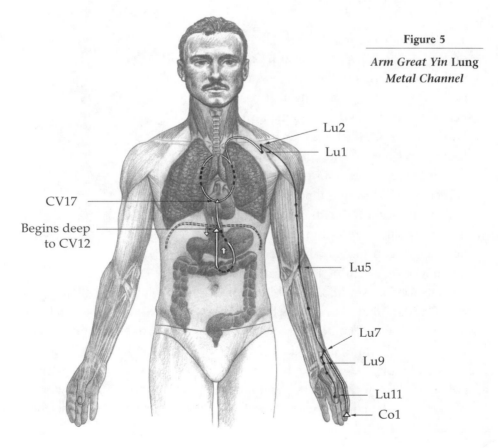

Figure 5

Arm Great Yin Lung *Metal Channel*

Lu2
Lu1
CV17
Begins deep to CV12
Lu5
Lu7
Lu9
Lu11
Co1

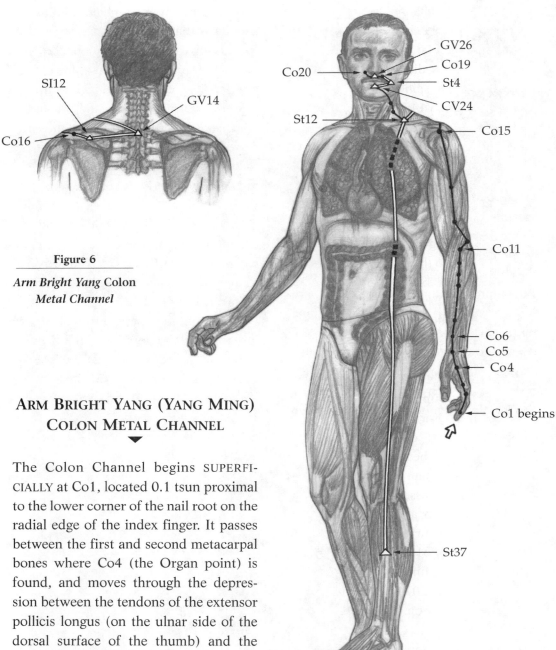

Figure 6

Arm Bright Yang Colon
Metal Channel

ARM BRIGHT YANG (YANG MING) COLON METAL CHANNEL

The Colon Channel begins SUPERFI-CIALLY at Co1, located 0.1 tsun proximal to the lower corner of the nail root on the radial edge of the index finger. It passes between the first and second metacarpal bones where Co4 (the Organ point) is found, and moves through the depression between the tendons of the extensor pollicis longus (on the ulnar side of the dorsal surface of the thumb) and the extensor pollicis brevis and abductor pollicis longus (on the radial border of the dorsum of the thumb). This is known as the "anatomical snuffbox," and it is here that Co5 is found. The channel ascends along the posterolateral border of the extensor digitorum, through Co6, over the supinator and toward the cubital crease. Co11 is located at the lateral end of the transverse cubital crease. The chan-

nel follows the lateral aspect of the triceps to the acromioclavicular articulation. Between the acromion and the head of the humerus lies Co15. From Co16, located on the superior aspect of the shoulder in the depression between the acromial extremity of the clavicle and the spine of the scapula, the channel moves DEEP to intersect with SI12, located in the center of the suprascapular fossa. From here the channel moves medially to GV14, which lies between the spinous process of C7 and T1. From GV14 it moves anteriorly to St12, located at the midpoint of the supraclavicular fossa, on the mammillary line. The channel splits here, a DEEP pathway descending into the thoracic cavity and a SUPERFICIAL pathway ascending into the neck and face. The DEEP branch descends, passing through the lung and the diaphragm to the flexure of the colon. (Each bilateral branch of the Colon Channel descends to the associated flexure, that is, the branch on the right passes to the hepatic flexure and the branch on the left passes to the splenic flexure.) The branch terminates its descent at St37.

From the supraclavicular fossa, a SUPERFICIAL branch moves upward through the neck, crossing the chin to CV24, located at the mentolabial groove. From CV24 the channel moves DEEP into the jaw, where it passes through the roots of the lower teeth and gums and intersects with St4. It curves around the upper lip, surfaces at Co19, and meets GV26, located at the philtrum. The channel crosses over to Co20 on the opposite side of the face. The Colon Channel ends at the ala of the nose at Co20, where it connects with a deep pathway of the Stomach Channel.

TRANSVERSE LUO: Co6 to Lu9

LEG BRIGHT YANG (YANG MING) STOMACH EARTH CHANNEL

▼

This channel starts DEEP at Co20 at the ala of the nose. It ascends the side of the nose to Bl1, and then passes laterally to emerge SUPERFICIALLY at St1, which lies vertically below the center of the pupil in a depression on the infraorbital margin. It moves through St2 and St3, and then moves DEEP to meet with GV28 at the labial frenum. It passes around the mouth, surfacing at St4, goes DEEP to CV24, and then moves laterally along the border of the jaw. The channel becomes SUPERFICIAL at St5, located at the inferior border of the mandible, anterior to the border of the masseter muscle in the depression appearing when the jaw is clenched and the muscle is contracted.

From St5 the channel splits, one branch ascending along the angle of the jaw and one branch descending into the torso. The ascending branch continues along the angle of the jaw, moving up the lateral aspect of the face and head, passing through GB3 and GB6 to St8, which is found at the corner of the forehead, 0.5 tsun within the anterior hairline and 4.5 tsun lateral to the Governing Vessel. The channel then moves DEEP to end at GV24. The descending branch from St5 moves down the neck into the supraclavicular fossa to St11, then moves laterally to St12. From here it moves DEEP to GV14 and then emerges once again SUPERFICIALLY at St12. It splits again here and descends into the torso with both a SUPERFICIAL and DEEP branch.

The SUPERFICIAL branch descends along the mammillary line to St18, where it moves medially to follow the lateral margin of the rectus abdominus. It passes lateral to the umbilicus through St25 and continues to the lower abdomen to St30, located superior to the inguinal groove, 2 tsun lateral to CV2. The DEEP pathway runs internally from St12, parallel to the

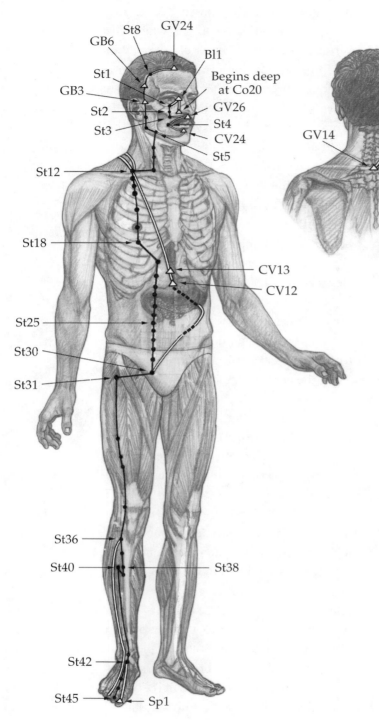

St8
GV24
GB6
Bl1
St1
Begins deep
at Co20
GB3
St2
GV26
St3
St4
CV24
St5
St12
CV13
CV12
St18
St25
St30
St31
St36
St38
St40
St42
St45
Sp1
GV14

Figure 7

Leg Bright Yang Stomach
Earth Channel

The channel leaves the abdomen at St30, moving laterally toward the anterior thigh, where St31 is found lying in the apex of the angle formed by the sartorious and tensor fascia lata. The channel continues in its descent, following the interstice between the vastus lateralis and rectus femoris. It descends to St36, where it again splits. St36 is located 3 tsun distal to the lower border of the patella and 1 tsun lateral to the anterior crest of the tibia. From St36 a DEEP branch descends lateral to the tibia, continuing over the dorsum of the foot to terminate at the lateral edge of the third toe. The SUPERFICIAL branch continues from St36 down the lateral border of the tibialis anterior. Note that St40 (the Luo point) is directly lateral to St38 as the channel descends. As the channel passes over the dorsum of the foot where St42 (the Organ point) is located, it continues between the second and third metatarsals and ends at St45, 0.1 tsun proximal to the lower corner of the nail root at the lateral side of the distal phalange of the second toe. A DEEP branch separates from St42 and terminates on the medial edge of the big toe, where it connects with the Spleen Channel at Sp1.

TRANSVERSE LUO: St40 to Sp3

SUPERFICIAL channel. It passes through the diaphragm, intersecting with CV13 and CV12, and then moves into the stomach, spleen, and large intestine. The DEEP and SUPERFICIAL channels join at St30.

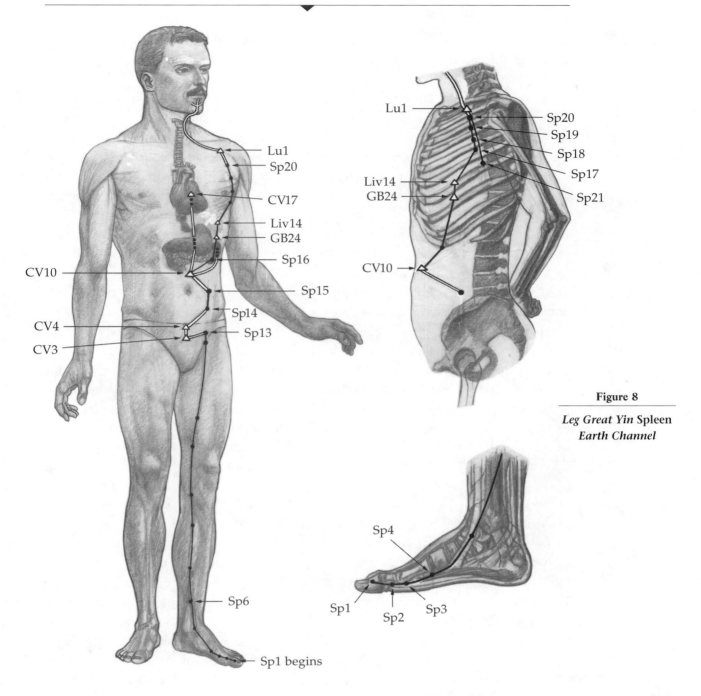

Lu1
Sp20
CV17
Liv14
GB24
Sp16
CV10
Sp15
Sp14
CV4
Sp13
CV3

Lu1
Sp20
Sp19
Sp18
Sp17
Sp21
Liv14
GB24
CV10

Figure 8

Leg Great Yin Spleen
Earth Channel

Sp4
Sp1
Sp2
Sp3

Sp6

Sp1 begins

LEG GREAT YIN (TAI YIN) SPLEEN EARTH CHANNEL

The SUPERFICIAL pathway originates at Sp1, located 0.1 tsun proximal to the lower corner of the nail root on the medial border of the distal phalange of the great toe. The pathway moves through Sp2 and Sp3 (the Organ point) and continues along the border of the foot at the meeting of the dorsal and plantar skins, where Sp4 can be found. It passes anterior to the medial malleolus, medial to the tendon of the tibialis anterior. The channel continues in its ascent up the medial leg to Sp6, located 3 tsun proximal to the vertex of the medial malleolus, on the posterior tibial border. From Sp6 the channel continues upward, running along the posterior aspect of the tibia to the patella, and ascends the anteromedial thigh, traveling anterior to the Liver Channel. The channel reaches the inguinal fold at Sp13, located on the mammillary line. Here the channel enters DEEP into the abdominal cavity. The pathway continues DEEP, intersecting with CV3 and CV4. It emerges SUPERFICIALLY at Sp14, continues to Sp15, and then moves DEEP once again to communicate with CV10. At CV10 one branch enters the spleen and another branch enters the stomach. The latter continues in its DEEP pathway, passing through the diaphragm and entering into the heart.

From CV10 a SUPERFICIAL branch passes through Sp16 to GB24 and then to Liv14. From here the channel continues through Sp17–Sp20, and then descends to Sp21. Sp21 is the endpoint of the SUPERFICIAL pathway. It is located on the midaxillary line 6 tsun below the axilla, midway between the axilla and the tip of the eleventh rib. Sp21 is called the Universal Luo, the Great Regulator. This point helps to regulate the flow of Qi and Blood throughout the body as they flow through the many small Blood Connecting Vessels.* A DEEP branch moves from Sp20 to intersect with Lu1, and then ascends along the esophagus, dispersing into the root of the tongue and lower lingual area.

TRANSVERSE LUO: Sp4 to St42

---

* The Blood Connecting Vessels are a subdivision of the Connecting Vessels (Luo Channels). They are the superficial blood vessels that can be seen with the naked eye. These tiny vessels transport Qi and Blood to the tissues and superficial regions of the body.

ARM LESSER YIN (SHAO YIN) HEART FIRE CHANNEL

▼

The Heart Channel begins DEEP, in the heart, traveling down through the major blood vessels and the diaphragm to connect with the small intestine. A branch separates in the heart and runs upward along the esophagus to the face, where it joins the tissues surrounding the eye. Another branch travels transversely from the heart to the lung, and then emerges SUPERFICIALLY at the axilla.

The channel surfaces (SUPERFICIAL) at Ht1, located in the center of the axilla on the medial side of the axillary artery. It passes along the medial aspect of the upper arm, traveling in the interstice between the biceps brachii and the medial head of the triceps. It then moves through the cubital fossa to Ht3. (To locate Ht3, flex the elbow. The point is between the medial end of the transverse cubital crease and the medial epicondyle of the humerus.) From here the channel continues along the medial aspect of the forearm in the space between the palmaris longus and the flexor carpi ulnaris through Ht7 (the Organ point) to the pisiform bone, proximal to the palm. The channel passes on the radial border of the hypothenar eminence, where it continues to the radial border of the fifth metacarpal. It ends at Ht9, located 0.1 tsun proximal to the lower corner of the nail root at the radial edge of the fifth digit.

TRANSVERSE LUO: Ht5 to SI4

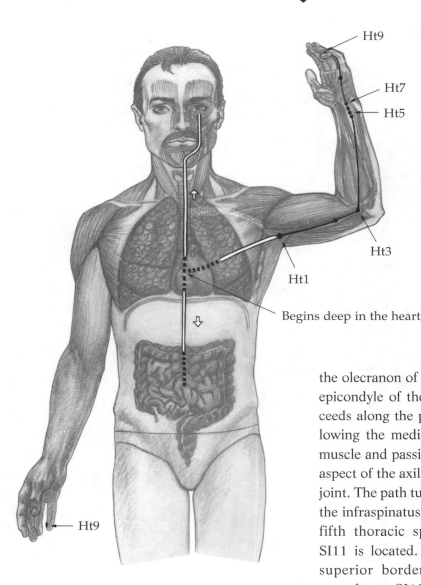

Ht9

Ht7

Ht5

Ht3

Ht1

Begins deep in the heart

Ht9

Figure 9

Arm Lesser Yin Heart
Fire Channel

ARM GREAT YANG (TAI YANG) SMALL INTESTINE FIRE CHANNEL

▼

This channel begins SUPERFICIALLY at SI1, located 0.1 tsun proximal to the lower corner of the nail root on the ulnar side of the fifth digit. It ascends along the ulnar side of the dorsal surface of the hand through SI4 (the Organ point) to the wrist, continuing to the styloid process of the ulna. It ascends the posteromedial forearm and passes between the olecranon of the ulna and the medial epicondyle of the humerus. It then proceeds along the posteriomedial arm, following the medial aspect of the triceps muscle and passing through the superior aspect of the axillary fold to the shoulder joint. The path turns toward the center of the infraspinatus fossa at the level of the fifth thoracic spinous process, where SI11 is located. It then ascends to the superior border of the spine of the scapula to SI12. The path continues medially, passing over the supraspinatus fossa to the medial border of the scapula and then ascends toward the neck. At the top of the shoulder it crosses the Bladder Channel (at Bl41) and continues to SI14, then to Bl11 and SI15. The path then intersects with GV14, located between the spinous processes of C7 and T1.

From GV14 it moves DEEP and then anteriorly to St12 at the supraclavicular fossa, then descends DEEP to intersect with CV17 and to communicate with the heart. The pathway continues in its

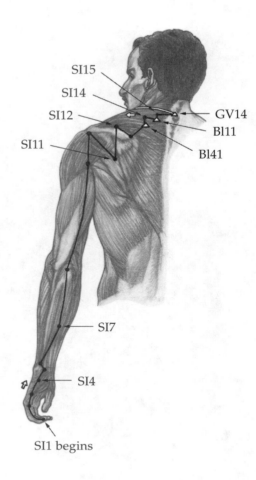

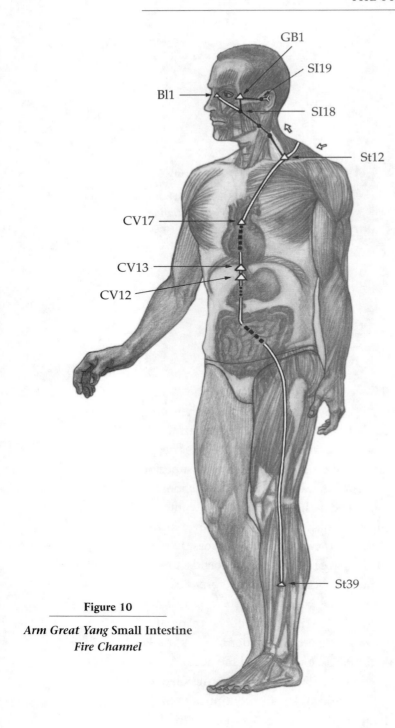

Figure 10

Arm Great Yang Small Intestine
Fire Channel

organ, the small intestine. The descending branch moves down the anterolateral aspect of the thigh and leg to terminate at St39.

A SUPERFICIAL branch ascends from St12 at the supraclavicular fossa into the neck and the cheek, where SI18 is found. It moves to the outer canthus of the eye where it meets GB1. The channel turns back across the temple and enters DEEP into the ear at its ending point, SI19, located in the depression between the tragus of the ear and the temporomandibular joint. Another DEEP branch separates from SI18 in the cheek and ascends to the inner canthus of the eye, where it meets with Bl1.

TRANSVERSE LUO: SI7 to Ht7

descent along the esophagus, passing through the diaphragm to connect with the Conception Vessel at CV13 and CV12. The channel then enters first into the stomach and then into its pertaining

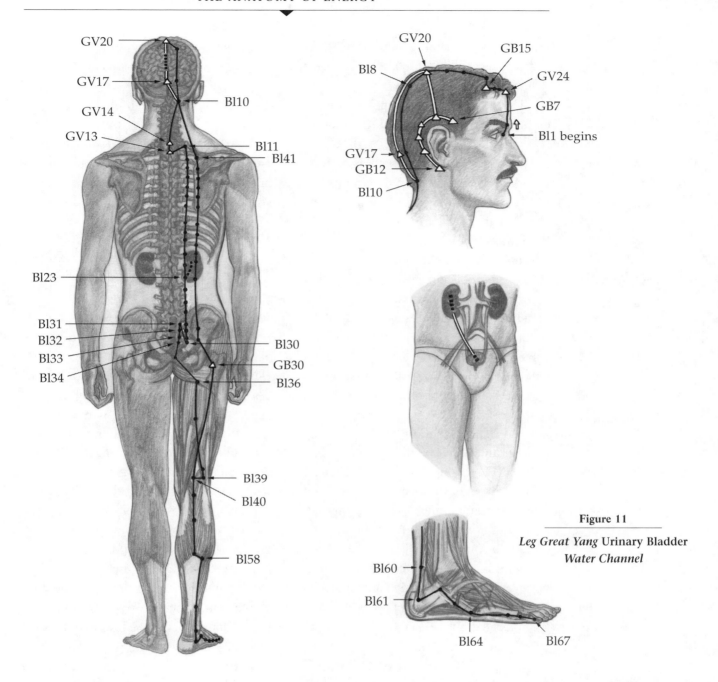

GV20
GV17
GV14
GV13
Bl10
Bl11
Bl41
Bl23
Bl31
Bl32
Bl33
Bl34
Bl30
GB30
Bl36
Bl39
Bl40
Bl58

GV20
Bl8
GB15
GV24
GB7
GV17
GB12
Bl10
Bl1 begins

Bl60
Bl61
Bl64
Bl67

Figure 11

Leg Great Yang **Urinary Bladder**
Water Channel

LEG GREAT YANG (TAI YANG) URINARY BLADDER WATER CHANNEL

▼

This channel begins SUPERFICIALLY at Bl1, at the inner canthus of the eye. It ascends the forehead, intersecting with GV24 and GB15. It then crosses to the vertex and intersects with GV20. From GV20 the SUPERFICIAL branch moves bilaterally across the cranium from Bl8 to Bl10. From GV20 a DEEP branch passes laterally to the area surrounding the ear, joining the Gall Bladder Channel from GB7–GB12. Another DEEP branch descends vertically from GV20 into the brain, and then emerges at GV17. The channel descends to Bl10, where it joins the superficial branch.

The SUPERFICIAL channel bifurcates at Bl10 and then descends the neck in two parallel branches. From Bl10, the medial branch descends to intersect with GV14 and GV13. It then moves upward to Bl11 before descending parallel to the spine to the lumbar region at Bl23. At Bl23 the channel enters DEEP into the internal cavity via the paravertebral muscles to communicate with the kidneys and with the channel's pertaining organ, the bladder. The channel resurfaces (SUPERFICIAL) at Bl23. It descends from the lumbar region to Bl30, which is located 1.5 tsun lateral to the Governing Vessel at the level of the fourth sacral foramen. From Bl30 the channel ascends to Bl31, located in the first sacral foramen midway between the posterior superior iliac spine and the Governing Vessel. The channel moves through the second, third, and fourth sacral foramen, passing through Bl32–34. It continues from Bl35, then crosses the buttock to Bl36, located at the midpoint of the gluteal crease. It continues over the posterior thigh and descends to the lateral side of the popliteal fossa at Bl39, located on the medial border of the biceps femoris tendon.

From Bl10 the second (lateral) branch descends parallel to the spine along the medial border of the scapula, from Bl41 to the gluteal region. It crosses the buttock, intersecting with GB30, and then descends along the posterior portion of the thigh, crossing the medial branch to Bl40, at the midpoint of the popliteal fossa. At the popliteal fossa the two branches join and continue as one pathway between the lateral and medial heads of the gastrocnemius muscle to the area posterior to the lateral malleolus, where points Bl60 and Bl61 are found. The pathway moves through Bl64 (the Organ point) and then follows the fifth metatarsal to end at Bl67, located 0.1 tsun proximal to the lower corner of the lateral nail root of the fifth digit.

TRANSVERSE LUO: Bl58 to Ki3

LEG LESSER YIN (SHAO YIN) KIDNEY WATER CHANNEL

The Kidney Channel begins DEEP, on the plantar surface of the fifth digit. It moves across the sole of the foot and surfaces (SUPERFICIAL) at Ki1, located in the depression appearing on the plantar aspect of the foot between the second and third metatarsophalangeal joints when the toes are flexed, one third of the distance from the base of the toes to the heel. The channel travels to Ki3 (the Organ point), located between the medial malleolus and the calcaneal tendon. From here it descends to Ki4 at the heel, proceeds to Ki5 and then to Ki6, located inferior to the medial malleolus. The channel then moves upward along the medial aspect of the lower leg to Sp6, where it unites with the Spleen and Liver channels. It ascends the medial aspect of the leg within the gastrocnemius muscle to Ki10, located at the medial aspect of the popliteal fossa between the tendons of the semitendinosus and semimembranosus muscles. The channel continues to ascend the posteromedial aspect of the thigh and then goes DEEP to the base of the spine, where it intersects with GV1. GV1 is located midway between the coccyx and the anus.

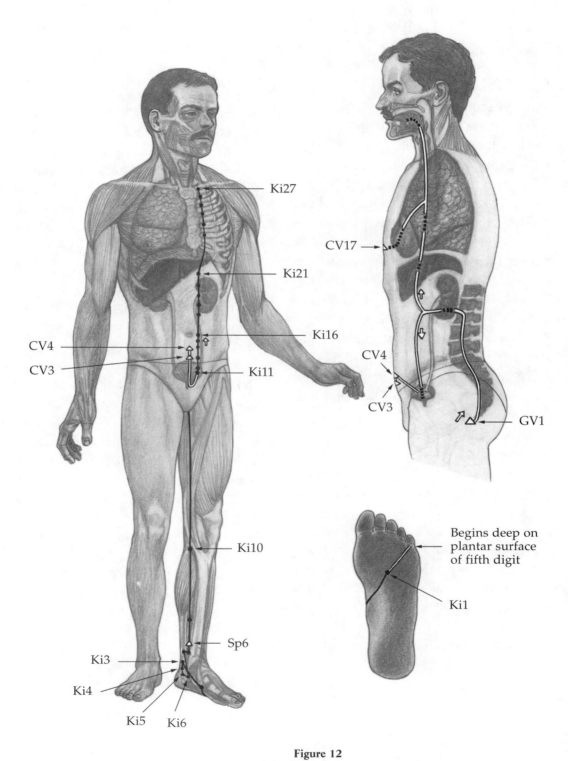

Ki27

Ki21

Ki16

CV4

CV3

Ki11

CV17 →

CV4

CV3

GV1

Ki10

Begins deep on
plantar surface
of fifth digit

Ki1

Sp6

Ki3

Ki4

Ki5   Ki6

Figure 12

Leg Lesser Yin Kidney
Water Channel

From GV1 the channel enters the spine, moving through the sacral and lumbar regions and entering its associated organ, the kidneys. Here the channel divides into two pathways. The ascending branch from the kidney passes through the liver and the diaphragm and enters the lung. It then passes through the throat to terminate at the root of the tongue. A branch separates from the lung, connecting with the heart and dispersing into the chest, where it connects with the Heart Envelope and CV17. The descending branch from the kidney travels down into the bladder. From the bladder the channel connects with CV4 and then CV3, and then descends to surface at Ki11. Here it unites with the Penetrating Vessel (Chung Mai). The Penetrating Vessel has a regulating effect on all twelve Primary Channels. It is known as the Sea of Blood for its governing effect on menstruation.

From Ki11 (SUPERFICIAL) the channel travels with the Penetrating Vessel to Ki21. The channel continues from Ki21, ascending over the most medial aspects of the intercostal spaces of the sixth, fifth, fourth, third, and second ribs to terminate at Ki27, located in the depression on the lower border of the medial head of the clavicle, 2 tsun lateral to the Conception Vessel.

TRANSVERSE LUO: Ki4 to Bl64

ARM ABSOLUTE YIN (JUE YIN) HEART ENVELOPE FIRE CHANNEL

▼

This channel begins DEEP, in the chest, intersecting with CV17. It descends across the diaphragm and into the abdomen, where it connects successively with the Upper, Middle, and Lower Burners of the San Jiao. A branch from the chest runs transversely toward the axillary region, where it emerges SUPERFICIALLY at HE1, located 3 tsun below the axillary fold, approximately 1 tsun lateral to the mammillary line in the fourth intercostal space. From HE1 the channel ascends to the axilla, where it then descends along the midline of the upper arm between the two heads of the biceps brachii, to the cubital fossa. From here it continues down the forearm between the tendons of the palmaris longus and the flexor carpi radialis, passing through HE7 (the Organ point) at the wrist. Entering the palm, it travels to end at HE9, located at the tip of the third finger. A branch separates in the palm from HE8 and runs DEEP along the fourth finger to the ulnar nail root, where it connects with the San Jiao Channel at SJ1.

TRANSVERSE LUO: HE6 to SJ4

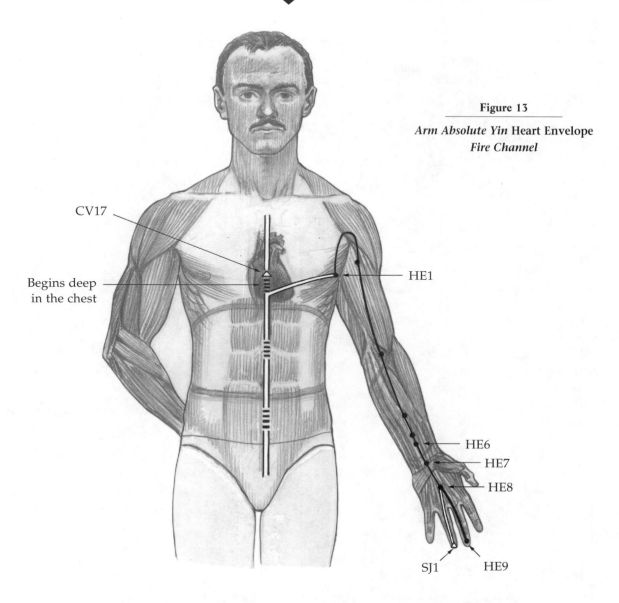

Figure 13

Arm Absolute Yin Heart Envelope
Fire Channel

CV17

Begins deep
in the chest

HE1

HE6
HE7
HE8

SJ1   HE9

ARM LESSER YANG (SHAO YANG) SAN JIAO FIRE CHANNEL

This channel originates SUPERFICIALLY at SJ1, located 0.1 tsun proximal to the lower corner of the ulnar nail root of the fourth digit. It proceeds between the fourth and fifth metacarpal bones on the dorsum of the hand, passing through SJ4 (the Organ point) and then ascending the posterior forearm between the ulna and the radius. It continues upward across the olecranon and along the posterior aspect of the upper arm, passing between the lateral and long heads of the triceps to the shoulder region. Here it intersects the Small Intestine Channel at SI12, moves to SJ15, and then goes deep to intersect with GV14. From GV14 the channel passes through GB21 and then enters into the supraclavicular fossa at St12. From here the channel descends DEEP into the chest region, to CV17. Here the channel divides into an ascending and a descending branch. The descending branch communicates first with the Heart Envelope, and

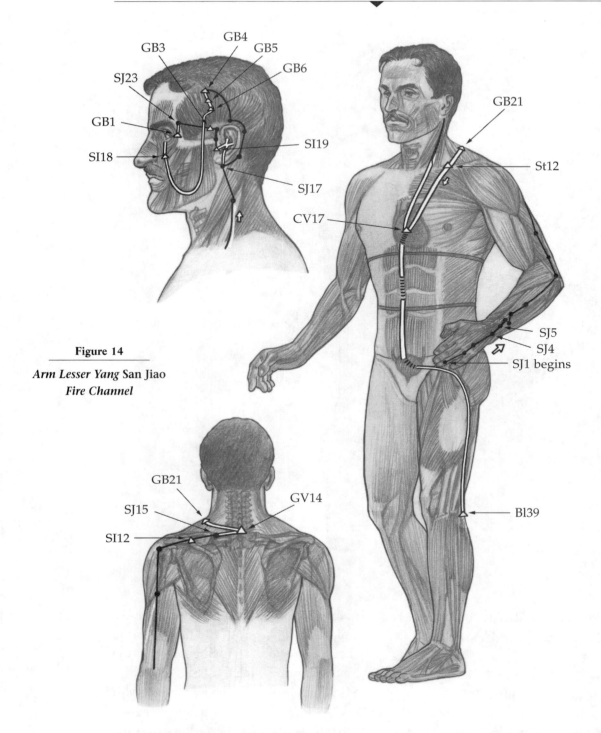

Figure 14

Arm Lesser Yang San Jiao
Fire Channel

then descends through the diaphragm to the abdomen, linking successively with the Upper, Middle, and Lower Burners of the San Jiao.

The ascending branch from CV17 emerges SUPERFICIALLY at the supraclavicular fossa. The channel proceeds up the neck to SJ17, which is located posterior to the lobule of the ear, in the depression between the mandible and the mastoid process. It then moves around the posterior ear to intersect DEEP with the Gall Bladder Channel at GB4, GB5, and GB6 before winding downward around the cheek, through SI18, to terminate below the eye in the infraorbital ridge.

Another branch separates from behind the ear at SJ17 and enters DEEP into the ear. It then emerges SUPERFICIALLY in front of the ear, where it intersects the Small Intestine Channel at SI19. From SI19 the channel moves up the anterior aspect of the ear and then crosses the Gall Bladder Channel at GB3. It traverses the side of the head to terminate at the lateral border of the eyebrow at SJ23. This branch then moves DEEP to GB1 at the outer canthus of the eye. A separate (DEEP) branch descends from the bladder in the Lower Burner to connect with BL39 at the lateral popliteal fossa.

TRANSVERSE LUO: SJ5 to HE7

LEG LESSER YANG (SHAO YANG) GALL BLADDER WOOD CHANNEL

▼

The Gall Bladder Channel begins SUPERFICIALLY at GB1, located 0.5 tsun lateral to the outer canthus of the eye, in the depression on the lateral side of the orbit. It traverses the temple region to the area slightly below the tragus of the ear, then ascends the temple to St8 at the superior hairline and continues to GB4. From here it descends to the level of the ear and then follows a path around the ear, intersecting with SJ22 and SJ20 along its course and continuing to the base of the occiput. GB12 can be found posterior and inferior to the mastoid process. The channel then ascends and crosses the cranium to GB14, which is located approximately 1 tsun above the midpoint of the eyebrow. The channel moves somewhat medially before crossing and descending the cranium to GB20, which lies in the depres-

sion between the sternocleidomastoid muscle and the lateral border of the trapezius at the base of the occiput. From GB20 the channel intersects SI17 before descending the neck. At the top of the shoulder it turns posteromedially through GB21 to intersect with GV14. From GV14 it intersects with Bl11 and then SI12 before moving anterior into the supraclavicular fossa to St12, where it divides into superficial and deep pathways.

A DEEP branch originating at GB20 passes through SJ17 before entering into the ear. The channel emerges at SI19. From SI19 a branch intersects with St7 before rejoining GB1 at the outer canthus of the eye. Another branch moves from GB1 to the jaw and then curves upward to the infraorbital region before descending again across the cheek and into the neck. Here it joins the original channel at St12 at the supraclavicular fossa.

From the supraclavicular fossa, a DEEP pathway descends into the chest, crossing the diaphragm and connecting with the liver before joining its pertaining organ, the gall bladder. It continues along the inside of the thorax before reaching the inguinal region of the lower abdomen. It winds around the genitalia, and then emerges SUPERFICIALLY at the hip at GB30.

The SUPERFICIAL pathway of the channel moves from the supraclavicular fossa anterior to the axilla along the lateral aspect of the chest. It moves through Liv13 before passing through the free ends of the floating ribs. It turns posteriorly toward the sacral region, intersecting with Bl31–Bl34 at the sacrum. The SUPERFICIAL channel joins with the DEEP pathway at GB30 at the hip joint. This

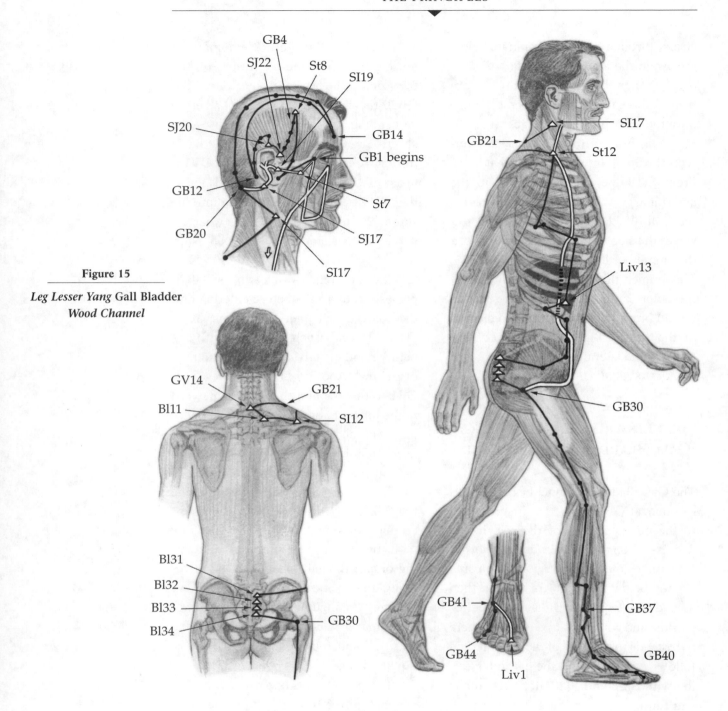

Figure 15

Leg Lesser Yang Gall Bladder
Wood Channel

union creates one SUPERFICIAL pathway that descends along the lateral aspect of the thigh to the knee. The channel continues to descend just anterior to the fibula. It crosses anterior to the lateral malleolus, passing through GB40 (the Organ point), and traverses the dorsum of the foot, moving between the fourth and fifth metatarsals before terminating at GB44, located 0.1 tsun proximal to the lower corner of the lateral nail root of the fourth digit. A DEEP branch separates from GB41 and runs between the first and second metatarsals to the great toe, where it communicates with Liv1.

TRANSVERSE LUO: GB37 to Liv3

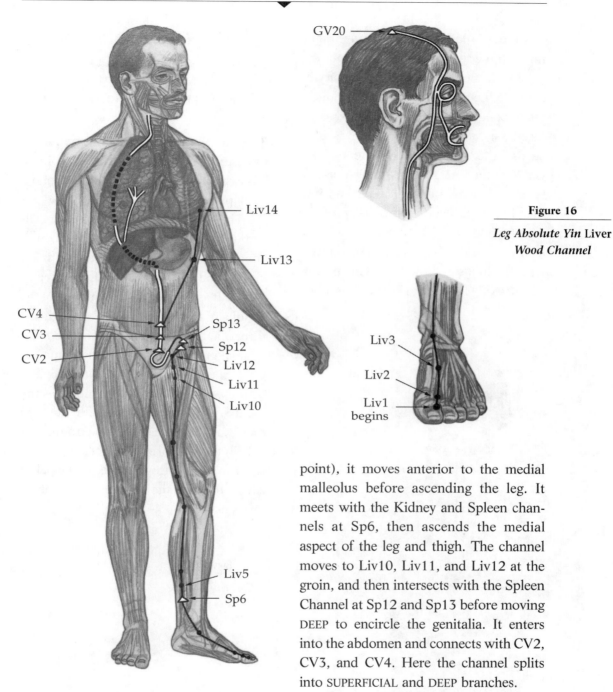

Figure 16

Leg Absolute Yin Liver Wood Channel

LEG ABSOLUTE YIN (JUE YIN) LIVER WOOD CHANNEL

▼

This channel begins SUPERFICIALLY on the dorsum of the foot, 0.1 tsun proximal to the lower corner of the lateral nail root of the great toe. Passing over the dorsum of the foot through Liv2 and Liv3 (the Organ point), it moves anterior to the medial malleolus before ascending the leg. It meets with the Kidney and Spleen channels at Sp6, then ascends the medial aspect of the leg and thigh. The channel moves to Liv10, Liv11, and Liv12 at the groin, and then intersects with the Spleen Channel at Sp12 and Sp13 before moving DEEP to encircle the genitalia. It enters into the abdomen and connects with CV2, CV3, and CV4. Here the channel splits into SUPERFICIAL and DEEP branches.

The SUPERFICIAL branch continues from CV4 to Liv13 at the tip of the eleventh floating rib, and then to Liv14 which is located on the mammillary line, two ribs below the nipple, in the sixth intercostal space. The DEEP branch ascends from CV4, then enters the stomach; its pertaining organ, the liver; and the gall bladder. From here the channel continues up through the diaphragm, through the lungs and costal region, traversing the neck posterior to the pharynx, entering the nasopharynx, and then moving to connect with the tissues surrounding the eye. Finally the channel ascends across the forehead and meets with GV20 at the vertex of the head. A branch separates below the eye to descend into the cheek and encircle the inside of the lips. An additional DEEP branch from the liver crosses the diaphragm and connects with the lungs and the Lung Channel.

TRANSVERSE LUO: Liv5 to GB40

EXTRAORDINARY VESSELS

CONCEPTION VESSEL (REN MAI)

▼

The Conception Vessel is the confluence of all the Yin channels. It consists of two pathways—a SUPERFICIAL pathway and a DEEP pathway.

The Conception Vessel arises SUPERFICIALLY in the lower abdomen, where it connects with the genital and urinary organs and emerges at CV1 at the perineum. It ascends along the midline of the abdomen and chest, passes through the throat, and crosses the chin to the mentolabial groove where CV24 is found. At CV24 the pathway goes DEEP and divides into two branches that encircle the mouth, both intersecting with St4 and then ascending the cheeks to terminate at St1, in the infraorbital ridge.

The DEEP pathway arises in the pelvic cavity. It enters the spine and ascends up the back.

Figure 17

Conception Vessel

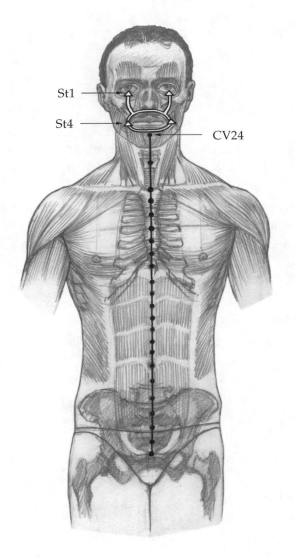

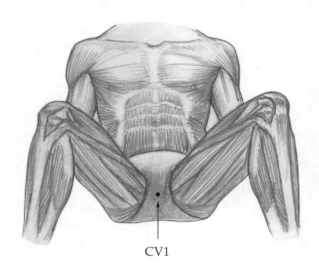

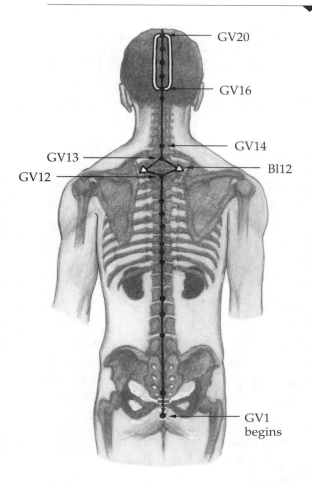

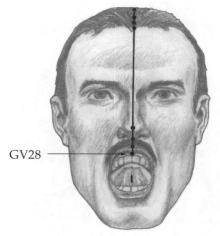

Figure 18

Governing Vessel

GOVERNING VESSEL (DU MAI)

The Governing Vessel is the confluence of all Yang channels. There are four pathways through which this vessel moves— one superficial Primary Channel and three deep pathways.

The Governing Vessel originates SUPERFICIALLY at the perineum. From CV1 the vessel moves posteriorly to GV1, midway between the coccyx and the anus. From here it ascends along the spine. At GV12 a branch diverts to intersect with Bl12, then unites with GV13. The vessel ascends to GV16, located directly below the inion. A DEEP branch enters into the brain, ascends to the vertex of the head, and emerges at GV20. The vessel then follows the midline of the forehead across

the bridge of the nose, terminating at the labial frenum at point GV28. Note that GV14 and GV20 are Intersecting points for all the Yang channels.

A DEEP pathway originates in the pelvic region. It descends to the genitals and perineum and passes through the tip of the coccyx, where it travels to the gluteal region and intersects with the Bladder Channel. It intersects the deep branch of the Kidney Channel at GV1, then returns to the spinal column and ascends to join the kidneys.

The origin of the second DEEP pathway begins bilaterally at Bl1 at the inner canthus of the eye. The branches ascend across the forehead and converge at GV20 at the vertex of the head, where the channel enters the brain, emerging at GV16. The channel divides again into two branches that descend along opposite sides of the spine to the waist. Here the pathways join with the kidneys.

The third DEEP pathway arises in the lower abdomen and ascends across the navel. It passes through the heart and enters the throat. Continuing an upward course, the channel crosses the cheek and encircles the mouth before terminating at St1 in the center of the infraorbital ridge.

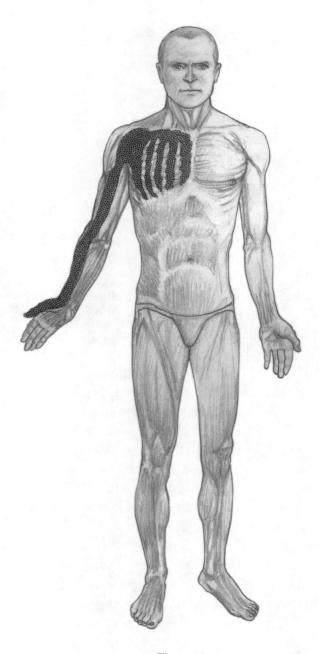

Figure 19

*Arm Great Yin
Tendino-Muscle Channel*

THE TENDINO-MUSCLE CHANNELS

ARM GREAT YIN (TAI YIN) TENDINO-MUSCLE CHANNEL (PERTAINING ORGAN—LUNG)

This channel begins on the palmar surface of the thumb and travels up along the thenar eminence to the radial aspect of the wrist. From here the pathway ascends the anterolateral forearm to connect at the elbow, and continues along the anterolateral aspect of the arm to the axilla, where it crosses medially through the anterior shoulder and into the chest. In the chest it connects with the clavicle and disperses downward, connecting with the ribs, sternum, and diaphragm.

Musculature Through Which this Channel Passes

Thenar eminence: opponens pollicis, abductor pollicis brevis, flexor pollicis brevis. **Forearm:** flexor pollicis longus, brachioradialis, flexor digitorum superficialis, flexor carpi radialis, pronator quadratus, pronator teres, supinator. **Arm:** biceps brachii, brachialis. **Shoulder:** coracobrachialis, anterior deltoid. **Chest:** pectoralis major, pectoralis minor, external intercostals, internal intercostals, diaphragm, transversus thoracis, subclavius.

ARM BRIGHT YANG (YANG MING) TENDINO-MUSCLE CHANNEL (PERTAINING ORGAN—COLON)

▼

This channel begins on the dorsal tip of the index finger and travels up the dorsum of the hand to connect at the wrist. It continues over the posterolateral forearm, connecting at the lateral elbow, and then ascends the lateral surface of the arm to the shoulder. From here the channel divides into two. A posterior branch disperses over the scapula and connects with the spine. An anterior branch travels through the supraclavicular fossa to the neck, where it crosses the sternocleidomastoid as it ascends to the angle of the mandible. Here the pathway divides again. One branch ascends across the cheekbone to the side of the nose. A second branch continues upward from the angle of the mandible to connect at the jaw, then passes through the temple region and over the top of the head to terminate at the angle of the mandible on the opposite side.

Musculature Through Which this Channel Passes

Hand: dorsal interosseous. **Forearm:** extensor pollicis brevis, extensor pollicis longus, abductor pollicis longus, extensor carpi radialis brevis, extensor carpi radialis longus, extensor digitorum superficialis, brachioradialis, supinator. **Arm:** lateral head of the triceps. **Shoulder/Back:** middle deltoid, upper, middle, and lower trapezius, supraspinatus, infraspinatus, rhomboid major, rhomboid minor, levator scapulae. **Neck:** sternocleidomastoid, suprahyoids, infrahyoids, platysma. **Head:** masseter, zygomaticus, levator anguli oris, levator labii superior, buccinator, risorius, medial pterygoid, lateral pterygoid, temporalis, galea aponeurotica.

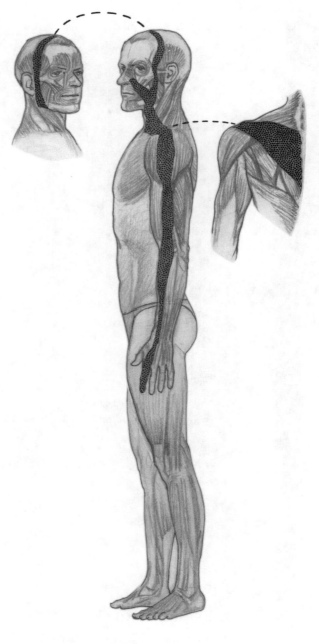

Figure 20

*Arm Bright Yang
Tendino-Muscle Channel*

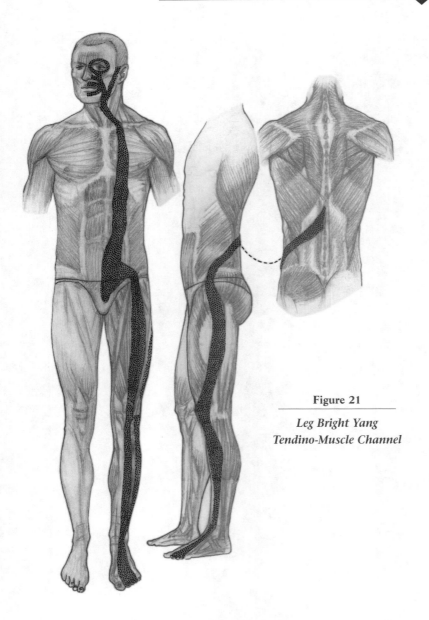

Figure 21

*Leg Bright Yang
Tendino-Muscle Channel*

LEG BRIGHT YANG (YANG MING) TENDINO-MUSCLE CHANNEL (PERTAINING ORGAN—STOMACH)

This channel arises from the dorsal surfaces of the second, third, and fourth toes and passes over the dorsum of the foot. It connects at the anterior ankle, where two branches continue to ascend the lower extremity. One branch ascends the lateral leg, connecting at the knee, then continues up the lateral thigh, crossing the Leg Lesser Yang Gall Bladder Tendino-Muscle Channel to connect at the hip and posteriorly with the lower thoracic spine. The main branch ascends from the ankle to the anterolateral leg, connecting at the knee and continuing up the anterolateral thigh to the inguinal region, where it travels medially to the genitals and lower abdominopelvic region. It ascends along the rectus abdominis muscles and runs parasternally in the chest to connect at the supraclavicular fossa. The channel crosses the sternocleidomastoid as it ascends to the angle of the mandible where the pathway divides. The posterior branch travels to the area anterior to the ear. The anterior branch moves medially to the mouth and nose and then forms a muscular net with the Leg Great Yang Bladder Tendino-Muscle Channel around the eye.

Musculature Through Which this Channel Passes

Foot: dorsal interosseous, extensor digitorum brevis, extensor hallucis brevis. **Leg:** extensor digitorum longus; tibialis anterior; peroneus brevis, longus, and tertius; extensor hallucis longus; soleus. **Thigh:** sartorius, rectus femoris, vastus lateralis, vastus intermedius, tensor fasciae latae, iliotibial tract. **Buttock:** gluteus medius and minimus. **Abdomen:** rectus abdominis, pyramidalis, external abdominal obliques, internal abdominal obliques, transversus abdominis. **Back:** latissimus dorsi. **Chest:** pectoralis major, subclavius. **Neck:** sternocleidomastoid, platysma, suprahyoids, infrahyoids. **Head:** masseter, orbicularis oris, depressor anguli oris, depressor labii inferioris, mentalis, levator anguli oris, levator labii superioris, risorius, orbicularis oculi, buccinator, zygomaticus, lateral pterygoids, medial pterygoids, temporalis.

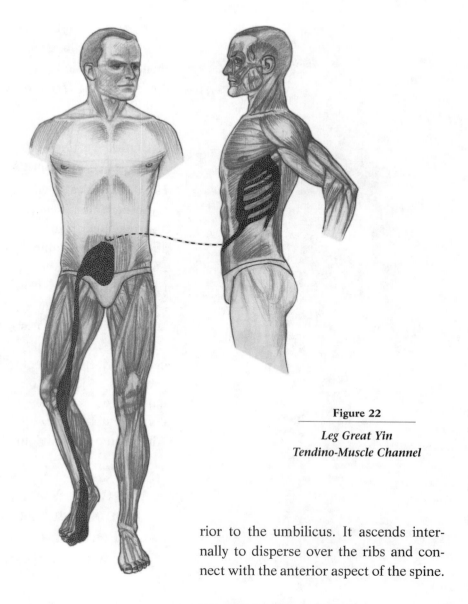

Figure 22

*Leg Great Yin
Tendino-Muscle Channel*

rior to the umbilicus. It ascends internally to disperse over the ribs and connect with the anterior aspect of the spine.

LEG GREAT YIN (TAI YIN) TENDINO-MUSCLE CHANNEL (PERTAINING ORGAN—SPLEEN)

This channel begins at the medial side of the great toe and travels up the medial aspect of the foot to connect anterior to the medial malleolus. It continues up the anteromedial leg to connect at the medial condyle of the tibia. The pathway ascends the medial thigh to the inguinal region, where it joins with the external genitalia and then enters the abdominal wall infe-

Musculature Through Which this Channel Passes

Foot: extensor hallucis longus tendon, tibialis anterior tendon, tibialis posterior tendon. **Leg:** soleus, gastrocnemius. **Thigh:** vastus medialis, sartorius, gracilis, adductor magnus, adductor longus, adductor brevis, pectineus, psoas, iliacus. **Abdomen:** rectus abdominis, pyramidalis, transverse abdominis, external abdominal obliques, internal abdominal obliques, psoas. **Chest:** external intercostals, internal intercostals, subcostals, serratus anterior.

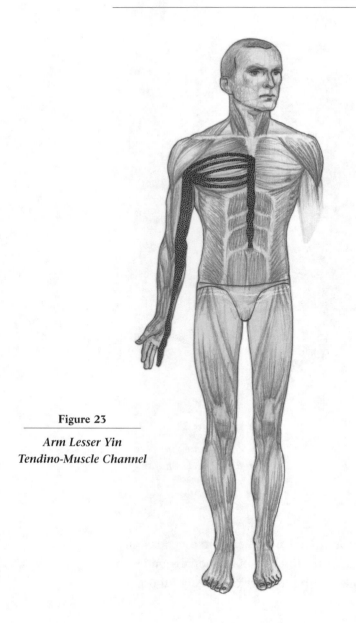

Figure 23

*Arm Lesser Yin
Tendino-Muscle Channel*

to the sternum, it crosses the Arm Great Yin Lung Tendino-Muscle Channel and then descends along the midline, crossing the diaphragm and connecting with the umbilicus.

Musculature Through Which this Channel Passes

Hand: lumbricals, palmar interosseous. **Hypothenar eminence:** opponens digiti minimi, flexor digiti minimi brevis, abductor digiti minimi, palmaris brevis. **Forearm:** palmaris longus, flexor digitorum superficialis, flexor digitorum profundus, flexor carpi ulnaris, pronator teres, pronator quadratus, flexor carpi radialis. **Arm:** biceps brachii, medial head of triceps, coracobrachialis. **Chest:** pectoralis major, pectoralis minor, external intercostals, internal intercostals, transversus thoracis, diaphragm. **Abdomen:** rectus abdominis, linea alba.

ARM GREAT YANG (TAI YANG) TENDINO-MUSCLE CHANNEL (PERTAINING ORGAN— SMALL INTESTINE)

This channel begins on the dorsal tip of the fifth digit and connects at the posteromedial aspect of the wrist. It ascends the posteromedial forearm to connect at the medial condyle of the humerus, and continues up the posteromedial arm to the axilla. From the axilla, a branch moves posteriorly to surround the scapula, where it then travels up the neck anterior to the Leg Great Yang Bladder Tendino-Muscle Channel to connect behind the ear. A branch enters directly into the ear and emerges at the apex of the ear, where it descends the cheek area

ARM LESSER YIN (SHAO YIN) TENDINO-MUSCLE CHANNEL (PERTAINING ORGAN—HEART)

This channel starts on the lateral aspect of the fifth digit and passes through the hypothenar eminence to connect with the medial aspect of the wrist. It continues to ascend the anteromedial forearm to connect at the elbow. It ascends the medial arm and enters the chest at the axilla. As the pathway continues to move medially

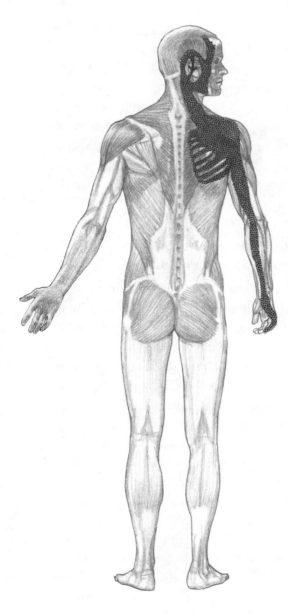

Figure 24

*Arm Great Yang
Tendino-Muscle Channel*

Musculature Through Which this Channel Passes

Hand: abductor digiti minimi. **Forearm:** extensor carpi ulnaris, flexor carpi ulnaris, anconeus. **Arm:** triceps. **Shoulder/Back:** posterior deltoid; supraspinatus; infraspinatus; teres minor; teres major; subscapularis; upper, middle, and lower trapezius; rhomboid major, rhomboid minor, levator scapulae, serratus anterior, serratus posterior superior. **Neck:** sternocleidomastoid, splenius capitis, splenius cervicus. **Head:** masseter, lateral pterygoids, medial pterygoids, zygomaticus, orbicularis oculi, temporalis, auriculares, temporoparietalis.

LEG GREAT YANG (TAI YANG) TENDINO-MUSCLE CHANNEL (PERTAINING ORGAN—BLADDER)

▼

This channel begins at the lateral aspect of the fifth toe and moves proximally to connect with the lateral malleolus, then ascends the leg to connect at the lateral knee. According to my observations, this branch continues up the lateral thigh to the base of the gluteal region. A second branch separates from below the lateral malleolus and connects at the heel, where it ascends to connect at the lateral aspect of the popliteal fossa. A third branch separates from the second at the head of the gastrocnemius muscle and continues up to connect at the medial aspect of the popliteal fossa. Both branches continue to ascend the posterior thigh to unite with the first branch at the base of the gluteal region. The united branches then travel over the buttocks and ascend the spine to connect at the occiput. From here, a branch separates and enters the

to connect at the angle of the mandible. From here, the channel continues to the outer canthus of the eye. Another branch begins at the angle of mandible, ascending around the teeth and anterior to the ear, where it reconnects with the outer canthus of the eye and the corner of the forehead.

and neck, connecting at the occiput. A second branch arises from the spine and connects at the lateral shoulder. A third branch separates from the spine and crosses over the shoulder, where it ascends the neck and travels across the cheek, uniting with the main pathway at the side of the nose. A fourth branch moves from the lower spine across the buttocks to the lateral hip.

Musculature Through Which this Channel Passes

Foot: dorsal interosseous, abductor digiti minimi, extensor digitorum brevis, flexor digitorum longus tendon. **Leg:** flexor hallucis longus, gastrocnemius, soleus, peroneus longus, peroneus brevis, peroneus tertius, tibialis posterior, flexor digitorum longus, popliteus, plantaris. **Thigh:** semitendinosus, semimembranosus, biceps femoris, iliotibial tract. **Buttock:** gluteus maximus, gluteus medius, gluteus minimus; piriformis. **Shoulder/Back:** erector spinae, latissimus dorsi, upper, middle and lower trapezius, serratus posterior superior, serratus posterior inferior, serratus anterior, teres major, rhomboid major, rhomboid minor, infraspinatus, supraspinatus, levator scapulae, levator costarum. **Chest:** pectoralis major, pectoralis minor. **Neck:** sternocleidomastoid, platysma, anterior scalene, middle scalene, posterior scalene. **Head:** occipitalis, galea aponeurotica, frontalis, orbicularis oculi, corrugator supercilii, compressor nares, dilator nares, zygomaticus, levator labii superioris, levator anguli oris, procerus, buccinator, risorius, masseter, medial pterygoid.

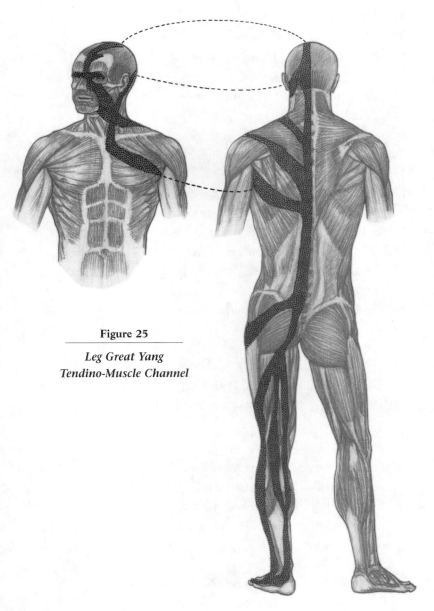

Figure 25

*Leg Great Yang
Tendino-Muscle Channel*

root of the tongue. The main branch continues from the occiput and crosses over the head to the bridge of the nose, where a branch spreads around the eye and continues downward to connect at the area lateral to the nose. A branch from the spine passes under the axilla to the chest

LEG LESSER YIN (SHAO YIN) TENDINO—MUSCLE CHANNEL (PERTAINING ORGAN—KIDNEY)

This channel begins on the plantar surface of the foot beneath the fifth toe. It travels to the area below the medial malleolus, where it converges with the Leg Great Yin Spleen Tendino-Muscle Channel, and passes posterior to connect at the heel, where it converges with the Leg Great Yang Bladder Tendino-Muscle Channel. The pathway continues to ascend the medial leg to connect at the medial knee, where it again unites with the Leg Great Yin Spleen Tendino-Muscle Channel. It continues to ascend the posteromedial thigh to unite at the genital region and lower abdomen. It enters the body inferior to the umbilicus and follows a DEEP pathway, where it connects with the anterior spine, then travels upward to connect at the occiput, where it unites with the Leg Great Yang Bladder Tendino-Muscle Channel.

Musculature Through Which this Channel Passes

Foot: all plantar muscles of the foot, tibialis anterior tendon. **Leg:** tibialis posterior, flexor digitorum longus, flexor digitorum brevis, flexor hallucis longus, soleus, gastrocnemius. **Thigh:** sartorius, gracilis, vastus medialis, adductor magnus, adductor longus, adductor brevis, pectineus, semimembranosus, semitendinosus. **Abdomen:** rectus abdominis, pyramidalis, psoas, iliacus. **Spine:** diaphragm, anterior longitudinal ligament, longus colli, longus capitis, rectus capitis anterior, rectus capitis lateralis.

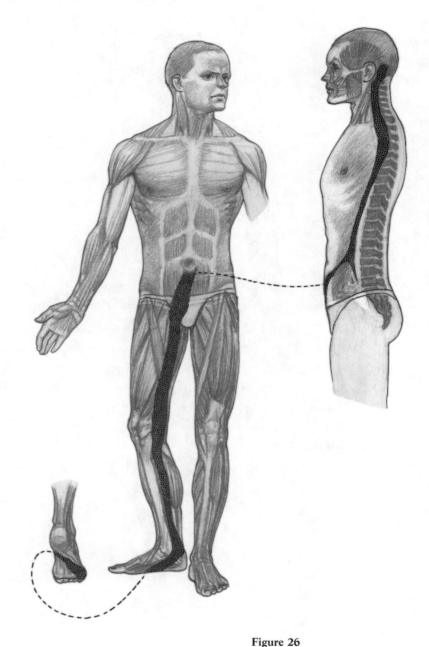

Figure 26

Leg Lesser Yin Tendino-Muscle Channel

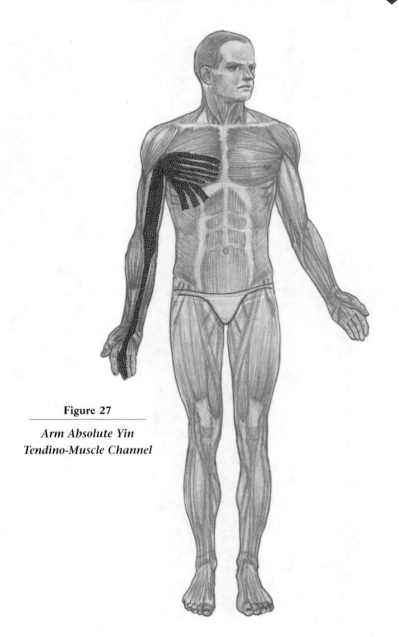

Figure 27

*Arm Absolute Yin
Tendino-Muscle Channel*

medial elbow, then continues up the anteromedial arm and connects to the area below the axilla. From here, the channel disperses across the chest and downward, connecting with the anterior and posterior surfaces of the ribcage. A branch enters the chest below the axilla and spreads over the chest to connect at the diaphragm.

Musculature Through Which this Channel Passes

Hand: lumbricals, palmaris brevis, palmar interosseous. **Forearm:** palmaris longus, flexor digitorum superficialis, flexor carpi radialis, pronator teres, pronator quadratus. **Arm:** biceps brachii, brachialis, coracobrachialis. **Chest:** pectoralis major, pectoralis minor, external intercostals, internal intercostals, transversus thoracis, diaphragm.

ARM LESSER YANG (SHAO YANG) TENDINO-MUSCLE CHANNEL (PERTAINING ORGAN—SAN JIAO)
▼

This channel begins at the tip of the fourth digit and travels up the dorsum of the hand to connect at the posterior wrist. It continues to ascend the midline of the posterior forearm to connect at the olecranon process of the elbow. The pathway ascends the lateral arm to the shoulder, where it converges with the Arm Great Yang Small Intestine Tendino-Muscle Channel as it travels up the neck. From the neck the channel travels to the angle of the mandible, where a branch separates to connect at the root of the tongue. Another branch ascends anterior to the ear, connects at the outer canthus of the eye, crosses the temple, and connects at the corner of the forehead.

ARM ABSOLUTE YIN (JUE YIN) TENDINO-MUSCLE CHANNEL (PERTAINING ORGAN— HEART ENVELOPE)
▼

This channel begins at the palmar aspect of the third digit and continues over the palmar surface of the hand to the wrist, where it joins the Arm Great Yin Lung Tendino-Muscle Channel. It ascends the anterior forearm to connect at the antero-

LEG LESSER YANG (SHAO YANG) TENDINO-MUSCLE CHANNEL (PERTAINING ORGAN— GALL BLADDER)

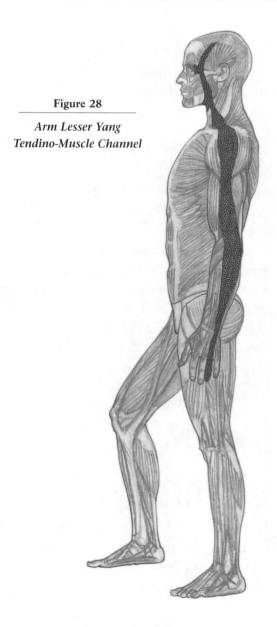

Figure 28

Arm Lesser Yang Tendino-Muscle Channel

This channel begins at the fourth toe and travels proximally to connect with the lateral malleolus. It ascends the lateral leg to connect at the lateral knee and continues up the thigh to the hip. A branch separates from the proximal fibula and continues upward along the anterior thigh. Another branch separates from the main pathway just above the knee, where it also travels upward along the anterior thigh. From the lateral hip, a horizontal branch separates and travels posteriorly to the buttock to connect at the sacrum. The main pathway continues up the lateral torso, passing over the ribs to the region anterior to the axilla, to connect at the lateral supraclavicular fossa. An anterior branch passes from the lower ribs. Crossing the pectoral region, it unites with the main pathway at the lateral supraclavicular fossa. The channel ascends the neck to the posterior ear and passes to the temple. From here, it travels to the vertex of the head, where it joins its bilateral counterpart. A branch descends from the temple, crosses the cheek, and connects with the bridge of the nose. A small branch separates from the cheek to connect to the outer canthus of the eye.

Musculature Through Which this Channel Passes

Hand: dorsal interosseous. **Forearm:** extensor digitorum superficialis, extensor digitorum profundus, extensor indicis, extensor carpi ulnaris, extensor digiti minimi. **Arm:** triceps brachii, biceps brachii. **Shoulder/Back:** middle deltoid, upper trapezius. **Neck:** sternocleidomastoid, suprahyoids, platysma. **Head:** masseter, temporalis, buccinator, orbicularis oculi, medial pterygoid.

Musculature Through Which this Channel Passes

Foot: dorsal interosseous, extensor digitorum brevis. **Leg:** extensor digitorum longus, peroneus longus, peroneus brevis, peroneus tertius, tibialis anterior, soleus. **Thigh:** tensor fascia lata, iliotibial tract, vastus lateralis, rectus femoris.

etalis, auriculares, masseter, buccinator, medial pterygoid, lateral pterygoid, zygomaticus, levator labii superioris, levator anguli oris, risorius, procerus, orbicularis oculi.

LEG ABSOLUTE YIN (JUE YIN) TENDINO-MUSCLE CHANNEL (PERTAINING ORGAN—LIVER)
▼

This channel begins at the dorsum of the great toe and travels up the dorsum of the foot to connect anterior to the medial malleolus. It continues up the medial leg to connect at the medial knee. The pathway ascends the medial thigh, passing above the genitals to enter the body inferior to the umbilicus, where it unites with the Leg Great Yin Spleen, Leg Lesser Yin Kidney, and Leg Bright Yang Stomach Tendino-Muscle channels.

Musculature Through Which this Channel Passes

Foot: dorsal interosseous, extensor hallucis brevis, tibialis anterior tendon. **Leg:** extensor hallucis longus, gastrocnemius, soleus. **Thigh:** gracilis, sartorius, adductor magnus, adductor longus, adductor brevis, pectineus, vastus medialis. **Abdomen:** rectus abdominis, pyramidalis, psoas.

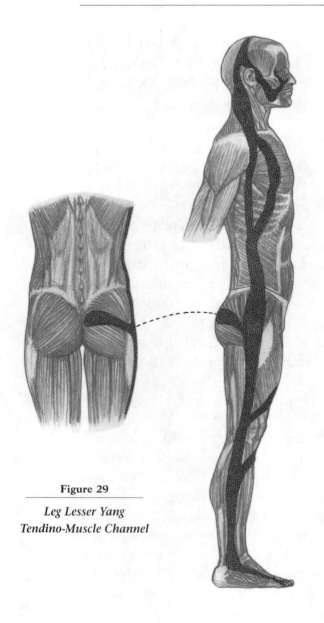

Figure 29

*Leg Lesser Yang
Tendino-Muscle Channel*

Buttock: gluteus maximus, gluteus medius, gluteus minimus, piriformis. **Abdomen:** transversus abdominis, external abdominal obliques, internal abdominal obliques. **Chest:** serratus anterior, pectoralis major, pectoralis minor. **Shoulder/Back:** anterior deltoid, upper trapezius. **Neck:** sternocleidomastoid, anterior scalenes, middle scalenes, posterior scalenes. **Head:** occipitalis, galea aponeurotica, temporalis, temporopari-

THE CUTANEOUS REGIONS

The channel system is a complex system of major and connecting channels that supply Qi, Blood, and Fluids to all the organs, bones, muscles, flesh, tissues, skin, and hair throughout the body, thus forming a unified, bioenergetic organism. There are seventy-two channels in all, twelve Primary Channels, sixteen Connecting Channels, eight Extraordinary Vessels, twelve Divergent Channels, twelve Tendino-Muscle Channels, and twelve Cutaneous Regions.

The twelve Cutaneous Regions, representing the division of the body's surface integument into twelve areas, are the most external extension of the Organ Channel orb of influence. These regions correspond to the Six Divisions of the primary Yin/Yang polarities. They are nourished by the superficial or Blood Connecting Vessels and represent the body's first line of defense against invasion by perverse energies. Exogenous pathogens can enter the body directly through the Cutaneous Regions and do battle with the body's Wei Qi. If the pathogen is stronger than the body's defenses, the pathogen will travel to penetrate into the corresponding Tendino-Muscle channel. Without appropriate treatment, it can proceed from there through the superficial pathway of the Primary Channel and Connecting Vessels into the deeper pathways, and ultimately to the organ itself.

This process can also be reversed; that is, a pathogen that has already found its way into the interior of the body can be moved from the deeper areas to the

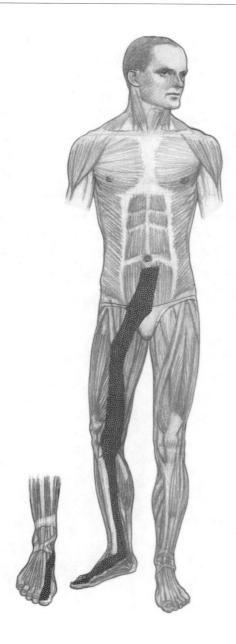

Figure 30

*Leg Absolute Yin
Tendino-Muscle Channel*

more superficial, and finally be expelled through the exterior regions. While many acupuncture texts state that only Defensive energy is to be found in the Tendino-Muscle Channels and Cutaneous Regions, this seems unlikely as there would then be no method for distribution of Nutrient Qi to the superficial areas of the body.

The study of the Cutaneous Regions can be of value in both diagnosis and treatment. For example, discoloration of the skin can be an indication of disease in the Organ channel that flows through the area; red skin is an indication of heat, purpleish blue skin is an indication of Stasis, and pale skin can be an indication of Cold or Deficiency. Edematous tissue that is visible or palpable also reflects an underlying pathology.

Manipulation and pressure techniques applied to the Cutaneous Regions and the Tendino-Muscle Channels will not only move the Qi and Blood of the local area, but can affect distal areas as well. They can also affect the superficial pathways of the Primary Channels and, through point manipulation, their deeper pathways and organs.

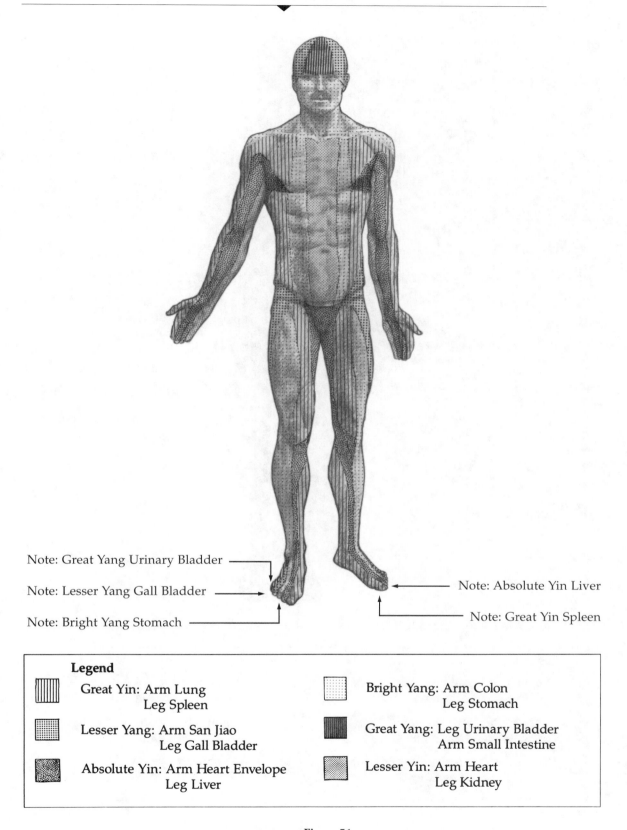

Note: Great Yang Urinary Bladder

Note: Lesser Yang Gall Bladder

Note: Bright Yang Stomach

Note: Absolute Yin Liver

Note: Great Yin Spleen

Legend

Great Yin: Arm Lung
Leg Spleen

Lesser Yang: Arm San Jiao
Leg Gall Bladder

Absolute Yin: Arm Heart Envelope
Leg Liver

Bright Yang: Arm Colon
Leg Stomach

Great Yang: Leg Urinary Bladder
Arm Small Intestine

Lesser Yin: Arm Heart
Leg Kidney

Figure 31

Cutaneous Regions—front view

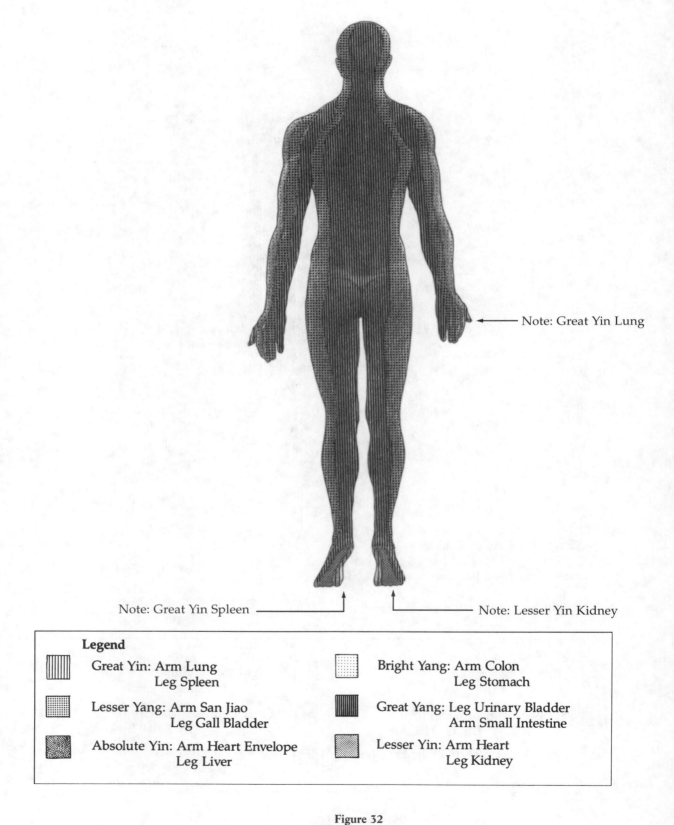

Figure 32

Cutaneous Regions—back view

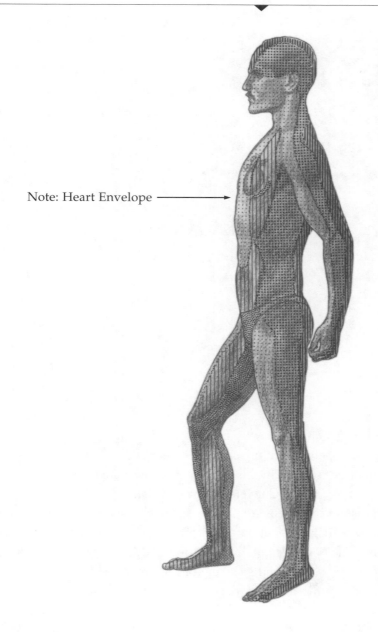

Note: Heart Envelope ──────────→

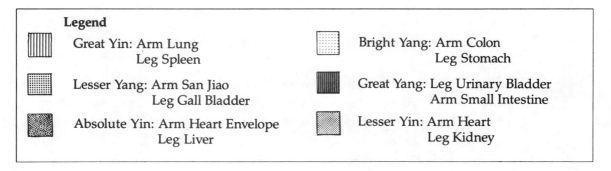

Legend

Great Yin: Arm Lung Leg Spleen		Bright Yang: Arm Colon Leg Stomach	
Lesser Yang: Arm San Jiao Leg Gall Bladder		Great Yang: Leg Urinary Bladder Arm Small Intestine	
Absolute Yin: Arm Heart Envelope Leg Liver		Lesser Yin: Arm Heart Leg Kidney	

Figure 33

Cutaneous Regions—side view

CHAPTER
7

ORIENTAL PHYSIOLOGY

In this chapter I will describe each of the Yin/Yang pairs of Organs as they are coupled in their pertaining channels. References to the Organ/function complex will be capitalized, such as in this statement: One of the main activities of the Lung is dispersing and descending. Conversely, the physical organ will be referred to without a capital, such as in this statement: The lung is in contact with the air and is easily injured by exogenous pathogenic factors. Similarly, syndromes as they are known in traditional Chinese medicine will be capitalized, as in Blood Stagnation; generalized references will appear in lower case. When speaking of the organs it should be understood that once the physical organ is affected, the Organ/function complex will also be disturbed.

LUNGS AND COLON

The Lung is often referred to in Chinese medical literature as the Delicate Organ because it is the first of the Organs to be injured by negative substances or energies (called Evil Qi) entering with air. Its pertaining sense organ is the nose. The Lung controls Qi and oxygen, and has the property of dispersing and descending; it therefore spreads Qi, Blood, and Vital Fluids throughout the body, and causes air and Qi to descend. The Lung also regulates water passages. Its dispersing function causes the excretion of sweat and thereby helps regulate temperature and detoxification, while its descending function causes fluids to pass down to the Kidney to be excreted as urine, again aiding in detoxification and basic elimination. The Lung dominates the skin and hair, dispersing the nutritive energy to the total body surface. Through the control of Protective Qi (Wei Qi), the Lung opens and closes the pores; the Lung is generally in charge of the first lines of defense of the organism. Since the Lung is involved with the processes of bringing Qi and oxygen into the body and dispersing them, and since the nose is the gateway of Qi and oxygen, the health of the Lung will be reflected in conditions of the nose and the paranasal sinuses. As well, since the Lung controls Qi and respiration, and Qi is necessary for the Heart to circulate the Blood, if the Lung Qi is strong, the circulation of Blood will be healthy. However, if the Lung Qi is weak, there will not be enough Qi to move the Blood, and consequently the extremities will be cold.

The main function of the Lung is to disperse and to cause to descend. The functions of respiration, control of the Vital Energy of the organism, and regulation of the metabolism and circulation of fluids are all activities related to dispersing and/or descending—moving energy and fluids throughout the body. Because the Lung is in charge of the water passages, it is responsible for sending the water down to the Kidney and the Urinary Bladder. The Lung is associated with the skin and the hair, reference being actually to the superficial part of the body, and especially the superficial defensive energy, the protection of the body. Because it is in charge of respiration and so is in intimate contact with the external environment through the air, the lung is vulnerable to the attack of exogenous pathogenic factors. (The other

organ that can be directly invaded by exogenous factors is the stomach, as it is in contact with the food that enters the body.)

Cough and asthma (in its technical meaning of "obstruction" and not necessarily the full-blown condition referred to as asthma in the West) are the most common symptoms of disturbed dispersing and descending functions of the Lung. In relation to respiration, dispersing is exhalation and descending is inhalation; any obstruction in the air passages will therefore impair the dispersing or descending functions. Cough and asthma are usually caused by exogenous pathogenic factors (Wind, Cold, Heat, Dry, or Damp, or some combination thereof) blocking the air passages. They can also be caused by endogenous pathogenic factors, such as Phlegm and Damp, usually from deficiency of the Spleen function; or Fire, usually from some disturbance of the Vital Energy of the Liver.

Sputum in the lung is a cause of cough and asthma, not the result as it is often misunderstood to be. Differential diagnosis—the determination of which one of two or more diseases with similar symptoms is the one from which the patient is suffering—is greatly assisted by considering the quality of the expectorated sputum. Expectoration of sputum in acute conditions, especially when it is accompanied by chills and fever, indicates an attack on the Lung by exogenous pathogenic factors. A common example is an attack of Heat, causing the fluid that is to nourish the lung to condense and be transformed into thick sputum. On the other hand, Cold promotes the secretion of thin sputum. Wind may also stimulate secretion of the lungs, and Dryness with

Wind renders the sputum sticky and scanty. In clinical practice we make distinctions between types of sputum and evaluate by these differentiations. Thin, whitish sputum suggests the presence of Cold and is called Cold sputum; thick, yellow, usually purulent sputum indicates Heat and is called Heat sputum; scant, sticky sputum implies the presence of Dryness and is called Dry sputum.

Expectoration of sputum in chronic cases is often caused by endogenous factors. Deficient Spleen Yang (hypofunction of the Spleen) is characterized by the failure of the Spleen to transport Fluid. This condition causes accumulation of Fluid in the Lung, resulting in Damp or Phlegm which will then appear as sputum. This may lead to persistent expectoration of large quantities of sputum, called Damp sputum. If the Damp is combined with Cold, copious quantities of thin sputum, called Cold Damp sputum, will be expectorated. If Damp is combined with Heat, large amounts of yellowish sputum, called Heat Damp sputum, will be present.

Functional insufficiency of the Lung itself may also lead to the formation of sputum, because if the dispersing function of the Lung is insufficient, Fluid may accumulate in the lung and turn into sputum. This is another case of sputum being caused by endogenous factors. It is usually thin and not very sticky because there is no Heat.

The Lung is instrumental in controlling the Vital Energy of the organism. This Vital Energy includes both the Vital Qi or Qi of Air and the Pectoral Qi, formed by the combination of Food Essence (Qi of Grain) from the Spleen and the Qi of Air. This Vital Energy formed in the Lung is stored in the chest, and is also sent throughout the body to the viscera as the Vital Energy of the body. Because the substance and function of the Lung also needs energy, some of the Pectoral Energy is used by the Lung. Therefore, if the Lung function is deficient in controlling the Vital Energy (a form of Deficient Lung Yang), the supply of Vital Energy for the function of the Lung will also be deficient.

Shortness of breath, a feeble and low voice, and weakness in coughing indicate weakness of the Lung function itself and are specific indicators of Deficient Lung Yang. Shortness of breath shows a deficiency of both the dispersing (exhalation) and descending (inhalation) functions. Since the Lung controls the voice, the voice quality reflects the Lung Yang. A weak voice is a clear indication of Deficient Lung Yang. Coughing indicates either Deranged Lung Qi, the normal descending function having reversed to an ascending function, or an effort to discard purulent material. In either instance, when the cough is weak it shows a disturbed and weakened Lung function. These conditions may be accompanied by indicators that point to other Organ involvements.

Other symptoms that indicate Lung involvement include Deficiency of Vital Energy all over the body, as evidenced by fatigue, lassitude, weakness, and so forth. Lassitude and weakness can also be caused by the impairment of other Visceral Organs, especially the Spleen. Deficient Spleen Yang will cause Deficiency of the Food Essence, leading to Deficiency of Vital Energy. (The distinction between Deficient conditions and Deficiency conditions is discussed on page 134.)

Part of the Vital Energy is sent to the Cutaneous Regions as Superficial Defensive Energy. A Deficiency of Vital Energy in the Lung will bring about Deficiency of Superficial Defensive Energy. Since the Defensive Energy controls the opening and closing of the pores, there will be spontaneous sweating with even the mildest exertion or cough. Spontaneous sweating can be seen in disturbances of other Viscera as well, especially the Heart. In the absence of other symptoms, spontaneous sweating is considered to be a condition of Deficient Wei (Protective) Qi.

Edema results when the Lung is invaded by exogenous pathogenic factors because the Lung function of dispersing and descending the Fluid is diminished. When the Fluid is thus prevented from flowing downward to the Kidney and to the Urinary Bladder, Fluid accumulates in the Lung and the upper portion of the body. This can be seen in acute nephritis (inflammation of the kidneys), in allergic reactions in which the lips and face become swollen, in common cold conditions, and in all forms of bronchial conditions. Edema can be caused by other Organ deficiencies as well.

The Colon, the Yang Bowel in paired functioning with the Lung, is in charge of the salvage of water from the impure matter passed on to it by the small intestine. Like the Lung, the Colon is involved in water metabolism, being responsible for regulating the fluid content and absorbing any nutrient content from the impure matter from the small intestine and discharging the resulting stool. Constipation or diarrhea often point to a disturbance in the Colon function, although bowel movement disturbances are often the result of the Spleen and sometimes the Kidney being in disorder. (It is interesting to note here that the functions of the superficial Yang Organs are described in more concrete terms, and in that way are closer to the conceptions of the Western-trained health professional.)

The Lung and Colon have the following diagnostically significant Five Phase correspondences as they are assigned to the Metal Phase: the season of autumn, the climatic condition of Dryness, the color white, the melancholy emotion, the pungent taste, and the sound of crying or sobbing.

SPLEEN AND STOMACH

The Spleen controls digestion while the Stomach receives the substances to be digested. Thus the Spleen is responsible for the transformation and transportation of Nutrient Qi. It is the source of Blood in that it is the source of both Qi and the Fluids that create Blood, and it is responsible for keeping the Blood in the vessels. The Spleen controls the limbs and the flesh, and its channel opens into the mouth.

The Spleen likes Dryness; it can easily become excessively Damp, which creates diarrhea. The Spleen Qi, also called Middle Qi, is responsible for keeping the organs in their places. Therefore when the Spleen is healthy there will not be any prolapses of the stomach, bladder, or rectum. Because the Spleen is responsible for keeping the Blood circulating in the vessels, unexplained bleeding, as well as hemorrhaging at the level of the skin, a symptom common to diabetes, are failures of the Spleen function. The classic Oriental medical texts say that the Spleen dominates the muscles, and that the density and strength of the muscles are the result of the Spleen's proper control of the transportation and transformation of nutrients. Oriental medical tradition also indicates the Spleen as the controller of the digestive functions. This is not as alien to the Western view as it may at first seem. Studies have shown that canine spleens hold extra quantities of blood, and that this extra blood is released as soon as the digestive process is stimulated.

Although traditional Chinese medicine did not have any specific knowledge of the pancreas, the function of the pancreas in relation to sugar metabolism and blood sugar balance was known, and it was considered to be controlled by the Spleen. The work of Dr. Reinhold Voll has shown that the right Leg Great Yin Spleen Channel acts as if it were a Great Yin Pancreas Channel, and certain points on the foot of the right Leg Great Yin Spleen Channel show specific effects on certain tissue and functions of the pancreas. The Spleen stores the soul, called Yi, which corresponds to the functions of reflection and intention.

When the Spleen is unable to extract the Qi of Grain and the food is not properly digested, the impaired transportation and transformation functions will lead to such symptoms as anorexia, poor appetite and abdominal distention (because the foodstuff retained in the Stomach is preventing further food intake), blood-free loose bowel movements (because fluids are not transported), and a sallow complexion.

Deficient Spleen Yang, manifesting as impaired transformation and transportation of nutrients, in long-standing cases leads to a lack of Vital Energy and insufficient Blood production. The absence of energy is noticeable in the common experiential sense as fatigue and lassitude; as the case progresses, anemia and malnutrition can result. The sallow complexion is a common factor in all Spleen dysfunctions.

Deficient Spleen Yang manifesting as disturbed distribution of Fluid in the body will result in water retention and eventually Dampness. The Damp symptoms take different forms in different areas of the body. The Middle Burner can be congested with nausea and lead to vomiting (Deranged Stomach Qi can accompany Spleen symptoms). Damp in the intestines will cause watery stools or diarrhea. Exudation in the pleural cavity is indicative of Damp. Ascites (serous fluid in the peritoneal cavities) is Damp in the abdominal cavity, while generalized edema is subcutaneous Damp. When there is Damp in the limbs there will often be a feeling of heaviness in the limbs. Deficient Spleen Yang from endogenous Damp and water retention will lead to a variety of Damp symptoms, such as pleurisy, ascites, diarrhea, and edema.

The dysfunctional Viscera causing edema can be differentiated in the following ways. Deficient Spleen Yang will show edema more marked in the limbs, accompanied by classic Spleen symptoms, such as malnutrition and indigestion. The Spleen pulse will be relaxed and loose. Deficient Kidney Yang will show edema primarily in the loins and lower extremities, with aching or soreness in the same areas; other indications of Kidney dysfunction, such as intolerance to cold and sexual dysfunction, will also be present, and the Kidney pulse will be weak. Deficient Lung Yang will result in a type of edema that shows mainly in the head and face, with accompanying upper respiratory symptoms or exterior syndromes, such as chills and fever. The Lung pulse will be superficial and floating.

Damp retained in the Lung (not to be confused with Western pulmonary edema) usually gives rise to expectoration of sputum. If there has been no obvious exogenous pathogenic attack on the Lung, then it is a dysfunction of the Spleen in transportation of Fluid. Even if a cough or constriction is present, such as in chronic bronchitis, the condition should still be treated through the Spleen.

The Spleen is responsible for keeping the organs in their places. Chronic Deficient Spleen Yang may bring about sinking symptoms, such as prolonged diarrhea, prolapse of the rectum or uterus, gastroptosis (downward displacement of the stomach), and so forth. It is interesting to compare Western and Oriental treatment protocols for a condition such as gastroptosis. All the symptoms that accompany gastroptosis, including poor appetite, indigestion, heavy downward pressure in the abdomen, weakness, and loss of body weight, point to Spleen Deficiency. Western medical treatment for a sinking organ generally involves invasive surgery to return the organ to its normal position. Oriental medicine uses herbs both for the particular organ that is affected and for strengthening the Spleen function of holding the organs in their places. Amma

therapy treatment also focuses on both the Spleen and the affected organ.

The Spleen is also responsible for keeping the Blood in the vessels. Chronic Spleen Yang Deficiency leads to hemorrhage. Bleeding from such deficiency is different than that caused by Heat or Fire, such as in hemoptysis (spitting of blood from the lungs) and epistaxis (nosebleed), which are caused by Liver Fire. It occurs in chronic cases where there is a deterioration of the Spleen function, which leads to weakening of the vascular walls because of failure of the production of Nutrient Qi. Such bleeding usually occurs in the lower part of the body, such as with excessive uterine bleeding, hematochezia (blood in the stools), and hematuria (blood in the urine), as well as in the leg ulcerations common to diabetics. The Spleen generally sends things upward; therefore, in Spleen dysfunction there is a downward tendency (as in sinking symptoms), and the lower part of the body will show the downward bleeding symptoms.

The character of the Stomach's function is descending in nature. The Stomach receives food and, under the control of the Spleen, separates the Qi of Grain from the substance. The Spleen transports the Qi of Grain up to the Lung for further processing, while the Stomach moves the substance down to the Small Intestine for further processing. In keeping with its Earth source, the Stomach likes Damp. Thus the Stomach is called Damp Earth and the Spleen is called Dry Earth.

When the Stomach does not send down the substance that remains after transformation by the Spleen, there will be indigestion and poor appetite or anorexia, nausea, and a stuffy feeling over the gastric region, since the food stays in the stomach. Deranged Stomach Qi is characterized by upward movement instead of the normal descending functions; this upward movement can result in belching, hiccough, vomiting, and even eructation of solid food.

Pain will result from stagnation in the flow of Qi and Blood. The stagnation, usually located in the epigastric region, may be due to either dysfunction of the Liver or to disharmony of the Liver and the Stomach. It may also be due to the congealing effect of Cold, either from an exogenous factor, such as exposure of the abdomen to cold, or an endogenous cause, such as Deficiency of Yang of the Stomach. The stagnation may also result from the retention of undigested food. The nature of the pain varies according to the cause. Fire of the Stomach may also cause epigastric pain. This Fire may be of the Excess type, such as Excess Yang, or may be due to Deficiency of Yin of the Stomach, with the relative Exuberance of Yang producing Heat or Fire. In this case, the pain is usually a burning pain. The pain caused by Stagnation of Qi is often accompanied by a sensation of distention; that caused by Blood Stasis is severe and stabbing or pricking in character, and is often accompanied by tenderness; that caused by Deficiency of Qi or Yang can be eased by pressure or the intake of food, and that caused by Deficiency of Yang of the Stomach can be relieved by warmth. Pain due to Stagnant Qi or Stagnant Blood cannot be relieved by the intake of food, since the syndrome is one of Excess and more food will only increase the Excess and thereby increase the pain. Pain caused by retention of undigested food is distending in character and is accompanied by belching with a fetid odor.

The Spleen and Stomach have the following diagnostically significant Five Phase correspondences as they are assigned to the Earth phase: the late stage of each season (that is, the interseasonal period), the climatic condition of Damp (although note that the Spleen tends toward Dryness), the color yellow, the pensive emotion, the sweet taste, and the sound of singing.

The pertaining channels of the two Viscera/Bowel pairs just described constitute the first four channels of the primary energy cycle. Beginning with the Great Yin of the Lung, the energy moves to the Bright Yang of the Colon. The energy manifests most actively in the Lung from 3 to 5 A.M., in the Colon from 5 to 7 A.M., in the Stomach from 7 to 9 A.M., and in the Spleen from 9 to 11 A.M. In looking at this cycle we begin to see the wisdom of the lifestyles of yogis, Buddhist monks, and other so-called ascetics. According to this cycle, one should awaken at 3 A.M. and do breathing exercises and postures until the day's bowel movement occurs, sometime between 6 and 7 A.M. The day's meal should be taken preferably before 9 A.M., and one should never eat after 11 A.M. It is obvious that in the hours before dawn, when the Lung Qi is at its strongest, the Lung will be most efficient in absorbing the Qi of Air and oxygen necessary for the creation of the body's various needs for Qi. This is also a time when meditative breathing in the calm of the morning, the purity of the Qi in the air, and the strength of the Qi of the Lungs can all interact to produce Ancestral Qi. The process of converting Ancestral Qi into the theoretically limited Prenatal Qi of the Kidney can thus be accomplished. This transformation of Qi was a major endeavor in the lives of the monks and yogis of whom we speak.

HEART AND SMALL INTESTINE

The Heart is responsible for the movement of the Blood in the blood vessels. The Heart also houses the Mind. The tongue, a part of the body that is used extensively in diagnosis and gives many indications related to Blood and the Heart, is considered to be a branch of the Heart. (It is interesting to note that Western medicine corroborates this association by its finding that, ontologically, the heart and tongue develop from the same tissue in the fetus.) Heart energy effects the speech; therefore speech problems, such as stammering and stuttering, are often treated through points on the Heart Channel. The condition of the Heart is reflected in the face. This is an obvious and common observation, as we often judge people's condition by the appearance of the face in terms of color, vivacity, muscle tension or flaccidity, and so forth.

Because the Heart governs Fire in the Five Elements, it is considered Sovereign Fire in relation to the other organs associated with Fire, such as the Small Intestine, Heart Envelope, and Triple Warmer. These Organs are considered to be Minister Fire in relation to the Sovereign Fire. The Fire is the Yang of the Heart and the Blood is the Yin of the Heart. Where the classics state that the Heart houses the Mind and the Spirit (Shen), it is meant that the Heart is involved with all mental activities, such as thought, memory, sleep, and so forth, as well as emotional activities. The Heart is thus the center of both the cardiovascular system and the central nervous system, especially the cerebral functions. The Brain is the Sea of Marrow and, although perfectly situated and designed as a switching center, it is at best a super computer. It is not the programmer.

In English we have many idiomatic expressions that indicate the same sphere of functional influence as the Oriental concept of the Heart: to "know by heart" suggests the function of memory, to "have a heart" suggests compassion, to "take heart" suggests having a positive outlook, to "have a heart-to-heart talk" suggests the experience of being honest and forthright, and listening and evaluating fairly.

In Chinese, the word *shen* has several meanings. A character that translates as "kidney" is pronounced *shen*. Shen as it is spoken of in reference to the Heart has at least two meanings. It refers to the human soul, or the emotional component that controls all mental activity. (Other Yin Organs are recognized as housing other "souls.") It also refers to the sense of being in good spirit or in poor spirit. The latter is the Shen that is referred to and evaluated when looking at the patient's condition as it is reflected in the face.

For obvious reasons, the Heart is referred to as the ruler of all the Organs. The Heart supplies True Yin (Blood) to the Kidney to generate Water in the Kidney, while the Kidney elevates True

Yang (Fire) to the Heart to generate Fire in the Heart. This reciprocity is called the Heart and Kidney communicating with each other. The relationship between the Heart, which represents Fire, and the Kidney, which represents Water, is fundamental to the body's harmonious balance. Since Fire is Yang and Water is Yin, disease will result when the Heart/Kidney relationship is out of balance. The Spirit of the Heart and the Essence of the Kidney together constitute the consciousness of the organism.

If the function of the Heart in housing the Mind is disturbed, there are neurotic symptoms as well as insomnia or dream-disturbed sleep. The symptoms will all appear to be of excitement or excess. This is an excellent example of an Apparent Yang condition arising due to Deficient Yin. Deficient Heart Yin, which itself can arise from a Deficiency of the Vital Essence of the Organ and/or Deficient Blood, will show symptoms of Exuberance of Yang, and the Heart will be hyperfunctional. Having no place to reside, the Mind wanders, resulting in absentmindedness, lack of concentration, a tendency toward distraction, poor memory, restlessness during the day, and insomnia or dream-disturbed sleep at night. Palpitations will commonly accompany the mildest excitation because the Heart is, in fact, deficient in Yang and therefore strains itself in order to function. Since most of the symptoms in Oriental medicine relate to the central nervous system, this deficiency is obviously not the same as Western medicine's concept of a heart deficiency, which would lead to heart failure.

The Heart may also be disturbed by pathogenic factors. Because the Heart houses the Mind, Excess Heart or Liver Fire will disturb the Mind by heating the Blood. The manifestations may be similar to those of failure to house the Mind due to a Deficiency of Vital Essence or a Deficiency of Blood, as stated above. If Phlegm, which is sticky and turbid, disturbs the Heart, it can cause disturbance of consciousness, lack of clarity, or blurring of the mind, and may even lead to a loss of consciousness or to a coma. This action is called Misting of the Heart by Phlegm. When Fire and Phlegm both attack the Heart at the same time, the manifestations are a combination of both impairment of consciousness and wandering of the mind, that is, mania. There will be symptoms of mental restlessness, which may then develop into extreme manic (but never depressive) behavior.

When the Vital Energy of the Heart is deficient there is not enough force to move the Blood in the vessels, and a series of symptoms appears. First, the Heart's functional activity will be insufficient, causing palpitations, and shortness of breath due to lack of Pectoral Qi. The Heart pulse will be thready and feeble. The face will show pallor or be ashen and the tongue will be pale, all signs of Deficient Heart Yang. The absence of Yang can lead to irregular heartbeat (arrhythmia).

Deficient Heart Yang can eventually result in Blood Stasis, which is the result of insufficient force to circulate the Blood. Obstruction causes pain; when the Blood Stasis is sufficiently developed, pain will occur. Stagnation of Blood in the vessels causes pain localized in the area of the heart, leading to angina pectoris. In mild cases the pain will be intermittent, but in more severe cases the pain can become persistent. Such pain will usually be accompanied by a purple tongue body or one with purple spots on its surface, both further signs of Blood Stasis. The veins on the underside of the tongue may be engorged and black, a sign of intense Blood Stasis. Deficiency of Blood of the Heart can also lead to a deficient blood supply throughout the body, with signs of pallor (lack of blood in the face), pale tongue (lack of blood to the tongue, a major diagnostic indicator), dizziness (lack of blood in the head), and other common symptoms of anemia. If the Deficiency of Blood continues over time there may eventually be Death of Blood, with the development of a virtually black complexion and a skinny, rather rigid body. The skin and hair begin to wither as well. This is a dangerous condition.

Worry will eventually deplete Heart Qi, leading to Deficient Heart Fire. In the Five Phase Cycle, Fire will then not create Earth, and the Spleen will be weakened. The flesh and muscles will not be supplied with Nutrient Qi, and decreased appetite, insomnia, and weight loss will follow. Deficient Heart Qi causes depression of spirit and great sadness.

Excess Heart Qi will show signs of reddened, subjectively hot, painful skin. If extreme, Excess Heart Qi will cause "spirits in excess," characterized by incessant laughter. Chest pain with coughing and pain in the ribs is not considered to be true pain in the Heart. (Pain in the physical organ that indicates failure or disturbance of the Western physiological function of the heart is, of course, recognized in Chinese medicine.) True heart pain is very severe and is generally accompanied by cold hands and feet (Stasis of Blood). Excess Heart pain is accompanied by a congested sensation in the ribs; pain below the ribs; and pain between the pectorals and in the back, scapula, and medial arm, all signs of excess and disturbance of the Heart Channel. Deficient Heart pain is accompanied by swelling in the chest and abdomen (Blood Stasis and Apparent Yang), pain below the ribs, and pain across the lumbar region, because True Yang is not sent down to the Kidney.

The Small Intestine extracts Pure Fluid from chyme, then sends the waste matter to the Colon and the remaining fluid on to the Kidney for further extraction of Pure Fluids. Heat accumulation or an attack of exogenous Heat may cause hemorrhoids through the complications of constipation as the Heat dries up the Small Intestine and then the Colon. An excess of Cold causes blood discharge from the Rear Yin (anus), which is often accompanied by pus. Traditional Chinese medicine assigns certain urinary tract problems to dysfunction of the Small Intestine; however, in light of the Yin/Yang relationship of the Heart and Small Intestine, it would be better to look to the Heart if there is a burning sensation upon urination and even mild hematuria. If there are Fire symptoms present you should treat the Heart, since it is the Heart Fire acting through the Small Intestine that is likely to be the cause of the urinary problem.

The Heart and Small Intestine have the following diagnostically significant Five Phase correspondences as they are assigned to the Fire Phase: the summer season, the climatic condition of Heat, the color red, the emotion of joy, the bitter taste, and the sound of laughter.

KIDNEY AND BLADDER

The Kidney in Chinese medicine is unquestionably a very special Organ. The Kidney is unique among all the Yin Organs because it supplies all the other Organs with both Yin and Yang energies. It is therefore referred to as the Root of Life. Although in the Five Element theory Water is the element ascribed to the Kidney, because the Kidney is the foundation of all the Yin and Yang energies, it is the real source of both Fire and Water in the body. Thus the Kidney's warming function becomes the source of Fire in the Heart. This warming function is called the Gate of Vitality.

As it was traditionally held that there was only one of each organ, the right Kidney was called the Gate of Life or Gate of Vitality (also Vital Gate, Life Door), and was considered the storehouse of the Prenatal Qi (the Qi of Prior Heaven), the primary life force of the body. In more recent times the Gate of Life is considered to be the area between the kidneys, and both anatomical organs are understood to be part of the Organ/Function complex called the Kidney.

The Qi of the Gate of Life is the Qi of Prior Heaven, which enters into the process of circulation of Qi. In its kinetic form of Yuan Qi, the Qi of Prior Heaven is in fact the driving force of this circulation; it also enters into all the processes of the body that involve the creation or modification of energy. Prenatal Qi is easy to lose through drug use, excessive sexual activity, insufficient or excessive sleep, improper diet, and living habits in general. Its total loss is the ultimate reason for death. Although easy to lose, Prenatal Qi is difficult to increase, except by engaging in certain specific meditation techniques, as well as by the proper and repeated practice of chi kung, the Taoist equivalent of hatha yoga's pranayama.

This Prenatal Qi combines with the Essence of Food to become the Acquired Essence of the Kidney. The Acquired Essence defines the cycle of growth, maturity, and decay and the cycle of reproduction. This Acquired Essence, called Jing Qi, also forms Marrow, which supplies the bones and the spinal column and forms the brain. Marrow is partly responsible for Blood formation. The other agents acting with the Marrow to form Blood are the Fluids from the Spleen, the Essence from the Kidney, the action of the Heart and Lungs, and the smooth functioning of the Liver.

The Jing has a specific manifestation as sperm and ovum. Jing and Post-Heaven (Nutrient) Qi form the foundation of the True Fire of the Kidney, otherwise known as the True Fire of the Gate of Vitality. The True Fire of the Kidney has the following functions: it warms the Heart and assists in housing the Spirit; it warms the Spleen and Stomach to aid in digestion; it warms the Bladder and Lower Warmer to assist in the transformation and excretion of Fluids; and it is the energy that activates reproduction. If the True Fire of the Gate of Vitality (the Gate of Life or Life Door) is Deficient, then the Heart and Spirit will be injured; the Spleen and Stomach will not digest food; the Lower

Burner will not transform Fluids; the Lung will not inspire nor spread Qi through the body; the Essence of the Kidney will turn Cold; the Uterus will become weak and Cold, resulting in infertility (or at least chronic leukorrhea) or impotence; and sexual desire will cease. With this deficiency a variety of symptoms will manifest, including chilliness, intolerance to cold, and cold limbs where the patient feels cold himself and is cold to touch. These are signs of failure in warming the body. Fluid stools containing undigested food, especially occurring daily before dawn, indicates its failure in heating the Spleen. (In TCM this condition is called fifth watch diarrhea or cock crow diarrhea, relating to the time of the fifth watch in old China, when watchmen wandered the city at night.) Dyspnea (difficulty in breathing) or asthma indicates failure in helping the Lung in inspiration. When the Kidney Yang is Deficient, that is, when there is not enough Heat from the Gate of Vitality, the Kidney will not be able to grasp the Qi descending from the Lung. This causes Rebellious Lung Qi, which manifests as asthma and breathing problems. Generalized weakness indicates failure in spreading Qi through the body. Oliguria (slight or infrequent urination) and edema indicate failure in regulating water metabolism. Dysuria (difficult or painful urination) or incontinence of urine indicates failure in assisting the Urinary Bladder. Impotence or hyposexuality indicates Deficiency of Minister Fire. (Just as the Heart is considered Sovereign Fire to the Minister Fire of the Small Intestine, Heart Envelope, and Triple Burner, the warming function of the Kidney is considered Sovereign Fire to the sexual energy, which is Minister

Fire. One can live without sexual energy, but without the warming function, the body will die.)

If the True Fire of the Gate of Life is in decline and the Kidney Yin is Deficient, there will be exhaustion of Original Qi (Prenatal Qi) followed by floating of Deficiency Yang (that is, temporary hyperactivity), and finally Yang prolapse (virtual cessation of function) and death. Kidney Yang Deficiency can result in swollen feet, diarrhea, night sweats, difficulty in standing, lumbago, cold sensations in the spine, and usually impotence.

Deficiency of Kidney Yin will produce Deficiency Fire Burning Upward, causing sore throat and hoarseness, weakness, and Deficiency Fire symptoms of hot sensations in the sole of the foot or the tibia, poor complexion, and pain in the heel. Amma therapists therefore treat the Kidney for all genitourinary disease conditions, prostatitis, uterine congestion, incontinence, lumbago, impotency, and inability to conceive.

The Kidney enters into a special relationship with the Heart, a fact not overlooked by Western allopathic doctors. It elevates True Yang to the Heart to generate Fire in the Heart, while the Heart sends True Yin to the Kidney to generate Water in the Kidney. This reciprocity is called the Heart and Kidney communicating with each other. The Kidney's sense organ is the ear. Not only does the slow creeping of deafness in older people reflect the loss of Prenatal Qi and the weakening of the Kidney, but, under non-degenerative conditions, deafness can be often effectively treated by using the Kidney as the basis of treatment.

The Kidney is the residence of Zhi, or

will, which helps in reflection and the ability to focus and recall. The Fire of the Gate of Vitality rises to the Heart to provide it with the Heat necessary for it to function, and thus feeding the Heart Fire. In this way the Kidney helps the Heart to house the Mind, and plays a role in thinking and influencing emotional and mental states. A strong Kidney results in will power and a strong mind.

The Kidney controls sex and urine; it also controls water metabolism, and therefore has a special relationship with the Colon. For these reasons, the Two Yin—the genital organs and the anus—are its outlets. By upsetting the Colon's function, Excess Kidney Yang or Kidney Fire is often the cause of constipation.

When Fear injures the Kidney, whether over time or from a sudden shock, neurasthenia and other generalized neuropsychological disturbances will occur as a result of disruption of the Yuan Qi, which essentially activates all the functions of the organism. Deficient Kidney Yang causes coldness in the limbs, while Exuberant Kidney Yang resulting from Deficient Kidney Yin often leads to generalized edema. Exuberant Kidney Fire, again as a secondary result of Deficient Kidney Yin, can lead to lumbar pain and stiffness and an inability to extend the back and limbs, causing difficulty in skeletal movement and possible loss of motility and range of motion. This condition is known as Paralysis of the Bones.

Of all the viscera, the Kidney is the only one that has no Excess syndrome. There is no Excess of the Kidney because it is the foundation of all the Yin and Yang energies of the body. You can never have too much Kidney energy. In fact, the more Yin you store through meditation and energy-building exercises, such as t'ai chi and yoga, the longer and healthier life you will live. The Taoist monks believed that, in this way, immortality could be gained.

There is also no basic excess in the functioning of the Kidney. When an organ is attacked by an exogenous pathogenic factor, there is hyperreaction of the function of the Organ. However, the Kidney can hardly be attacked by exogenous pathogenic factors, which usually attack the Lung, the Spleen, and the Stomach first, as these take in elements from the outside environment. Similarly, endogenous pathogenic factors may attack or invade the internal viscera, though they usually do not attack the Kidney, and when they do, the primary cause is still Deficiency.

Excessive Minister Fire can arise due to Deficiency of Yin. While initially Excessive, if protracted it will become a Deficiency syndrome because the excessive sexual activity will consume the Yin, the Essence. When there is only sexual hyperactivity without subsequent complication, the patient is not sick.

Because it is so important to human life, the Vital Essence stored in the Kidney can never be pathogenic. The more Essence the Kidney stores, the healthier the person is. An excess of Yin or Vital Essence stored in the Kidney gives an elderly person vital spirits and extraordinarily keen intelligence. Such a person would generally be much healthier than others his or her age. The same applies to the vital function of the Kidney—hyperactivity just makes one stronger. It may lead to unusual cold resistance, tremendous vital capacity, and extremely good digestive functioning.

The Kidney is said to open into the ears. The ear needs Essence and Fluids from the Kidney. Weak Kidney Qi results in hearing loss, deafness, and tinnitus. These problems are often seen in the elderly as their Kidney Jing begins to wane. The hair is also dependent on nourishment from the Kidney. Hair loss, graying hair, or dry, dull hair is a sign of weak Kidney Essence.

The major function of the Urinary Bladder is the temporary storage and excretion of impure Fluids in the form of urine. The Bladder also transforms the turbid Fluids passed to it from the Small Intestine into urine. The functions of the Bladder are controlled by the Kidney. The Kidney is associated with the Water element, and works with the Spleen in the transformation and transportation of Fluids. The Kidney is said to "open and close," controlling the flow of urine to the Bladder. This can malfunction when Kidney Yin and Kidney Yang are out of balance, leading to scanty urination from Kidney Yin Deficiency (not enough Fluid being produced) or excess urination from Kidney Yang Deficiency (failure to close properly). The Kidney provides Qi to the Bladder so it can store urine and transform the turbid Fluids into urine. Thus, dysfunction of the Urinary Bladder will lead to an inability to either store or excrete urine, symptoms seen in such conditions as polyuria, dysuria, and incontinence. However, most urinary tract symptoms are related to Organs other than the Urinary Bladder.

It should be noted that the Kidney also takes some of the Fluids descending from the Lung function, excreting some Fluid and returning some to the Lung to keep them moist, a process called "misting."

Failure to excrete Fluids can cause Fluids to stagnate and affect the Stomach. On the other hand, insufficient Stomach Fluids will cause the Stomach to draw excessively upon the Kidney, leading to a Kidney Yin Deficiency.

The Kidney and Urinary Bladder have the following diagnostically significant Five Phase correspondences as they are assigned to the Water Phase: the winter season, the Cold climatic condition, the color black, the emotion of fear, the salty taste, and the sound of groaning.

The Arm and Leg Lesser Yin channels of the Heart and Kidney relate to the Great Yang channels of the Small Intestine and Urinary Bladder. They are the second set of four channels in the primary energy circulation. The energy is most prominent in the Heart from 11 A.M. to 1 P.M., in the Small Intestine from 1 to 3 P.M., in the Bladder from 3 to 5 P.M., and in the Kidney from 5 to 7 P.M.

HEART ENVELOPE AND TRIPLE WARMER

The Heart Envelope is also known as the Heart Constrictor, Pericardium, Hsin Pao Lao, and Xin Bao Lao. The Triple Warmer system is also known as Triple Burner or Triple Heater, Three Heaters or Three Burning Spaces, and San Jiao. These two channels have no Western organ counterparts. Of the Heart Envelope the classics say "It has Name without Shape." Although they are assigned to the element Fire, the Fire is of lesser consequence than the other pair of Fire Organs (the Heart and Small Intestine), and so they are considered to be Minister Fire to the Heart/Small Intestine Sovereign Fire.

The Heart Envelope, which is primarily concerned with the circulatory system, is the Organ pertaining to the Arm Absolute Yin Channel. The sphere of influence of this channel extends deeply into the circulatory function, which accounts for the channel's effects on sexual function, one of the first correspondences noted by early Western students of Chinese medicine.

According to *The Yellow Emperor's Classic of Internal Medicine,* the Heart Envelope is the Sea of Energy situated in the chest, and it spreads Joy from the Heart. According to the *Nan Ching* (known in English as *The Classic of Difficult Ideas*), there are only five Viscera and six Bowels. The five Viscera—Lung, Spleen, Heart, Kidney, and Liver—are paired with the six Bowels—Colon, Stomach, Small Intestine, Bladder, Gall Bladder, and Triple Warmer. The Triple Warmer is not paired with a visceral organ because it is considered to be different from the other Yang Organs. The Triple Warmer does not pertain to an organ per se, but rather to a division of the torso and head into three centers of activity. A later chapter in *The Classic of Difficult Ideas* actually refers to only five Yang Bowels, omitting the Triple Warmer, and thus confusing the issue.

We know that, in the development of channel theory, the Triple Warmer and the Heart Envelope were paired to make twelve Primary Channels, and that since it has no actual pertaining physical organ, the significance of the Heart Envelope lies more in its influence on the channel's pathway and its role in effecting and protecting the Heart. The Heart Envelope is thus the paired "Viscera" to the Triple Warmer, for it has a channel pertaining to it that surfaces on the chest, and it is the Sea of Energy that surrounds the Heart. The Sea of Energy could be seen as the tremendous force of the pumping of the physical heart and its large powerful surrounding arteries whose muscular walls contract rhythmically, driving the Blood as the messenger of the Heart to every area of the organism.

Traditional practitioners treated most symptoms described under the discussion of the Heart through the Heart Envelope Channel. They held that if the Heart itself was diseased, the patient would die. In modern times, the Heart Channel is treated directly.

The Three Heater or Triple Warmer system refers to three groupings of Organs. The Lung and Heart are the Upper Warmer, the Stomach and Spleen are the Middle Warmer, and the Kidney, Bladder, and Intestines are the Lower Warmer. (The Liver is sometimes included as part of the Lower Warmer.) Besides the diagnostic use of the Triple Warmer Channel in relation to other Organ groups, there are specific functions that can be treated through the San Jiao. Disturbances to the processes of digestion, assimilation, and elimination are usually facilitated by use of the Three Heater Channel points in conjunction with other Organs. Emotional problems are sometimes treated through this channel as well. Dr. Reinhold Voll, a German physician who did much to expand the study of acupuncture, has devised very effective treatments for the endocrine glands using points on the San Jiao channel.

The Heart Envelope and Triple Warmer have the same Five Phase correspondences as the Heart and Small Intestine.

LIVER AND GALL BLADDER

Strong negative emotions, such as anger, rage, and deep depression, are states that are both the result and the cause of difficulties in this Organ pair. Such extreme states are often the result of Liver Yang Upsurging or Abundant Liver Fire. In America, anger and self-righteous behavior are met with the phrase, "You've got a lot of gall." In Germany, short-tempered and self-righteous behavior is described by a phrase that translates as "A flea must have crawled over his liver." These two expressions from two distinct cultures indicate the common awareness of the Liver/Gall Bladder relationship to strong negative states.

The Liver Channel opens into the eyes, and Liver conditions are reflected in the eyes. The condition of exophthalmia is indicative of Excess Liver Fire Rising. In addition to its other clinical implications, this condition is a clear indication of emotional instability. Whenever a person is either in the process of manifesting negativity or is repressing strong negative emotions, the pulse of the Gall Bladder will be pounding relative to the other pulses. Headaches are often associated with Excess Liver Fire, and dizziness may be the result of Liver Yang Upsurging or Liver Fire Rising. Depression and frustration upset the major function of the Liver, which uses its ascending and outward-spreading energy to provide for the smooth flow of Qi and Blood throughout the body. When this function

is upset, the result is further depression and frustration, with the addition of bad temper. The smooth flow of Qi and Blood is essential to emotional well-being.

The Liver stores Blood and is responsible for nourishing and moistening. Failure of this moistening function is reflected in dry and painful eyes with blurred vision, difficulty in movement (including joint pain or stiffness), and dry skin. The Liver stores and regulates the volume of circulating Blood, holding part of the Blood when the body is at rest. It cooperates with the Heart in this Blood-controlling function.

The Liver shares responsiblity for the distribution of Qi with the Lung (it smoothes and regulates the flow of Vital Qi), thereby controlling certain vital functions, including emotional changes, the functioning of the channels and the Organs, bile secretion by the Gall Bladder, and particularly the digestive functions of the Spleen and Stomach. The Liver tends toward upward movement of Qi. If it is unable to extend up (a condition known as Liver Oppressed), it will tend to injure Earth, causing a Deficiency of Spleen and Stomach. This will tend to produce pain in the ribs, a feeling of congestion in the chest, vomiting, swollen stomach with no appetite, diarrhea with undigested food and "plum-pit throat." Note that these are basically Spleen- and Stomach-related symptoms. Pain in the ribs and congestion in the chest are, however, related to the path of the Qi of the Liver and Gall Bladder Channels, and are generally reliable indicators of oppression of the Liver Qi.

The Liver controls the lower abdomen (the Lower Warmer), and is therefore important in the healthy functioning of the menstrual cycle. It is the residence of the aspect of Spirit called the human soul (Hun), which rises to Heaven after death. It is Yang to the Po, the animal soul in the Lung. Its health is reflected in the condition of the nails, with thin and weak nails indicating a weakness in the Liver Yang. The Liver controls the sinews (the joints, and particularly the tendons and ligaments), and the ribs on both sides; it is called the Root of Tendon Fortitude. The Liver therefore controls the movement of the limbs and the skeletal muscles. Symptoms from minor trembling to extreme stiffness and spasms all are indicative of Liver dysfunction, usually Liver Excess. Sudden cowardice or congenital extreme cowardice are generally considered to be signs of severe depletion of Liver/Gall Bladder Yin.

Liver is Wood and Wind is Wood. Oppressed Wood (Liver) may transform into Wind and Fire. All Wind signs tend toward movement and change. Liver Wind causes vertigo, spasms, apoplexy, and a numb sensation in the tongue. Liver Fire causes pain in the ribs, hiccough, loss of blood, and acid regurgitation (both upward movement and burning qualities relate to Fire). Deficient Liver Yin with Abundant Liver Yang causes dizziness, ringing in the ears, spots before the eyes, and a bitter taste in the mouth (also Fire signs but less intense than those from a real abundance of Fire).

Several serious conditions occur as a result of the dysfunction of the Liver in smoothing and regulating the flow of Qi and Blood. Generally speaking, pain caused by obstruction or stagnation of the flow of Vital Energy is distending in character, unlike the pain caused by Blood Stasis, which is sharp or pricking in character. Since Vital Energy is the dynamic force in the circulation of blood, long-standing Stagnation of Vital Energy may cause Blood Stasis, the symptoms of which usually occur in the lower abdomen, especially in the uterus. When the Liver is diseased, the Qi of the Liver is usually stagnated in the areas where the Liver Channel passes; therefore, the common areas of distending are the hypochondriac region, the mammary and pectoral areas, the lateral abdomen, and the inguinal region. The pain may be bilateral but is often on the left side, consistent with the TCM view that the Liver arises on the left side even though the physical organ is on the right.

Since energy manifests on a continuum from most fine to most dense, there are varying degrees of formations that arise due to the stagnation of Qi, Blood, and Fluids. Stagnation of Qi that is immaterial can be palpable in spite of the fact that it does not have a definite shape. A long-standing stagnation or stasis situation can ultimately lead to congealing, and form masses that are defined and materialistic.

Stagnation of either Vital Energy or Blood due to dysfunction of the Liver may give rise to mass formation, where the mass itself has no definite shape; it may change from time to time, coming and going unpredictably and accompanied by pain without definite location. For example, if the patient is suffering from intestinal spasm, a mass may be felt in the abdomen, accompanied by the movement of gas through the intestines. In this case, the mass that is palpable may be due to either Qi Stagnation causing muscle spasm or intestinal muscle spasm causing Qi Stagnation. Amma therapy manipulations will both relax the muscles and relieve the stagnation of Qi. Often the mass will disappear within minutes, and so will the symptoms of gas movement and belching. Conversely, the masses formed by Blood Stasis, such as an enlarged liver or spleen, gynecological tumors, tumors in the abdomen, and so forth, have a definite shape, and are usually accompanied by fixed pain of a pricking or even stabbing nature. In conditions of Blood Stasis, the pain may be very severe.

Stagnation of Vital Energy in the extreme may transform into Fire. As a rule the Fire flames upward, so the Fire symptoms of the Liver are usually manifested in the head, giving rise to headaches, dizziness, bloodshot eyes, tinnitus, impaired hearing, and a constant bitterness in the mouth.

Fire of the Liver may transform into endogenous Wind. Vertigo, tremor, convulsion, certain kinds of stroke, and pain that moves and cannot be pinpointed (as in certain kinds of arthritis) all show extremes of Fire and the constant movement characteristic of Wind.* Liver Wind can also be caused by high fever, as in the convulsions suffered by a febrile patient. This is particularly noticeable with infants, since infants suffer convulsions easily when the body temperature is elevated.

The Liver function of smoothing and regulating the flow of Vital Energy also facilitates the digestion of food by the Stomach and the Spleen. Therefore, depression of the Vital Energy of the Liver may affect the function of the Stomach and the Spleen, and there may be digestive symptoms, such as loss of appetite, belching, nausea, and even vomiting. Anorexia may also be related to

depression of the Vital Energy of the Liver. When such symptoms of the Stomach manifest, there is a disharmony of the Liver and the Stomach. Depression of Vital Energy of the Liver may also have an influence on the function of the Spleen, giving rise to abdominal distention and diarrhea. When the distention and diarrhea are severe, the problem is considered to be one of disharmony between the Liver and the Spleen.

The Liver may be attacked by exogenous Damp. The first symptoms to show will be symptoms of Damp Heat, and later, as the Yang Qi weakens, Damp Cold. Since the Liver and the Gall Bladder are a Yin/Yang pair, dysfunction of the Liver in smoothing and regulating the flow of Qi may also involve bile secretion and excretion, pain in the right hypochondriac region, jaundice, digestive system reactions related to a failure in the ability to digest fat, and other Damp symptoms. These symptoms may correspond to Western diseases such as hepatitis, cholecystitis (inflammation of the gall bladder), and cholelithiasis (formation of gall stones). All physical activities, especially of the skeletal muscles and eyes, depend upon the supply of Blood that is stored in and released from the Liver. If the Blood stored in the Liver is deficient, symptoms related to Liver Blood Deficiency, such as pallor, blurred vision or dryness of the eyes, spasms of the sinews and skeletal muscles, numbness of the limbs, sensory disturbance, and scanty menstrual flow with a prolonged cycle will be present.

Liver Fire may injure the blood vessels and cause internal bleeding, leading to such conditions as hematemesis (the vomiting of blood), epistaxis (nosebleed), and

---

* Dizziness is a symptom of Liver Fire, and vertigo is a symptom of Fire transformed into Wind.

profuse uterine bleeding during menstruation. Such bleeding is characterized by the sudden onset of massive hemorrhage, and may occur after an emotional upset. This type of hemorrhage results from the mobilization of the large amount of stored Liver Blood by the pathological Fire of the Liver.

The Gall Bladder contains pure Fluid (as bile) and is thus unlike other Bowels. Along with the Womb and the Brain, the Gall Bladder is considered an Odd and Constant Organ as well as a Yang Bowel. The Gall Bladder is considered to be involved with the Heart in decision-making processes. It is interesting to contemplate the effect of this involvement. Could the angry influence of the Western Gall Bladder, unhealthy due to the excess of fat ingestion in the Western diet, lead to the highly charged and far-reaching negative decisions that are so often made by our leaders?

Frequent indecision will lead to Deficient Gall Bladder, with overflowing bile causing a bitter taste in the mouth. Heat from long-standing Liver Qi Stagnation can be transferred to the Gall Bladder, causing unnatural hunger accompanied by an exhausted feeling in the arms and legs. Swelling of the Gall Bladder, which is not a form of edema but rather an indication of Gall Bladder Deficiency, produces symptoms of pain and swelling below the ribs, a bitter taste in the mouth, and constant sighing.

The Liver and Gall Bladder channels show the following diagnostically significant Five Phase correspondences as they are assigned to the Wood Phase: the spring season, the climatic condition of Wind, the color green, the angry emotion, the sour taste, and the sound of shouting.

The Absolute Yin of the Arm and Leg Heart Envelope and Liver channels relate to the Lesser Yang channels of the San Jiao and the Gall Bladder. These constitute the last set of four channels in the primary circulation of energy. The energy is at "high tide" in the Heart Envelope from 7 to 9 P.M., in the Triple Warmer from 9 to 11 P.M., in the Gall Bladder from 11 P.M. to 1 A.M. and in the Liver from 1 to 3 A.M. The cycle begins again in the Lung at 3 A.M. The Organ Clock, as this Nutrient Cycle is often called, is concerned with the prominent tides of energy in each of the functional areas of the orbs, and these are as has been indicated in this chapter. It should be noted that the time of weakest energy of any one orb is during the period of eleven to thirteen hours after the period of maximum activity.

In contrast to the nourishing energy that circulates through the Nutrient Cycle, Wei Qi (Protective Qi) flows through the Tendino-Muscle Channels, circulating twenty-five times during the day through the exterior portion of the body, moving from the Great Yang to the Lesser Yang to the Bright Yang channels. At night it circulates twenty-five times through the Yin Organs, following the Five Element Cycle of Creation, beginning with the Kidney.

THE CREATION OF ENERGY, PURE FLUIDS, AND BLOOD

In the Chinese medical model, the processes involving the production, transformation, and circulation of Qi and the production, transformation, and circulation of Fluids are the two major processes that define, from a medical standpoint, most of what the organism is about. These processes involve all the organs and define all their functions. The method of diagnosing disease basically involves an assessment of the dysfunction of these two processes and an evaluation of how the dysfunction occurred. Because they are key to the evaluation methods, we shall describe each process in detail, with a subsidiary description of the movement of the dregs.

Ingested food and drink first enters the Stomach, where the process of rotting and ripening of food begins. The Spleen extracts the Gu Qi (the essence of the foodstuff) from the ripened food substance in the Stomach, and sends the Gu Qi to the Lung for further processing. Under the activating influence of the Yuan Qi (the active essence of the Kidney), the Lung, which has extracted the Da Qi from the inspired substance during inhalation, combines the two substances, the Gu Qi and the Da Qi, to form the Ancestral Qi or Zong Qi that will be used throughout the system.

The Ancestral Qi, so-called because it is the ancestor of all the energies that follow (also known as Pectoral Qi for its location), is used by the Lung for the control of the voice and the spreading of Qi through the organism, and by the Heart for the pumping of the Blood throughout the organism. It is also used by the Envelope of the Heart to spread Joy through the system. Under the influence of Yuan Qi, some portion of the Ancestral Qi is transformed into True Qi (Zhen Qi), which will be used throughout the system as Nutrient Qi and Protective Qi. Ying Qi, the nutrient sub-stance, flows in the vessels with the Blood. Wei Qi, the defensive energy, flows outside the Primary Channels and the blood vessels through the soft tissue and skin, enlivening the Tendino-Muscle Channels and the Cutaneous Regions.

Another portion of the Ancestral Qi is used or transformed, again under the influence of Yuan Qi, into three additional substances—Organ Qi (Zang-Fu Qi), Channel Qi (Jing Luo Qi), and Organ Essence (Jing Qi). Organ Qi is the energy used by the Organs, and by all the constituents of the Organ's orb of influence. Channel Qi or Jing Luo Qi is the Qi that flows in the channels, beginning with the Lung Channel and following the Nutrient Cycle. Organ Essence or Jing Qi, which is the Yin substratum of the Organ, under healthy conditions will be produced in excess, and the excess stored in the Kidney as Acquired Essence. The remaining Jing Qi and other substances (Organ Qi, Channel Qi, Nutrient Qi, and Defensive Qi) are passed on in the Five Phase Cycle, where each Viscera in turn produces a similar set of transformations.

The Organ Qi is differentiated by the Element aspect of the Organ, and its qualities are thus explained. For example, the Qi of the Liver is Wood. In excess, the Wood burns, producing Liver Fire. If the Fire is active and grows it transforms to Wind. (Note that, with the exception of the Stomach, the Yang Bowels are not mentioned in this explanation. Generally, the Bowels are involved primarily in the temporary storage and discharge of the dregs and the impure fluids from this process.) Another example of energetic transformation is seen in the communication between the Heart and the Kidney. The Kidney sends True Yang to the Heart for the Heart to transform into Fire; the Heart sends True Yin to the Kidney for the Kidney to transform into Water. (Remember that these are energetic qualities and not a reference to actual substances of fire and water.)

The process involving the extraction, transformation, and transportation of Fluids is more complex. The Yang Bowels become more significant in this process, as they are intimately connected to Fluid transformation and transportation. Again, the ripening and rotting of food in the Stomach is the first step. In this process the Spleen extracts all the Fluid from the rotting and ripening food, and then separates a large portion of the pure Fluid from the impure Fluid. The impure Fluid is then sent by the Stomach to the Small Intestine, where further extraction of pure Fluids occurs. The dregs sent down from the Stomach are sent to the Colon, where the final extraction of Fluid from the dregs occurs. The Colon eliminates the dregs through the Rear Yin (the anus), and sends the Fluid to the Kidney for further processing. The Kidney then extracts the balance of the pure Fluid and transforms the remnants into urine, which is eliminated by the Urinary Bladder through the Front Yin. The pure Fluid from the Spleen is sent to the Lung and the Heart. Part of the pure Fluid in the Lung is sent to lubricate the skin and the muscles; the balance is sent to the Kidney for the beginning of the transformation cycle.

The Kidney receives pure Fluid from the Small Intestine, the Colon, the Lung, and from its own extraction process. Some of this Fluid is sent to moisten the Lung, some may be sent by the Kidney to help moisten the skin and muscles, some is transformed into serous fluid, and the balance is sent on through the Five Phase Cycle, where each Organ transforms part of the Fluid for its use and sends the rest on in the cycle. The Liver produces tears (the Liver Channel opens into the eyes) and synovial fluid (the Liver is in charge of the sinews). The Liver also produces bile, which is stored in its Yang partner, the Gall Bladder. The Heart produces sweat, often resulting from increased work and thereby increased Heart function. The Spleen produces saliva, the first digestive substance. (One can assume that all digestive substances are controlled by the Spleen.) The Lung produces mucus, implying also that the Lung controls all mucous membranes in the body.

The pure Fluid sent by the Spleen to the Heart combines with Nutrient Qi from the Lung. Under the influence of Yuan Qi of the Kidney, these substances initiate the production of Blood by the Heart. (It is often written that the Spleen produces Blood. This is actually a reference to the Spleen as being the source of both the Qi and the Fluids that make up Blood.) The Spleen keeps the Blood in the vessels, the Heart and Lung move the Blood throughout the system, and the Liver smoothes the flow of both the Blood and the Qi and controls the volume of Blood flow in the vessels.

Figures 34 and 35 provide a graphic depiction of the processes described above. Note that, although the Organs are placed according to the Three Burner concept, it should not be read as though the actual substances of Qi, Fluids, and Blood are moving physically in the manner described. The exception to this is when it is obviously a physical function that is being depicted, particularly a function of the Bowels.

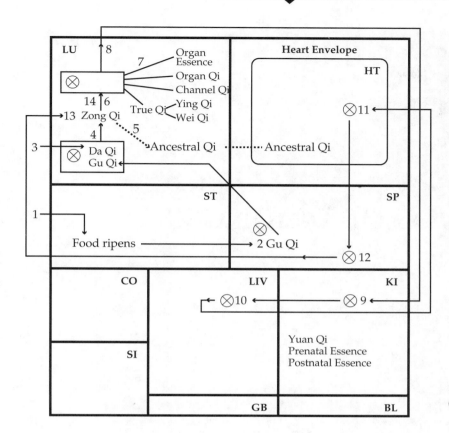

Figure 34

The process of the transformation of Qi under the influence of Yuan Qi. This transformation of Qi into the various energies depicted in the square representing the Lung (LU, upper left) occurs in each of the Viscera in turn in the Five Element Creation Cycle.

⊗ = Yuan Qi

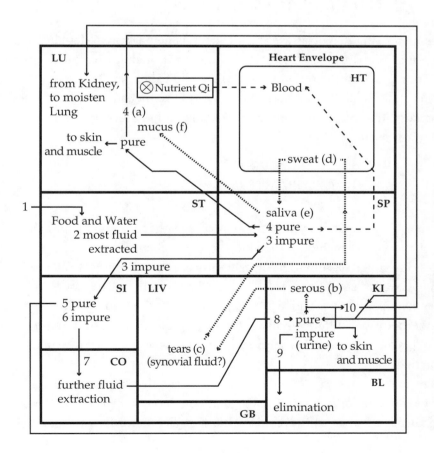

Figure 35

Based on the Five Element Creation Cycle, the separation of pure and impure Fluids by the Organs into various fluids utilized by the body

———— (1–10) Shows the movement of pure and impure Fluids in the extraction of pure Fluids and the elimination of impure Fluids.

·············· (a–f) Shows the transformation of pure Fluids into various thin fluids. This cycle starts in the Lung (a), however the transformations likely begin in the Kidney. It is the pure Fluid that is passed on, not the specific transformation product. (It is probable that the Liver produces synovial fluid, though this is still debated.)

– – – – – Shows Fluid and Qi movement for Blood production by the Heart.

⊗ = Yuan Qi

CHAPTER
8
METHODS OF DIAGNOSIS

EIGHT PRINCIPLES

The Eight Principles underlying diagnosis are the most fundamental way of looking at disease conditions in traditional Chinese medicine. The Eight Principles seek to characterize the essential qualities of the condition, which then allow the practitioner to successfully evaluate the condition and to act properly to harmonize the system. The Eight Principles describe a condition as being Interior or Exterior, Hot or Cold, Excessive or Deficient, and finally, Yin or Yang.

EXTERIOR/INTERIOR
▼

Exterior conditions are characterized by the invasion of a pathogenic agent into the superficial aspects of the body—including the skin, muscles, channels, and sinews—from seasonal excess, improper seasonal Qi, or general weakness. Generally, Wind is the primary Evil Qi of Exterior conditions; Heat and Cold are usually carried by Wind. Wind will also carry Damp and Dry, and will attack alone. As the pathogenic agent moves deeper into the body, half-Interior/half-Exterior symptoms, such as alternating fever and chills, may appear, indicating that the attacking agent is overcoming the superficial defenses of the body.

Interior conditions may be the result of an invading pathogen that has lodged within the Zang-Fu. It may be the result of an internal pathogenic condition, such as Liver Wind. It may also be an imbalance between entities or energies, such as Interior Excess Cold, as seen in such conditions as Damp Spleen and retention of Cold in the chest; Interior Excess Heat, as seen in such conditions as Heart Fire Upsurging and Abundant Liver Fire; and Blood Stasis and Phlegm, both conditions of Interior Excess.

HEAT/COLD
▼

Heat and Cold specify the kind of Qi that characterizes the pathogenic agent. Heat conditions show all the characteristics of something being heated—fluids dry up, and the patient feels hot, runs a fever, sweats, craves cold liquids, is flushed, and so forth. Cold conditions are characterized by exactly the opposite symptoms, including aversion to cold, little or no thirst, no sweating, tightly closed pores, long streams of clear urine from bladder constriction, and so forth.

EXCESS/DEFICIENT
▼

For many people, this is the most difficult aspect of the Eight Principles to comprehend. Excess conditions are not explained simply. When the pathogen is strong and the Wei (Defensive) Qi is strong, the battle will show Excess. As the pathogen migrates deeper into the body and the Wei Qi gets weaker, the Excess symptoms will change to Deficient symptoms.

While almost all Exterior conditions can simply be considered Excessive, Interior conditions present a more complex picture. While most internal conditions of long duration, no matter what their origin, are generally Deficient conditions, internal conditions can also be Excess. Hot or Cold conditions can manifest

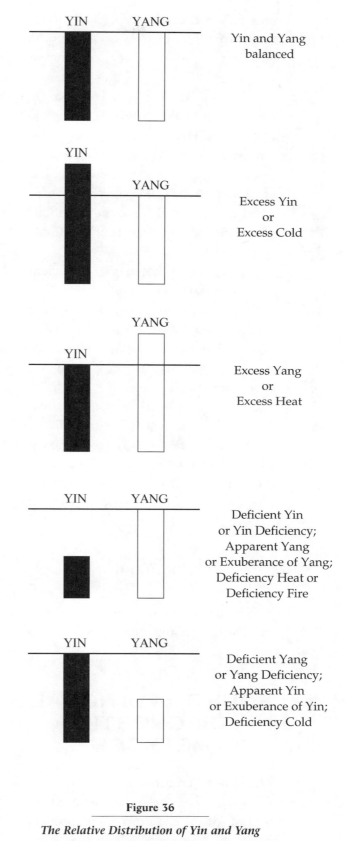

Yin and Yang balanced

Excess Yin
or
Excess Cold

Excess Yang
or
Excess Heat

Deficient Yin
or Yin Deficiency;
Apparent Yang
or Exuberance of Yang;
Deficiency Heat or
Deficiency Fire

Deficient Yang
or Yang Deficiency;
Apparent Yin
or Exuberance of Yin;
Deficiency Cold

Figure 36

The Relative Distribution of Yin and Yang

internally as Excess or Deficient. Hot can result from a true Excess of Yang in the Heart, Kidney, or Liver, or from a Deficiency of Yin in those or their controlling Organs. The first condition is Excess Heat or Fire, while the second is Deficiency Heat or Deficiency Fire. Similarly, Excess Yin can produce true Cold symptoms, but Yang Deficiency can cause Deficiency Cold symptoms. There are also Excess and Deficient conditions of specific Zang-Fu aspects of Qi, Blood, Yang, and Yin.

It should be noted that Deficient Yang (Yang Deficiency, Apparent Yin) indicates that there is not enough Yang energy present, while Deficient Yin (also called Deficiency Fire or Apparent Yang) indicates that there is not enough Yin energy present. It looks like Yang is in Excess when in fact it is not. Apparent Yin implies a Deficient Yang condition, making it appear that Yin is in Excess when in fact it is not. Figure 36 illustrates the patterns produced—with a complete set of alternate names—when Yin and Yang are out of balance.

YIN/YANG

▼

This relates to the generalized results of the diagnosis of the other principles.

FOUR TRADITIONAL DIAGNOSTIC METHODS

The Four Traditional Methods of Diagnosis have been the mainstay of medical diagnostic procedures throughout time. These methods include diag-

nosis by listening and smelling, by asking, by looking, and by touching. Only in modern Western allopathic medicine practices does the physician step out of the picture and rely on so-called objective tests to diagnose the patient. Due to the erroneous view that disease is patently the result of "little animals," such as bacteria and viruses, attacking the body, the art of diagnosis is relegated to the decision of a machine. Traditional Chinese medicine relies exclusively on the results of traditional diagnostic techniques and the health practitioner's assessment of the implications of that diagnosis.

DIAGNOSIS BY LISTENING AND SMELLING

▼

Diagnosis by Listening and Smelling includes listening to respiration, speech, and cough and noting the odor of the patient's breath, gynecological odors, and other smells emanating from the body.

Respiration

Shallow, weak breathing usually indicates Deficiency of Vital Energy, while coarse, rapid breathing usually indicates Excess.

Acute asthma with sputum rattling in the throat and/or chest is the result of pathogens invading the Lung, and is an Excess condition. Chronic asthma with weak wheezing and shortness of breath is usually due to Deficiency of Vital Energy of the Kidney or Lung.

Cough

Dysfunction of the dispersing and descending function of the Lung (Deranged Lung Qi) is the usual cause of coughing. A coarse cough is usually caused by an invasion of exogenous pathogens and is an Excess condition. A weak cough usually indicates a Deficiency condition. A dry cough or unproductive cough is often due to the invasion of exogenous Dryness. It may also result from endogenous Dryness caused by Deficient Yin (Fluid in the Lung).

Odor

Fetid breath usually points to Heat in the Stomach, but may also indicate Heat in the Lung. Sour breath simply indicates indigestion, pointing to a Spleen/Stomach dysfunction.

Extremely offensive odor of excrement indicates an Excess Heat syndrome usually related to a Spleen/Stomach disfunctioning, but possibly related to another of the digestion-related Organs. This odor may be reported by the patient; it may also be noticeable from the patient's breath. An insipid odor of excrement is a weak odor, with none of the overpowering qualities of the prior example. It indicates a Deficient Cold syndrome, usually of the Stomach/Spleen. Again, this odor may be reported by the patient. It may also be noticeable from the patient's breath, although not nearly as obvious as the odors mentioned previously.

Gynecological odors as reported by the patient are useful in differentiating gynecological syndromes.

DIAGNOSIS BY ASKING

By employing specific questions about certain processes, Diagnosis by Asking allows the practitioner to make an effective assessment and differential diagnosis leading to proper treatment. The questions include requests for information about fever and chills, perspiration, expectoration of sputum, food and drink intake, appetite and taste, bowel movements, urination, pain, and bleeding.

Fever and Chills

Simultaneous chills and fever usually indicate the early stage of invasion by an exogenous pathogen. If the chills predominate, this and other clinical signs indicate that the pathogen is Wind Cold. If the feverishness predominates, this and other clinical signs indicate that the pathogen is Wind Heat.

Alternate chills and fever indicate a half-Interior/half-Exterior condition. Although usually caused by exogenous pathogen invasion, this symptom can indicate Liver/Gall Bladder dysfunction. This internal dysfunction is accompanied by bitterness in the mouth, dry throat, a sense of bloatedness, and a congested sensation in the ribs.

A sustained high fever accompanied by a surging, rapid pulse and extreme thirst usually indicates Excess Interior Heat. A tidal fever appearing only in the afternoon, accompanied by flushed cheeks and feverish sensations in the palms and soles, usually indicates Yin Deficiency.

A tidal fever that appears daily, with no flushed cheeks but possible redness of the face, accompanied by constipation and a sensation of fullness with pain in the abdomen, usually indicates Excess Heat accumulated in the Intestines.

Chills with no fever usually result from Yang Deficiency and can be alleviated by warm clothing or blankets. Sometimes an exogenous Cold pathogen may be the cause. If this is the case, no clothing or blankets can alleviate the subjective sensation of cold.

Perspiration

Spontaneous sweating with no apparent cause usually indicates a Deficiency of Protective Qi and/or Deficiency of Lung Qi. Night sweats shows Deficient Yin with Deficiency Heat, a condition known as Exuberance of Yang. Severe sweating accompanied by other symptoms of Heat may indicate exogenous Heat invading the Interior.

In all conditions wherein the patient has been sweating, it is incorrect to use techniques to cause sweating. This will debilitate the patient.

Expectoration of Sputum

Thin, whitish sputum is called Cold sputum and usually indicates the presence of Cold. Thick, yellow sputum is called Heat sputum. It is usually purulent, and indicates the presence of Heat. Scanty, sticky sputum is called Dry sputum and usually indicates the presence of Dryness.

Food and Drink, Appetite and Taste

No appetite usually indicates impaired (Deranged, Excess, or Deficient) function of the Stomach and Spleen. Thirst with no desire to drink indicates Deranged Spleen function, not Deficiency of Fluids. In this situation, the Spleen does not transport Fluid and is therefore (along with the Stomach) holding the Fluids. Severe thirst with the desire to drink cold fluids indicates either an exogenous pathogen turning to Heat in the Interior, or an Interior Excess Heat condition.

A bitter taste in the mouth indicates Excess Fire. If it is present even when eating food, it is indicative of hyperactivity of the Liver and Gall Bladder. A sweet taste in the mouth is indicative of Damp Heat in the Spleen. A sour taste in the mouth usually results from indigestion.

Bowel Movements

Constipation indicates Excess Heat in the Intestines. In debilitated or elderly people, and in postpartum women, constipation may indicate Deficient Vital Qi or Deficient Fluids in the Intestines. Loose or watery stools usually indicate Deficient Spleen Yang (hypofunction of the Spleen). Diarrhea often indicates Deficiency of the Spleen; diarrhea upon awakening indicates Kidney Yang not warming the Spleen, a Kidney Yang Deficiency. Acute diarrhea with burning in the rectum indicates Excess Damp or Damp Heat in the Intestines.

Urination

Urine in short streams, difficult urination, diminished urine, red and yellowish urine, urine containing blood, gravel in the urine, suppression of urination with rapid pulse and yellow tongue coating indicate Damp Heat attacking the Bladder.

For diagnostic purposes the basic types of urine are condensed, dilute, turbid, and red-tinged (hematuria). Condensed and dark yellow urine usually indicates Heat. Diluted and clear urine usually indicates Cold. Turbid urine usually indicates Damp. Hematuria is usually caused by Heat. Hematuria may result from Deficiency Fire caused by Deficient Kidney Yin. This is an Interior Deficient syndrome. Hematuria with turbidity usually indicates Damp Heat in the Kidney and Bladder (with other clinical signs), and is an Interior Excess syndrome. Both of these syndromes indicate a fairly severe level of hematuria. Chronic but mild hematuria may be caused by Deficient Spleen Qi, wherein the Spleen does not properly keep the Blood in the blood vessels.

Pain

Pain is caused by obstruction of the proper flow of Vital Qi or Blood. Cold pain is relieved by warmth. Hot pain is relieved by cold. Yin pain or Deficient pain is relieved by pressure. Yang pain or Excess pain is aggravated by pressure. Distending pain usually indicates Stagnation of Vital Qi. Pain with accompanying heavy sensation usually indicates Damp accumulation. Stabbing or pricking pain, often severe and accompanied by tenderness, usually indicates Blood Stasis. Colicky pain usually indicates obstruction of the Yang by Phlegm, Damp, undigested food, or even gall stones (called visible pathogens). Migratory pain usually indicates Wind. Burning pain usually indicates Fire (or Heat). Epigastric pain is usually caused by Fire of the Stomach. Pain with cool sensation usually indicates coagulation of Yang Qi by pathogenic Cold. Dull persistent pain usually indicates a Deficiency syndrome.

Bleeding

Bleeding caused by external injury and hemorrhoidal bleeding are not considered signs of dysfunction of the Organs.

Severe bleeding and hemorrhage usually indicate Excess Liver Fire possibly burning the blood vessels. Hemoptysis (spitting blood from the lungs) and epistaxis (nosebleed) are indications of Fire of the Liver. Mild chronic bleeding in the lower part of the body often points to Deficient Spleen Yang not keeping the Blood in the vessels. Excessive uterine bleeding, hematochezia (the passage of bloody stools), and hematuria (the presence of blood in the urine) usually indicate Deficient Spleen Yang. Bruising easily usually indicates hypofunction of the Spleen.

DIAGNOSIS BY LOOKING

Diagnosis by Looking includes observation of edema, observation of the expression of the patient, observation of the complexion (facial colors), observation of the appearance, and tongue diagnosis. (Tongue diagnosis will be discussed in a separate section.)

Observation of Edema

Edema appearing primarily in the head and face or around the lips and mouth usually indicates impairment of the Lung function. Edema appearing primarily in the loins and lower extremities usually indicates impairment of the Kidney. Edema appearing primarily in the feet indicates Deficient Kidney Yang. (If the Gate of Vitality is in decline and Kidney Yin is Deficient, there will be exhaustion of Original Qi followed by Floating of Deficiency Yang, and finally Yang Prolapse.) Edema appearing primarily in the limbs usually indicates impairment of the Spleen.

Observation of Expression

The patient's expression is a general indicator of the condition of the spirits. If the patient is in good spirits, with bright eyes, and is aware and precise in responses, then the prognosis of the disease is good and the patient is not seriously ill. If the patient appears listless and in poor spirits, with dull eyes and sluggish responses, the illness is serious and difficult to cure. Sometimes, when the patient is critically ill, there may be signs of false vitality.

Observation of Complexion

Since Qi and Blood are sent to the face by virtually all the channels, it is reasonable that the face reflects the general condition of the Vital Energy and Blood. The condition of the Heart is particularly reflected in the condition of the patient's expression, as discussed above, and not necessarily only in terms of complexion.

According to the Theory of Five Elements, the colors of the complexion point toward dysfunction of the specific Organs as follows: Heart (Fire) shows as red, Spleen and Stomach (Earth) show as yellow, Lung and Large Intestine (Metal) show as white, Kidney (Water) shows as black, and Liver (Wood) shows as green (or blue). (The spectrum is divided differently in the East and the colors that Orientals call green are often called blue by Occidentals.)

White

Pallor may indicate a deficiency in the supply of Qi and Blood. This may point to deficient Blood production (Deficient Yin), or a condition of Deficient Yang not circulating the Blood. Endogenous Cold will also cause pallor by constricting and thereby interfering with the circulation of Fluids, Blood, and Qi. Deficient Blood pallor usually shows pallor of the lips as well. Deficient Qi pallor usually shows puffiness of the face and little pallor of the lips.

Red

Reddening of the face (and the skin in general) is usually due to the presence of Heat or Fire which tends to promote blood circulation, resulting in engorgement of the capillaries. Flushing of the whole face is often caused by exogenous Heat as well as Excess endogenous Heat. Flushing on the cheekbones only (malar flush), which will tend to produce a brighter red and may occur only in the afternoon, accompanied by a mild fever (again a symptom of Deficiency Fire), indicates endogenous Deficiency Heat resulting from a Deficient Yin condition.

Yellow

A sallow complexion indicates Deficient Spleen/Stomach Yang and accumulated Damp. The Spleen Earth tends to avoid Damp, and when Damp accumulates, the Spleen function has either failed to transport Fluids leading to the Damp accumulation or the Damp has entered into the Spleen and made its function sluggish.

In Western medical tradition, a yellow skin tone indicates jaundice. In TCM, jaundice is said to be caused by Dampness obstructing the passage of bile, and presents in two different ways: a bright yellow complexion indicates Yang jaundice caused by Damp and Heat; a lusterless or dark yellow complexion indicates Yin jaundice, which is caused by Damp and Cold.

Green (Blue)

A greenish hue to the skin may indicate retardation of the flow of Blood and Qi. It may also indicate Blood Stasis, which is often due to the Liver's failure to maintain harmony in the flow of Blood. Severe pain and convulsions will also lead to a blue or greenish hue to the skin.

Black (darkening)

A gray-black appearance to the skin indicates long-standing Blood Stasis. When the Yang of the Kidney is deficient, the general low metabolic function will cause a variety of symptoms, including Blood Stasis. A bronze color, as in Addison's disease, indicates Deficient Kidney Yin.

Observation of Appearance

The gait, posture, quality of movement, and the build of the body are considered when looking at the appearance. A strong build will usually indicate a positive prognosis. Emaciation will indicate a Deficient Yin condition, with a poorer prognosis.

Edema setting in suddenly, particularly in the upper part of the body, indicates an external attack by Wind or another element, and it is usually the Lung that is invaded. Edema in the lower part of the body is usually related to the dysfunction of the Spleen or Kidney.

The tendency to lie in a fetal position is usually indicative of Internal Cold, often arising from Deficient Yang. Lying on the back with no desire to cover the chest usually indicates Excess Heat syndrome.

Sudden severe convulsions and/or abnormal limb movement usually indicates an attack of Excess Wind either from outside, or from Excess Liver Fire with Damp. Chronic tremor is usually indicative of Interior Deficiency Wind. This usually results from Deficient Liver Yin and Exuberance of (Deficiency) Fire leading to Wind.

DIAGNOSIS BY TOUCHING

Diagnosis by Touching includes palpation of the skin, subcutaneous tissue, musculature, bone, abdomen, and points. It also includes Pulse Diagnosis, which will be discussed in a later section.

Palpation of the Skin and Abdomen

A patient's skin that at first contact feels warm then increases in heat as you continue to palpate indicates an Interior Heat syndrome. Warm skin that does not increase in temperature as you continue to palpate indicates a syndrome of Exterior Heat. Palpation of the abdomen will indicate the presence of masses, and helps to uncover areas of tenderness that may indicate blockages in the channels, or may be Mu points indicating particular Organ dysfunctions. (Mu points are special diagnostic points. They are discussed further in chapter 14.) This type of palpation over the skin surface can tell much about the disturbances in the channels.

Whenever encountering tender or painful areas that may suggest channel or Organ involvement, the response of the patient is diagnostically significant. If pain is alleviated by pressure, it is Deficiency Pain and points to a Deficiency syndrome. If the pain is aggravated by pressure, it indicates Excess.

TONGUE DIAGNOSIS

Reading the signs of the tongue is one of the most remarkable contributions the Chinese have made to medical diagnosis. It is a practice that is not matched in any other system of medical diagnosis. Although recognized in Western medicine to some small extent, the tongue is really studied only as an anatomical structure with limited pathologies and is virtually unused for diagnosis after the doctor leaves school. Tongue diagnosis is without peer in differential diagnosis and syndrome indication. It is much more important than the diagnosis of the pulse, since it is far more objective in use. The aspects of tongue diagnosis include looking at the "spirit" of the tongue, or color vitality, the color of the tongue, the shape of the tongue, the tongue coating, the presence of moisture on the tongue, and the surface features of the tongue.

"THE SPIRIT OF THE TONGUE," OR COLOR VITALITY
▼

No matter what the condition of the tongue and no matter what other symptoms and signs may be present, if the color of the tongue—whether it appears bright or pale—can be said to be vital, the prognosis of disease is good, and the patient, if treated properly, will soon recover. If, however, the tongue has a dark and withered appearance, the prognosis is poor and the patient's healing may be difficult and protracted. The tongue with vital color is called the Tongue of Life and one that is dark and withered is called the Tongue of Death. These terms are not to be taken literally, but should be regarded as figurative dichotomies. It is primarily the root of the tongue that is carefully scrutinized in considering the vitality of the tongue color.

BODY COLOR OF THE TONGUE
▼

This is the color of the tongue beneath any coating that may appear (and naturally after ruling out the ingestion of any substances that may color the tongue.) It reflects the conditions of the Viscera, Blood, and Nutritive Qi. Clinically it reflects Hot or Cold; Yin, Yang, Qi, or Blood Deficiencies; and Stagnation.

BODY SHAPE OF THE TONGUE
▼

The physical shape of the tongue—whether it is thin or swollen, long or short, has specific swollen areas, and so forth—are considered. Other condsiderations are features on the surface (pits, cracks, ulcers, etc.), texture (supple or stiff), and involuntary movement (quivering, trembling, side-to-side movement, curling or shifting in any particular direction). Clinically the shape of the tongue reflects conditions of Organs, Qi, and Blood. This aspect in particular helps to distinguish Excess and Deficient conditions.

COATING OF THE TONGUE
▼

There are four aspects of the coating of the tongue that must be considered, and each should be observed over the area from the tip to the root of the tongue. The color of the coating accurately reflects Hot or Cold influences, with a white coating indicating Cold influences and a yellow coating indicating Heat.

The thickness of the coating correlates with the strength of the pathogen, and indicates Excess or Deficiency. The coating should appear to grow out of the tongue, as though it had roots in the tongue body itself. Such a healthy condition is said to be a tongue with roots that has a "true" coating. Such a coating cannot be readily scraped off. If the coating appears to be sprinkled or dropped on to the surface of the tongue and can be readily scraped off, it is said to be a tongue without roots.

The roots of the coating reflect the strength of the Qi and the Excess or Deficiency of Qi. Distribution of the coating indicates the progression of the disease in conditions caused by exogenous factors, and the location of the pathogen or imbalances in conditions caused by endogenous factors.

MOISTURE ON THE TONGUE
▼

A slightly moist tongue is the normal condition while a wet tongue indicates an accumulation of body Fluids and a dry tongue indicates insufficient body Fluids. The moisture factor therefore reflects the relative state of Yin/Yang and Hot/Cold.

The normal tongue has spirit. It therefore has vital color, particularly at the root. It has a pale red color with a fresh look, not unlike fresh meat, which indicates that it has a sufficient supply of Heart Blood. If the tongue is a darker shade of red than expected, it has an insufficient supply of Stomach Fluids. (The Stomach sends Fluids to the tongue and forms the coating of the tongue.) The

tongue should be supple and straight without quivering, swelling, thinning, ulcerations, and cracks. Because the Stomach, while digesting food and transforming Qi, produces a certain residual Turbid Damp which rises up to coat the tongue, there should normally be a thin white coating growing out of the tongue, with a slight thickening of the coating on the root of the tongue. The tongue should be moist, leaning toward neither dry nor wet. This moisture also reflects the proper functioning of the Stomach.

SURFACE FEATURES
▼

Two major schemes have evolved to map the Organs in regard to the surface of the tongue, and a third scheme tracks the movement of disease. Figure 37 shows all three schemes. The first is useful in discovering the specific Organ or Organs involved in the disease condition. The second gives the location of the disease according to the Three-Burner breakdown, and is useful in tracking the movement of the disease in or out of the system. The third scheme is also used in some cases to track the movement of disease.

The tables on pages 142 and 143 describe tongue-diagnosis differentiation according to the Eight Principles. The first table lists various aspects of the tongue and their clinical implications. The second table describes more specific signs on the tongue and their significance. These tables give a good overview of tongue presentations, although they are not exhaustive.

The text that follows the tables will examine in greater detail how the Eight Principles relate to tongue diagnosis.

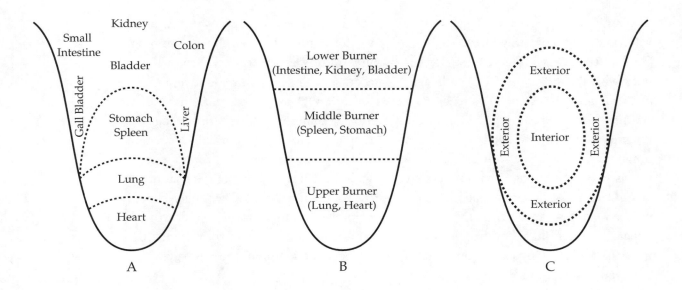

Figure 37

*The surface features of the tongue related to
(A) the Organ involved, (B) the location within
the Three Burners, and
(C) movement of the disease*

TONGUE DIAGNOSIS DIFFERENTIATION

TONGUE CHARACTERISTICS	GENERAL APPEARANCE	IMPLICATIONS	EIGHT PRINCIPLES
Tongue spirit	Tongue of Life	Good prognosis	
	Tongue of Death	Poor prognosis	
Tongue body	Color	Viscera, Blood, Nutritive Qi	Cold/Hot
	Shape	Organs, Blood, Qi	Deficiency/Excess, Yin/Yang
Tongue coating	Color white	Cold	Cold/Hot
	Color yellow	Hot	Cold/Hot
	Coat thickness	Strength of pathogen or weakness of Qi	Deficiency/Excess
	Area of surface with additional symptoms	Exterior—Disease progression Interior—Organ(s) disturbed by pathogens	Exterior/Interior
	Root of coating	Strength of Qi—primarily Qi of Stomach and Kidney	Deficiency/Excess
Tongue moisture		Condition of Fluids	Cold/Hot Yin/Yang

EIGHT-PRINCIPLE INDICATIONS BY TONGUE DIAGNOSIS

SIGNS ON THE TONGUE	PATHOGEN OR INJURED ORGAN	AFFECTED ENERGY/FLUID	8-PRINCIPLE CONDITION
Coat thin and white (normal)—thickens over time	Wind Cold	N/A	Exterior
Coat thin and white—yellows and thickens over time	Wind Hot	N/A	Exterior
Coating is thick*	Non-specific	N/A	Exterior Excess
Coating white on one side or white coating at the anterior portion and gray or black near the root	Non-specific	N/A	Half-Interior/ Half-Exterior
Body color and shape altered*	Non-specific	Non-specific	Interior
Body is pale; coating is white, thick, and slippery	Cold	Usually Damp; Fluid accumulates	Interior Excess
Body is red; coating is yellow and thick*	Hot	Non-specific	Interior Excess
Body is purple*	Blood Stagnation	Non-specific	Interior Excess
Coating is thick, slippery, and greasy*	Phlegm	Non-specific	Interior Excess
Body is red; coating is yellow*	Non-specific	Non-specific	Hot
Coating is white*	Non-specific	Non-specific	Cold
Body color is pale (or even bluish)*	Non-specific	Non-specific	Deficiency Cold
Body somewhat flaccid with some anterior swelling	Lung	Qi	Deficiency
Body is tooth-marked	Spleen	Qi	Deficiency
Coating is absent in the center of tongue	Stomach	Qi	Deficiency
Body color is pale*	Heart	Qi	Deficiency
Body color is pale (in Yang Deficiencies)*	Non-specific	Yang	Deficiency
Body color is pale; coating is white and wet	Spleen	Yang	Deficiency
Body color is pale; body is swollen; coating is white	Kidney	Yang	Deficiency
Body color is pale; tends toward bluish-purple as condition grows severe	Heart	Yang	Deficiency
Body color is pale (in Blood Deficiencies)*	Non-specific	Blood	Deficiency
Body color is pale and slightly dry	Spleen	Blood	Deficiency
Body color is pale; tip is paler than balance of tongue body	Heart	Blood	Deficiency
Body color is pale; sides are paler than the balance of tongue body	Liver	Blood	Deficiency
No coating in center; dry; wide crack in center	Stomach	Yin	Deficiency
Body color is red; (in all Yin Deficiencies except Stomach)*	Non-specific	Yin	Deficiency
Body color is red; no coating; dry; with cracks	Kidney	Yin	Deficiency
Body color is red; tip is redder; no coating on Heart area (and possibly Lung area, i.e., anterior is redder)	Heart	Yin	Deficiency
Body color is red; no coating; anterior cracks (Lung area)	Lung	Yin	Deficiency

* indicates that other signs are necessary for diagnosis.

EXTERIOR/INTERIOR

EXTERIOR CONDITIONS
▼

Exterior conditions arise from invasion by a pathogenic factor into the superficial regions—the skin, muscles, channels, and sinews. Initial pathogen action will cause little or no change in the tongue.

Wind Cold Attacks

The coating is white due to Cold, thin because the pathogen is just beginning to affect the system and therefore not yet having a strong effect, and probably overly moist since Cold will block the proper movement of fluids in the skin and muscles, leading to a slight accumulation on the tongue. The coating is possibly limited to the anterior portion of the tongue, and is easily scraped off, but returns shortly thereafter. If the coat becomes white and dry, covers the tongue, and is not easily scraped off, the pathogenic Cold is about to enter deeper into the system and turn to Fire. If the Coat is thin, white, and has dry prickles, the Cold is about to transform into Heat. The dry prickles indicate that the Fluids in the Lung have been injured. If Damp Cold is present the coat will be thin, white, and greasy. The greasy quality always indicates the presence of Damp.

Wind Heat Attacks

The coating is white because Heat has had little chance to affect the system, thin because the pathogen is just beginning to affect the system and therefore is not yet having a strong effect, and dry because the Heat is drying the body fluids. As the pathogen begins to penetrate deeper, the coat will turn yellow. In severe attacks of Heat the coat may be gray or black, and have prickles on the surface.

Often the changes will only show on the front of the tongue. Sometimes the front and edges turn red. Unlike Heart Fire signs, the whole anterior tongue will change, not just the tip. Clinical symptoms will point away from Liver Fire, which will be indicated by red edges.

INTERIOR CONDITIONS
▼

Interior conditions indicate that the pathogenic factor is in the internal Organs. The pathogen may be an externally contracted one that has worked its way deep into the body. It may be an internally evolved condition from emotional, dietary, sexual, or other excesses or deficiencies, leading to Liver Fire, Abundant Heart Fire, and so forth. Finally, it may be an imbalance between Organs or Yin and Yang functions.

Interior conditions are reflected in a multitude of ways, and no generalization can realistically be made. Most Interior conditions are characterized by a yellow coating, as they are usually the result of transformation of an external Cold pathogen or long-standing internal development. After a time, these pathogens usually transform to Heat in the Interior since, in all long-standing conditions, the Essence will tend to deplete, showing, if not true Excess, then Deficiency Fire symptoms.

HEAT/COLD

COLD
▼

Generally there will be a pale tongue, white coating, and moisture.

Excess Cold

Excess Cold blocks the Yang Qi's transportation (circulation) of Blood, producing a pale tongue body, as well as Yang's transportation of Fluids, leading to an overly moist and possibly slippery coating. The coating is thick, which is the primary differentiation of an Excess condition. When there is chronic retention of Cold, the tongue body may appear blue. A purple-blue tongue body indicates prolonged retention of Cold with obstructed circulation and Blood Stasis.

Deficiency Cold

Deficiency Cold, an Internal condition, is the result of Deficient Yang Qi. A pale tongue body results from the Deficient Yang Qi's failure to transport Blood to the tongue. The thin coating results from the absence of a pathogenic agent to show on the tongue, and the moist white coating indicates that the Deficient Yang Qi fails to transport Fluids so they accumulate on the tongue producing moisture. The Apparent Cold (Deficiency Cold) makes the color white. Should the Yang Qi Deficiency reach extreme proportions, as in a long-standing Deficiency Cold syndrome, there may be no Fluid transformation and transportation at all, and the tongue coating will be dry.

HEAT
▼

A Heat condition shows as a red tongue body. There will be a yellow coating in Excess Heat conditions and no coating or a peeled coating in Deficiency Heat conditions. Different areas of Heat concentration show on the tongue according to the traditional view of the topography of the tongue. A dry tongue with red tip and red points indicates Heart Heat. A dry tongue with red sides and bilateral yellow coating indicates Liver Heat. A dry tongue with a thick yellow coating and (usually) red points around the center of the tongue indicates Heat in the Stomach. A dry tongue with a thin yellow coating on the anterior tongue indicates Lung Heat. A very dry tongue with a brown or black coating indicates Extreme Heat in the Stomach and Intestines, with retention of stool.

Excess Heat

Heat will inevitably produce Excess Yang Qi activity, with the result that the Blood will be excessive in the tongue and the tongue body will always be red or dark red. The tongue will be dry as a result of the Heat burning up the body's fluids. If the Heat is Excess, the coating will be yellow and the thickness of the coating will indicate the degree of severity of the pathogen.

Deficiency Heat

If the Heat is Deficiency Heat from Deficient Yin, there will be no coating, as there is no pathogenic factor to reflect.

EXCESS/DEFICIENT

There are four major aspects of the organism that can become Deficient and thereby disturb the normal functions of the organism. These are Qi in general, showing neither Hot nor Cold symptoms; Yang or Yang Qi, showing a deficiency of functions with symptoms of Deficiency Cold; Yin or Yin Qi (Essence), showing a deficiency of substance with symptoms of

Deficiency Fire; and Blood, which can be deficient, in stasis, coagulated, or stagnant.

Deficient Qi

The tongue body will be slightly flabby and may have no other signs in mild conditions. The location of the Deficiency is shown on the tongue as follows.

Lung Qi Deficiency will usually manifest as shortness of breath because the Lung Qi cannot take in air and Da Qi properly; weak voice because the Ancestral (Pectoral) Qi is not strong enough to activate the voice; and spontaneous sweating because the Wei Qi is out of control, may be depleted, and cannot properly control the pores. If the tongue appears normal other than slight flabbiness and possible swelling on the anterior tongue (not including the tip), Deficient Lung Qi is indicated.

The Spleen controls the processes of transformation and transportation of Fluids and Gu Qi and is prone to Deficiency. Spleen Qi Deficiency is characterized by lethargy resulting from the general depletion of Fluids and Qi, and by poor appetite and abdominal distention because the Spleen does not transport the contents of the Stomach as the digestive function falters. Drowsiness follows from the general depletion of the body functions. The tongue body will be flabby and show tooth marks, particularly on the anterior sides. Although no Cold symptoms are showing, the tongue may be pale. A mild condition may show no symptoms at all.

Stomach Qi Deficiency will fail to properly transform food and therefore there will be no Turbid Damp to produce the white coating of the tongue. Instead there will be a thin coating at the center of the tongue, or a coating without root.

Heart Qi Deficiency will manifest in circulatory irregularities, since the Heart controls the Blood and the blood vessels. There will be palpitations and shortness of breath during exertion. No symptoms of Cold will show, but the tongue body will be pale as the Deficient Heart Qi fails to carry Blood to the tongue. In severe cases the tip of the tongue will be swollen. Emotional trauma dispersing Heart Qi often accounts for this syndrome.

Deficient Yang

Blood not carried to the tongue produces a pale tongue body and one that is overly wet because the Deficient Yang Qi fails to transform and transport Fluids through the body, and it instead accumulates on the tongue. The coating is thin and white because of Deficiency Cold resultant from Deficient Yang.

Spleen Yang Deficiency shows symptoms of Spleen Qi Deficiency (which it is, but not a general Deficiency of Qi) which include lethargy from general depletion of Fluids and Qi; poor appetite and abdominal distention because the Spleen does not transport; and drowsiness from the general depletion of the body functions. The tongue body will be flabby and show tooth marks, particularly on the anterior sides. In addition there will be chills and very loose stools, because the Fluids are not properly transported and so accumulate in the Spleen, causing Wet Spleen diarrhea. The tongue body will be pale, and the coating will be white and thin, all from the Deficiency Cold. Since there is a likely accumulation of Dampness, the tongue may be very wet and swollen (thick). This condition is commonly caused by excessive eating of cold and/or raw foods.

Kidney Yang Deficiency often accompanies Spleen Yang Deficiency, indicating a much more severe condition. It exhibits the signs of Spleen Yang Deficiency—lethargy, poor appetite, abdominal distention, drowsiness, chills, loose stools—and further displays sore back and chills in the low back, resulting from the Deficiency Cold in the Kidneys. The tongue body is very pale, overly wet, and with a thin, white coating. In order to distinguish between these syndromes it is necessary to make a differential diagnosis based on pulses and clinical symptoms.

Deficient Blood

This will always show as a pale and slightly dry tongue, because the Blood will hardly reach the tongue. The Fluids will also be impaired. Clinical signs of Blood Deficiency include a pale face (since there is insufficient blood), numbness, and dizziness, common symptoms in all Western disease syndromes resulting from blood deficiency.

Since the Spleen is the origin of Blood (it controls both Fluid and Qi metabolism in the primary stages), a disturbance of that function may lead to general Deficiency of Blood, called Spleen Blood Deficiency. If Heart Blood Deficiency accompanies Spleen Blood Deficiency, palpitations and insomnia will occur from derangement of the spirits. The tip of the tongue is paler than the body in conditions of Heart Blood Deficiency.

Since the Liver stores the Blood and controls the harmony of its flow, Deficiency of Blood will affect the Liver,

causing Liver Blood Deficiency, with the same symptoms of a pale face, numbness, and dizziness, as well as brittle nails. Women will have very little blood discharge during menstruation. The sides of the tongue are paler than the body, and in severe cases which give way to Deficient Yin, may even have an orange shade.

Deficient Yin

When chronic conditions occur from excessive sexual activity, excessive labor, or excessive cold or raw foods and other dietary improprieties, the body will be depleted of Vital Essence, the underlying substance that becomes the active energy of Yang. This is Yin Deficiency, and it is a dangerous and serious condition. It can also occur from an external pathogen entering as Heat or becoming Heat in the Interior. The extreme Heat burns up the fluids and can cause the muscles and sinews to become shriveled and atrophied, as seen in some high febrile diseases.

Stomach Yin Deficiency is usually the first stage of the evolution of a general Yin Deficiency syndrome. When the Essence of the Stomach is deficient, it does not properly digest the incoming food and drink and Fluids are not properly passed down to the small intestines, resulting in epigastric pain; fullness; thirst with no desire to drink, or the desire to drink warm fluids in small sips; loss of appetite; and dry stools. In early stages the tongue will have a rootless coating, because the Stomach Yin does not produce Turbid Damp. Eventually the center of the tongue will be without coating.

As the condition progresses, the absence of Fluids will often stimulate the arousal of Deficiency Fire in the Kidney. This will produce the signs of Kidney Yin Deficiency with Reckless Fire, wherein the tongue body will be red and dry from Heat and absence of Fluids, and peeled (without a coating) because of Deficiency Fire. There will often be a deep crack lengthwise in the center of the tongue reaching the tip. The deeper the crack, the worse the condition. Some of the symptoms that often accompany this condition include tinnitus; vertigo; deafness, because the outlet of the Kidney is the ear; nocturnal emissions and night sweats, because the Reckless Fire causes excessive and uncontrolled sexual function, and water metabolism is disturbed; insomnia and impaired memory, because the Deficient Kidney does not raise True Yang to the Heart, causing derangement of the spirits; sore back; afternoon and evening feverish sensations from the Reckless Fire; dry mouth (particularly at night) and dry throat. Kidney Yin Deficiency with Reckless Fire is almost inevitably followed by Deficient Heart Yin, adding mental restlessness and palpitations to the symptoms. The tongue will be red, peeled, and dry, and the tip will be redder. If the condition exists independently, the peeled area will be only at the tip.

Deficient Lung Yin may follow upon or be a cause of Deficient Kidney Yin. Heat will manifest as hot sensation or sweating on the sternum and the palms (Five Palm Heat) and soles, and there is likely to be a feverish feeling in the afternoon and evening, weak cough with little sputum, dry throat, and sputum possibly containing blood. The tongue will be red, peeled, and dry, with possible cracks in the Lung area.

EXCESS

Interior Excess

Exterior Excess conditions have already been discussed under Wind Cold and Wind Heat attacks. In addition to Interior Excess Cold and Interior Excess Heat, there are two other Interior Excess conditions: Blood Stasis and Phlegm.

Blood Stasis can occur from either a Deficiency or Excess condition, such as Qi Stagnation (which may give rise to masses), Qi Deficiency, Blood Deficiency, Heat in the Blood, or Interior Cold. Some of the major signs and symptoms are a fixed pain, usually stabbing or pricking in nature; bleeding, often with dark purple clots; and a taut (wiry) or hesitant pulse. The tongue is purple in color and may have purple or dark red spots, which can be an indicator of which Organ is affected.

Phlegm is an Excess condition usually caused by a Spleen Yang Deficiency. When the Spleen fails to transform and transport Fluids, they can stagnate and coagulate, turning into Phlegm. Other Organs involved in the production of Phlegm are the Kidney and Lung. Phlegm is characterized by a slippery or greasy tongue coating and a slippery or taut pulse.

Phlegm can take many forms. It can manifest as sputum in the lungs or it can mist the Mind, disturbing the Shen and causing emotional illness. It can form stones, such as kidney or gall bladder calculi; it can also accumulate in the joint spaces and give rise to different forms of arthritis. Phlegm can also form cysts, fibroids, tumors, and other swellings, and it can block the channels, causing numbness and possible stroke. Phlegm can combine with different pathogens, giving rise to Hot Phlegm, Cold Phlegm, or Wind Phlegm.

The tables on pages 149 through 152 give detailed information regarding the clinical importance of the color of the tongue body, the shape of the tongue, and the various coatings that can appear on the surface of the tongue.

INDICATIONS OF TONGUE-BODY COLOR

COLOR OF TONGUE BODY	ADDITIONAL CHARACTERISTICS	INDICATIONS
Pale	Dry	Blood Deficiency
	Wet	Yang Deficiency
	Bright and shiny	Qi and Blood Deficiency, especially of Stomach and Spleen
Red	Usually yellow coating	Heat (Fire) at the Nutritive or Blood level
	Without coating	Yin Deficiency with Exuberant Fire
	Dry with (yellow) coating	Excess Fire burning up Fluids
	Dry without coating	Deficiency Fire from Deficient Yin and Fluid Exhaustion
	Wet	Damp Heat
	Smooth and bright	Deficient Stomach Yin and/or Kidney Yin
	Scarlet	Deficient Lung Yin and/or Heart Yin
	Dark red with a dry center	Stomach Fire Blazing or Fire from Deficient Stomach Yin
	Reddish purple	Fire with Stagnant Blood
	Reddish purple, swollen and distended	Excess Fire and Stagnant Blood with (alcohol) poison injuring the Heart
	Red points or spots	Fire with Stagnant Blood
	Prickles	Fire at the levels of the Nutritive Qi, Upper Burner, or Middle Burner
	Purple spot in center	Stagnant Blood with Fire in the Stomach
	Peeled	Deficiency Fire from Deficient Stomach Yin and Deficient Kidney Yin
Blue		Excess Internal Cold with Stagnant Blood
	Purple	Stagnant Blood from Internal Cold
	Purple and moist	Stagnant Blood from Internal Cold stiffening the tendons and bones
	Without coating	Excess Internal Cold with Stagnant Blood and Blood Exhaustion
	Blue in center of tongue	Spleen Yang Deficient and Phlegm retained in Chest
	Pregnancy	Impending miscarriage
Enlarged veins on either side of the frenulum		Deficient and Stagnant Qi
Dark (deep blue to black) enlarged veins on either side of the frenulum		Stagnant Blood

149

INDICATIONS OF TONGUE-BODY SHAPE

SHAPE OF TONGUE BODY	ADDITIONAL CHARACTERISTICS	INDICATIONS
Thin	Body color pale	Deficient Blood
Thin	Body color red	Deficient Yin
Swollen	Non-specific	Deficient Spleen Yang and/or Kidney Yang and Damp; Damp Heat in Stomach and Spleen; or poisoning
Swollen	Body color red	Heat in the Heart and Stomach or alcohol poisoning
Swollen edges		Deficient Spleen Qi
Swollen sides		Liver Fire Rising or Ascendant Liver Yang
Swollen tip	Body color red	Blazing Heart Fire
Swollen tip	Body color pale red (normal)	Deficient Heart Qi
Swollen between tip and center		Deficient Lung Qi with congealed Phlegm
Body half-swollen		Deficient Qi and Blood in channels on swollen side
Localized swelling	Body color normal	Deficient Qi in corresponding area of body
Localized swelling	Body color red	Stagnant Qi in corresponding area of body
Surface half-swollen		Deficient Lung Qi on corresponding side of body
Hammer-shaped		Deficient Spleen, Stomach, Kidney
Stiff		Heart Fire Blazing
Stiff	Body color normal	Internal Wind (Liver Wind)
Stiff	Body color red	Extreme Heat injuring Fluids
Stiff	Body color red or dark red	External Fire invading Heart Envelope
Flaccid	Body color pale	Qi and Blood Depletion
Flaccid	Body color red	Extreme Heat injuring Fluids
Flaccid	Body color deep red	Deficient Kidney Yin with Deficiency Fire
Long		Heart Fire Blazing or Phlegm Fire in the Heart
Short	Body color pale	Deficient Spleen Yang/Internal Cold
Short	Body color red	Liver Wind moved by Heat
Short	Body color red, with coating	Excess Fire causing Fluid Deficiency
Short	Body color red, no coating	Deficiency Fire
Short	Body color pale, slippery coating	Deficient Spleen Yang with Damp and Phlegm
Fissures	Deep fissure in the center with smaller cracks	Deficient Kidney Yin with Deficiency Heat
Fissures	Horizontal fissures	Deficient Yin
Fissures	Cracks like broken tiles	Deficient Yin from aging
Fissures	Irregular fissures	Deficient Stomach Yin
Fissures	Vertical fissures in center	Deficient Heart Yin or Blazing Heart Fire
Fissures	Transverse fissures in center	Deficient Lung Yin
Fissures	Transverse fissures on sides	Deficient Spleen Qi
Flabby	Body color pale	Deficient Heart Qi
Flabby	Body color red	Internal Excess Fire
Flabby	Body color red, slippery coating	Phlegm Fire clouding Heart

INDICATIONS OF TONGUE-BODY SHAPE (CONTINUED)

SHAPE OF TONGUE BODY	ADDITIONAL CHARACTERISTICS	INDICATIONS
Deviation	Body color normal	External Wind invading channels
Deviation	Body color normal or red	Internal Liver Wind
Deviation	Body color pale	Deficient Heart Qi
Movement	Body color red	Heart Fire with Internal Wind
Movement	Body color red and dry	Spleen Heat and exhausted body Fluids
Tremulous	Body color red	Excess Heat causing Internal Wind
Tremulous	Body color pale	Deficient Spleen Qi
Tremulous	Body color pale	Heart and Spleen Qi Collapse
Tremulous	Thin body with pale color	Yang Collapse
Numb	Body color pale	Deficient Heart Blood
Numb	Body color normal or red	Liver Wind
Tip rolled up		Excess Heat in the Heart
Tip rolled under		Deficiency Heat in the Heart
Tooth-marked		Deficient Spleen Qi
Ulcerated	Body color red	Heart Fire Blazing; Kidney Heat; Spleen Heat
Tongue Sores	Body color red	Hot poison in Heart
Tongue Sores	Body color red and peeled	Deficient Heat

INDICATIONS OF THE COATING ON THE TONGUE

COATING QUALITY	ADDITIONAL CHARACTERISTICS	INDICATIONS
White and thin		Normal coat or early attack of Wind, Cold, or Damp
White, thin, slippery		Exogenous Cold Damp
White, thick, slippery		Damp in the Middle Burner or Cold Stomach with food retention
White, thin, dry	Body color normal	Exogenous Wind Cold, Wind Heat, or dry and injured Lung Fluids
White, thin, dry	Body color pale	Blood Deficiency or Yang Deficiency
White, thick, wet	Body color pale to normal	Internal Cold Damp in Middle Warmer
White, thick, wet	Body color normal	Exogenous Wind Cold
White, thick, dry		Damp or Phlegm in the Interior with Excess Fire
White, thick, greasy		Deficient Yang with Dampness or food retention
White, thick, greasy, slippery		Deficient Spleen Yang with Damp Cold or Phlegm Damp
White, thick, greasy, dry		Damp Heat or Damp with depletion of body Fluids
White, rough, cracked		Summer Heat injures Qi
White, sticky, greasy		Damp or Phlegm in Middle Burner
White like fine dust	Body color; slight red tip or sides	Exogenous Heat attack

INDICATIONS OF THE COATING ON THE TONGUE (CONTINUED)

COATING QUALITY	ADDITIONAL CHARACTERISTICS	INDICATIONS
White like fine dust	Body color red	Heat in the Three Burners
White like fine dust	Body color red to dark red	Internal poison
White and moldy		Deficient Stomach Yin and Kidney Yin or Internal Damp poison
Half-white, slippery	Right side white	Pathogen half-Exterior/half-Interior
Half-white, slippery	Left side white	Liver Heat
Yellow or pale yellow		Exogenous Wind Fire; or Wind Cold turning to Heat; or Damp Heat in the Chest and Middle Burner
Yellow, slippery		Damp Heat
Yellow, turbid		Damp Heat in the Stomach, Colon, and Small Intestine
Yellow, sticky, greasy		Heat and Phlegm
Yellow, dry		Fluids injured by Excess Fire
Yellow root, white tip		Exogenous Pathogen turning to Heat and reaching internal regions
White with bilateral yellow stripes		Exogenous Pathogen penetrating to internal regions or Heat in the Stomach, Colon, or Small Intestine
Yellow with bilateral yellow stripes		Liver and Gall Bladder Fire
Half-yellow and half-white (lengthwise)		Liver and Gall Bladder Fire
Gray		Damp Cold in the Spleen
Gray, wet, slippery		Damp Cold in the Spleen
Gray, dry		Excess Heat
White and gray	Moist	Internal Damp Cold
White and gray	Dirty	Damp Cold or Phlegm of long duration
Half-white, half-gray		Half-exterior/half-interior Cold
Black		Damp Cold in the Stomach, Colon, and Small Intestine
Black, slippery, greasy		Damp Cold in the Stomach, Colon, and Small Intestine
White with black points		Exogenous pathogen penetrating to the interior regions and turning to Fire
White, with black prickles		True Cold with False Fire or Cold turned to Heat
White center with yellow surrounding		Exogenous pathogen moving to the interior regions and turning to Fire
Yellow center with white surrounding		Internal Heat starting to be driven out
Yellow center	Black, slippery, greasy surrounding	Damp Heat in Spleen
Yellow, dry	Black from center to tip	Heat in the Stomach, Colon, and Small Intestine
White center	Gray and black surrounding	Spleen Damp
Yellow center	Gray surrounding	Damp Heat with Heat-injured Fluids

PULSE DIAGNOSIS

For the Amma therapist, one of the most important skills in diagnosis is touching. Touching basically consists of two processes—palpation (particularly of the skin and abdomen) and pulse diagnosis. The Amma therapist uses palpation to assess muscular tone, body temperature, fluid retention, fluid movement, the quality of skin and flesh (which gives an indication as to the condition of the Spleen), and the abdomen (looking for masses). The Amma therapist also palpates particular points, the sensitivity of which indicates the condition of specific Organs and some degree of pathology.

Through pulse diagnosis the Amma therapist can assess the energy body and receive important information on Qi, Blood, and the condition of the Organs and their channels. The pulse can also provide information on the overall constitutional well-being of the patient. A practitioner with highly evolved palpatory skills can actually glean more information from pulse diagnosis than tongue diagnosis. Pulse diagnosis is more subjective than tongue diagnosis.

Because tongue diagnosis relies on objective signs, such as the shape of the tongue, the color of the tongue body, and the color of the coating, practitioners can more readily agree on the information being observed. However, because pulse diagnosis relies on well-developed sensitivity, which is difficult to learn and requires many years of practice, it is often difficult for practitioners to agree on what they are feeling. A practitioner should first be able to feel the acupuncture points before beginning the more difficult analysis of the Zang-Fu at the pulse.

The Amma therapist takes the patient's pulse while the patient is in the supine position. The patient's wrist is relaxed and supinated, with the arm resting on the table to promote the circulation of Qi and Blood. It should be noted that men's pulses are generally stronger than women's, and those who are more physically active will have stronger pulses than those who are more sedentary. As well, the pulse can be influenced by external events; for example, if a patient is late for his appointment and has been rushing to arrive on time, his pulse will feel very rapid. If the therapist is not aware of the situation, he may misinterpret this as a sign of Heat. In the same way that it is necessary to see a patient over several visits to ascertain the normal state of his tongue, it takes several visits for the therapist to become familiar with the normal state of the patient's pulses.

Traditionally the three places on the wrist where the pulse is taken are called inch (cun), bar or pass (guan), and cubit (chi). They are more easily remembered as the distal, middle, and proximal positions. The pass (bar) pulse lies along the Lung Channel, where the radial artery crosses the styloid process. The distance from Lu5 to the cubit position is approximately one cubit. The distance from Lu10 to the inch position is approximately one inch. Thus the derivation of the names.

There are several different ways that the pulse may be read at the radial artery at the wrist. The most popular way that the pulse is read in the West today is rather sophisticated, and derives from the insights and skills of Chinese medical practitioners. The method commonly employed in China is less difficult to

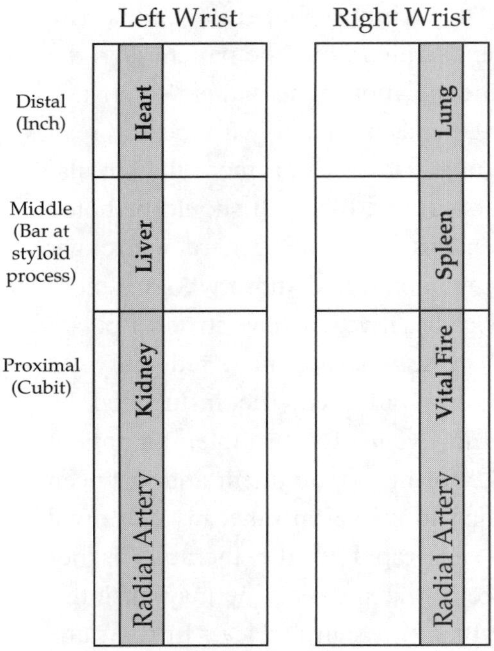

Figure 38

The ancient format for pulse diagnosis as used by traditional Chinese medical doctors in China

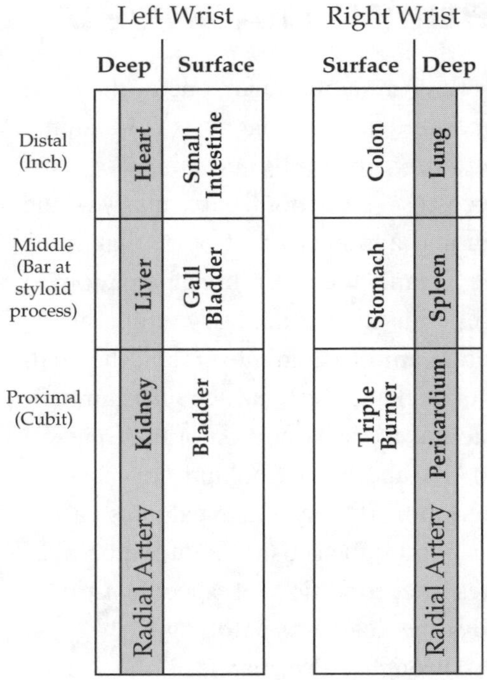

Figure 39

The modern format for pulse diagnosis, most commonly taught in the United States

master, and once the practitioner is skilled at this method, the subtleties of the American method will seem less esoteric.

Figure 38 shows the pulse diagnosis format as generally used by traditional Chinese medical doctors in China and is the method that should be studied first. (The diagrams here should be viewed as though the reader was looking at his or her own wrists.) It is based on the principle that the Yang Bowels (Fu) are generally not significant in disease syndromes, and are therefore not considered apart from the syndromes of the Yin Viscera (Zang). The Viscera are read at five pulse positions; the sixth position (right proximal) gives the condition of the Fire of the Gate of Vitality or Vital Fire, not the condition of the Minister Fire of the Kidney. The Fire of the Vital

Gate can never be in Excess, though Minister Fire in the Kidney, read from the left proximal pulse, can be in Excess from an underlying Deficiency. Depth and superficiality in this method are not indications of Zang and Fu Organs but rather of the superficiality or depth of the syndrome.

Figure 39 shows the method often taught in the United States. This method reads the Yang Bowels from superficial pulses and the Yin Viscera from the deep pulses, and does not consider the Fire of the Vital Gate. It is my considered opinion that, without long and sophisticated training in sensitivity, the second method is far less accurate and falls far short of the accuracy of the ancient method, although the newer method appears to give more information.

A normal pulse is smooth and forceful, with a regular rhythm. When reading the pulse, we read not only each position reflecting the condition of the Organ, but we also read what is called the pulse of the Stomach (a pulse with Stomach Qi). The pulse of the Stomach is qualitative, as opposed to an actual pulse. In other words, it is not the pulse position of the Stomach Organ but rather it indicates whether or not Stomach Qi, that is, the fundamental energy for feeding the organism, is present in sufficient quality and quantity. The pulse of the Stomach can therefore be felt throughout all the pulse positions. When there is strong Stomach Qi, the prognosis is good. When there is weak Stomach Qi, the prognosis is poor.

The pulse that is read by a practitioner will be a combination of normal and abnormal types of depth, frequency, strength, and shape. The location of the pulse will indicate the affected Organs, particularly in Interior syndromes. Since the Zang and Fu Organs are not indicated in superficial syndromes unless the Lung is involved, the pulse is read in general; that is, there is no differentiation of affected Organ by pulse observation.

The ancient texts simply listed up to seventy-two different types of pulses. We will categorize the pulse types so that they will have a certain order, and shall confine our studies to nineteen types.

DEPTH
▼

The depth of the pulse refers to whether the pulse is superficial or deep. This is distinguished by light or heavy pressure. Remember that, since the Fu are not being considered, the reading in any position reflects the Viscera. Fu Organ involvement is noted by tongue diagnosis and overall symptoms.

Floating (Superficial) Pulse

Felt easily with a light touch and tending to disappear on pressure—this is a common pulse quality in Exterior syndromes. Chills will be simultaneously present with this pulse quality if the condition arose from an attack by an external pathogen. If the patient presents in a debilitated condition and has been suffering for a long time, the pulse may be floating but will also be very weak. There is a poor prognosis in such cases.

Sinking (Deep) Pulse

The pulse is not felt on light touch and only appears when pressed firmly. This indicates an Interior syndrome, usually of the Deficiency type.

FREQUENCY
▼

The speed of the pulse is indicative of Cold or Hot syndromes, and is based on the normal pulse being between sixty and ninety beats per minute.

Slow Pulse

If the pulse is less than sixty beats per minute and the patient is not a serious athlete whose pulse is normally in the range of fifty beats per minute, it suggests an endogenous Cold syndrome, which indicates a hypofunction of Yang and a slowing or congealing of the flow of Vital Energy. Exogenous Cold does not cause significant slowing of the pulse.

Rapid Pulse

A pulse rate of more than ninety beats per minute usually indicates a Heat syndrome, but it does not indicate whether the condition is one of Excess or Deficiency.

VOLUME OR STRENGTH

In addition to the depth and frequency of the pulses, we are also to be concerned with different strengths to be read in the pulse, which can help to distinguish specific aspects of the syndrome encountered.

Surging Pulse

This pulse feels like a strong ocean wave dashing up against the finger and then slowly falling away. It is commonly seen in the second or Qi stage of the four stages of febrile disease resulting from attack of exogenous Cold. It is commonly present with a rapid pulse and indicates Extreme Heat often with high fever.

Forceful (Replete) Pulse

This pulse is felt as forceful on first encounter, and continues to feel forceful even to very heavy pressure. Such a pulse usually indicates an Excess syndrome.

Overblown Pulse

If the pulse feels forceful at first but becomes empty with an increase of pressure, it often suggests a Deficiency syndrome, indicating an Exuberance of Yang if it is Deficient Yin and Apparent Cold if it is Deficient Yang. This is usually only found in Interior syndromes.

Weak Pulse

This pulse shows no strength under varying pressures. It remains weak (feeble, empty) from first encountering the pulse with light pressure until you have applied strength sufficient to read deep pulses. This pulse indicates a Deficiency syndrome, often of both Vital Energy and Blood.

Thready (Thin) Pulse

This pulse is quite clear and easy to read but feels very thin. It usually indicates a Deficiency syndrome, particularly of Vital Essence, Blood, or Fluids.

Faint Pulse

This pulse is even thinner and weaker than a thready pulse, to the degree that it is difficult to read at all. It indicates an extreme Deficiency of Vital Qi and Blood.

FORM (SHAPE, TENSION)

String-tight (Taut, Wiry) Pulse

Unlike English, the Chinese words for *string* and *cord* imply two different entities. Think of *string* as a guitar string, stretchable but quite tight or firm. This type of pulse usually indicates syndromes involving the Liver and is seen in syndromes involving severe pain. Hypertensive patients with blood pressure of 200/120 or more will also show the string-tight pulse, as will patients with Phlegm or Blood Stasis patterns.

Cord-tight (Tense) Pulse

A cord is made of cotton, and although it may be stretched tight, one still feels the softness of the cotton, especially relative to a tight string. This pulse feels somewhat hard but not nearly as hard as the string-tight pulse. It will occur in Cold syndromes, with severe pain, and in Exterior Cold syndromes, where it will accompany a floating pulse.

Relaxed (Loose) Pulse

This pulse is related specifically to the right middle pulse position, and is therefore related to the Spleen. It feels softer than a normal pulse but is not extremely soft, and has a moderate frequency. In the presence of appropriate clinical symptoms, it confirms Spleen Yang Deficiency with Damp accumulation. It may be seen in normal persons of slight build.

Soft Pulse

This pulse is even softer than the thready (thin) pulse and has the quality of a thread floating on water. It is quite delicate and so requires a very light touch— it floats and grows even fainter on pressure, possibly disappearing. It suggests an accumulation of Damp and often indicates extreme Damp syndromes.

Slippery Pulse

This is a rather forceful, smooth-flowing pulse, described in the classics as though small round beads were rolling under the practitioner's finger. It points to Damp or Phlegm syndromes, and is often seen in pregnant women as early as the second

month. This can be accounted for by the fact that there is increased fluid volume, particularly blood volume, in pregnancy.

Hesitant (Uneven) Pulse

Try drawing the blade of a dull knife across a piece of hard wood. You will feel a kind of choppy or bouncing sensation in your fingers. The hesitant pulse feels similar to this. It indicates slowing of the blood flow, particularly from Blood Stasis but also from Deficiency of Blood and Vital Essence or Stagnation of Vital Energy.

Knotted Pulse

A knotted pulse is felt as a slow pulse with distinct pauses, but the pauses are at irregular intervals. It indicates a severe weakening of the Vital Energy, suggesting endogenous Cold or retention of Cold Phlegm. It can also suggest a Heart Qi or Heart Yang Deficiency.

Intermittent Pulse

This pulse is similar to the knotted pulse, except that the pauses occur at regular intervals. This indicates a serious Deficiency of Qi and Blood and may reflect an underlying Heart pathology.

Running Pulse

This is a very rapid version of the knotted pulse, and shows exhaustion of Blood and Essence. A very poor prognosis is indicated.

PART THREE

THE MAKING
OF AN
AMMA THERAPIST

CHAPTER
9

THE DEVELOPMENT OF THE AMMA THERAPIST

The evolution of an Amma practitioner can be divided into three plateaus: that of the novice Oriental bodywork therapist, the Amma therapist, and the healing sensitive. To the untrained eye, each level can look the same—the practitioner appears to be treating a patient by manipulating the soft tissues of the body by utilizing various bodywork techniques. Yet there is a great difference between the work of the beginning practitioner of Oriental bodywork and the Amma therapist, and in turn between the Amma therapist and the healing sensitive. This evolution, from the beginning stages of learning Oriental bodywork through the development of an Amma therapist to the attainment of healing sensitive, consists of many small steps along the way. Progression through these successive levels is predicated on the development of the practitioner's sensitivity to the patient as a physical, emotional, and bioenergetic system, combined with the practitioner's ability to integrate his knowledge of Oriental and Western medicine with this growing sensitivity. Thus what evolves is not simply technical skill, which is demonstrated at each level by increased palpatory sensitivity and the use of increasingly difficult treatment techniques, but also the degree of subtle sensitivity to the flow of the bioenergy and to the complex of signs and symptoms that are presented.

A beginning practitioner of Oriental bodywork relates to a patient from a viewpoint that focuses mainly on the physical organism, utilizing and incorporating some basic knowledge of the energy system. Much of the focus is on muscle tissue and blood and lymphatic circulation. An Amma therapy treatment at this level involves general manipulation of the primary channels and major points. The practitioner can produce a state of increased Qi and Blood circulation, lymphatic drainage, and muscular relaxation that can leave a patient feeling revitalized and refreshed. The outcomes of even the most basic manipulations often result in alleviation of the pain and discomfort that accompany many common ailments. From headaches, muscular tension, and common digestive disturbances to temporary relief of back and neck pain or the pain due to arthritis, the positive effects of such treatments can last for quite some time.

The balance and proper flow of various levels of energy in the patient is the primary concern of the Amma therapist. According to the homeodynamic model, disease can result from the effects of either endogenous or exogenous factors that disturb the energy system to such a degree that the ability of the organism to heal itself becomes severely limited. The causes of these imbalances are numerous and varied, but the result of all imbalance is the same—some level of dis-ease or disturbance to the energy system.

Amma therapy is used effectively in the treatment of both chronic and acute disorders that affect all areas of human physiology. The therapist directly manipulates not only the musculature but also the energy pathways that move through the muscles, tendons, ligaments, joints, and skin. This direct activity—movements designed to strengthen the body's innate ability to achieve physiological and energetic balance—indirectly affects the energy pathways that connect to and move through the organs and deeper areas of the body. The Amma therapist has studied Oriental and Western medicine to a much more advanced degree than the neophyte practitioner of Oriental bodywork and actively utilizes that knowledge in the assessment and treatment of his or her patients. Becoming an Amma therapist requires more education in the theory, principles, and practical application of Oriental and Western medicine, and a great many more hours of intensive practice, integration, and application of one's growing knowledge to the treatment of patients seeking preventive therapy as well as those with the most serious medical conditions. Patients receiving Amma therapy can experience pain relief; reduction of edema and swelling; greater range of motion; increased freedom of movement; less stress and tension; stronger resistance to both endogenous and exogenous pathogens; better digestion, respiration and circulation; help with genitourinary problems and elimination difficulties; and some basic measure of balancing to every system in the body. Patients experience a sense of vitality and well-being, increased awareness during activities of daily living, more restful sleep and decreased sleeping needs, and diminished symptoms or complete remission of their primary complaint. Because Amma therapy increases the functional energy level within the body through reducing stress, increasing the efficiency of energy production and utilization, and directly activating and balancing the energy system, the patient is able to respond more effectively to the environment and the stress of daily life experiences.

The highest level of accomplishment

for the practitioner is the healing sensitive, one who has evolved to the point of experiencing empathy with the condition of other living beings. A healing sensitive feels or senses the patient's energy system, sometimes even from the moment of first encounter. By directing attention specifically to the patient, the healing sensitive can feel any physical and emotional imbalances. The patient's pain, discomfort, illness, and even the patient's emotional distress can be directly experienced by the healing sensitive.

While some people are born with such sensitivities fully developed, others can evolve this ability through years of intense, dedicated practice accompanied by constant attention and correction. To insure the correct development of the physical and energy bodies as proper vehicles for the manifestation of healing sensitivities, I created a set of guidelines early in my training of Amma therapists that, when carefully followed, resulted in the development of sensitivities and intuitive abilities among my closest students. These guidelines became the fundamental principles for the training of future Amma therapists, and have been incorporated into the New Center College's advanced Amma therapy program.

The development of a therapist begins with training the physical body. Amma therapists must be able to treat the tenth patient of the day with the same attention, sensitivity, and strength as their first; therefore, the Amma practitioner must have stamina as well as strength. The hands are the practitioner's primary tools. Most basic to this physical development, the strength and sensitivity of the hands must be enhanced through intensive and sometimes strenuous exercises. Further training of the physical body is designed to produce direct experiential understanding of the body's internal functioning. Good physical health is a requisite condition for any person preparing to treat the ailments of another. There is no better way to study living anatomy than by learning to understand one's own organism. In training Amma therapists, several techniques are employed to develop this combined academic and experiential knowledge of the human body. Included among these are hatha yoga exercises and t'ai chi chuan.

Traditional hatha yoga is a system of exercise in which various muscle groups are stretched or strengthened by developing and maintaining specific postures for short periods of time. Once the posture is accomplished, the practitioner focuses attention on the specific areas of tension and concentrates on the muscles and tendons that are being used. The practitioner then focuses on relaxing these tensed areas. By directing attention to the muscle groups and attempting conscious control of their responses, a heightened awareness of the location and function of the various muscles is developed. At the New Center College many hatha yoga exercises are incorporated into t'ai chi classes, where the study of anatomy and myology can be applied as a living experience through exercise. Hatha yoga helps the practitioner develop muscular strength and coordination, flexibility, balance, and concentration. All of these physical qualities are essential for one who will be engaged in the rigorous activity of the application of Amma therapy. In addition, the postures of hatha yoga lead to a healthier and more physically fit practitioner. Digestion, elimination, and circulation are all improved through the practice of these exercises.

T'ai chi chuan, a Taoist form of exercise and active meditation, is studied to increase the practitioner's level of awareness and to establish control over one's own energy system. The practice of t'ai chi chuan is undertaken in an effort to create a mind-to-energy-to-physical-body pathway—that is, to establish mind control over the energy so that the energy may properly control and move the body. The mind moves the energy and the energy moves the body. As a result of the concentration and practice of subtle awareness required to master t'ai chi chuan, the movement of energy becomes a cognitive experience for the practitioner. Under appropriate conditions of instruction and effort, the practice of t'ai chi chuan can ultimately lead the Amma therapist to a point of direct conscious experience of energy deficiencies and excesses as they exist in the physical body of the patient.

It is through this focused effort of mind and body that a real understanding of the capabilities and functioning of the human body can be attained. The practice of t'ai chi chuan expands the individual's awareness to include the internal as well as the surface aspects of the physical body. Most people have little or no awareness of the three-dimensional, living physical body. Most tend to sense the body as a two-dimensional surface, with the primary focus of awareness encompassing only the face and upper chest. A growing level of internal awareness is essential for the proper development of an Amma therapist. Correct posture and spinal alignment and the effects of posture on physical processes become part of

this internal awareness. Such an awareness is the basis of the evolution of a much greater understanding of the physical difficulties that patients encounter in both stress and illness. Clearly those practitioners who know themselves deeply in relation to the physical body can more fully know their patients' physical pains and experiences and know what steps must be taken to alleviate patients' discomforts.

Equally essential to the evolution of the Amma practitioner from a technician to a healing sensitive is emotional development. As discussed in relationship to the homeodynamic model (chapter 3), emotions are part of the bioenergy system and as such are often responsible for many of the diseases that people experience. In order to treat a condition we must know its emotional component, which means that we must be able to understand the way the patient experiences the world. To see and feel another's physical and emotional experiences, diligent effort must first be made to see and to feel one's own emotional experiences. Therefore, a fundamental part of becoming a master therapist is the evolution of one's own self-awareness.

Caring and compassion are the primary attributes of a good therapist. When seeing patients who suffer from a multitude of problems, the personal emotional problems and needs of the therapist must necessarily be left outside the treatment room. A true health professional is one who cultivates concern for the well-being of her patients far beyond the normal levels of human concern. This requires that practitioners first undergo personal exploration of their emotional natures in order for them to be able to suspend their own emotions during treatment and give the patient the caring and support that is needed. Since the advanced Amma therapist treats all levels of physical problems, the therapist must be able to put aside any aversions he or she may have to the patient or the patient's condition. Practitioners must also be aware of physical and psychological responses they may have to touching another human being and the problems patients may have with being touched. The subject of ethics in bodywork is a very complex issue and is discussed at length in chapter 12.

Sometimes it is necessary to use a professional guide to help us learn to see who we are as emotional beings. Just as we need teachers to help us train our physical and energy bodies, we also need guides to help us gain an objective understanding of our emotional world. Through this direction we can learn to deal with those aspects of our inner world that are psychologically painful and prevent us from seeing others clearly. The discipline of our emotional nature is the primary means of energy conservation. Since an Amma therapist must work directly with the energy of a patient, personal awareness becomes one of the most important and basic efforts of the aspiring Amma therapist.

The major concern of Amma therapy is the harmonization of the energy system, directed at the attainment of a homeodynamic state of balance. Energy from the practitioner can be transmitted to the patient during the course of a bodywork session. This transmission is amplified by the techniques of Amma therapy and their direct affect on the energy body. The fact that the physical,

psychological, and emotional conditions of the practitioner can directly effect the concomitant areas in the patient clearly underscores the need for the clarity, balance, and internal alignment of these three centers on the part of the therapist. During the administration of an Amma therapy treatment by a skilled and evolved therapist, powerful effects upon the same three-part nature of the patient can result. In order to bring such effects to their maximum potential, the practitioner of Amma therapy must learn to directly experience his own energy body as well as the energy body of the patient. Subsequent control of the energy systems of both the practitioner and the patient leads to the very advanced and sometimes profound results seen in the work of some of my senior students. Thus, as physical strength, subtlety, and sensitivity develop, the practitioner is guided to focus on the internal workings of his or her own energy system. This personal familiarity with the feel and flow of energy helps in learning to experience the energy system of another. Concentration must be trained until laserlike attention can be focused upon the patient. Only after these skills are developed can intuitive ability evolve.

The third aspect of the development of the therapist is the importance of the practitioner as a role model. This begins with simple standards of hygiene. Personal cleanliness is an important prerequisite for any health professional, as poor hygiene is one of the primary contributing factors to ill health and disease. In order to maintain health, one must keep one's body clean internally as well as externally. This includes daily showering or bathing and internal cleansing practices, and the cleansing of hands and nails before and after each treatment. For the comfort of both practitioner and patient, clothing must be clean and free of perfumes and unpleasant odors.

As well, since many aspects of health relate to diet and bowel habits, it is important for the practitioner to keep his digestive system functioning effectively for the proper assimilation of nutrients and the elimination of waste products. Diet should consist of unprocessed whole grains, fresh organic fruits and vegetables, fish, poultry, and lean meat from animals that were not fed antibiotics or hormones. Processed foods should be avoided; dairy, salt, and sugar intake should be extremely limited. Foods that contain chemical additives and preservatives should also be avoided. Clean water should be part of the diet, both in drinking and for use in cooking. Distilled water or spring water is preferable to tap water in most areas of the United States. In general, this natural, whole foods diet is the same type of diet that should be recommended to patients. By adopting this diet the therapist will become healthier and better able to think and reason clearly. The other benefit of such a diet is that it allows the practitioner to produce more energy. By changing to such a diet the therapist will also be better able to understand the difficulties that patients may have in converting their own eating practices. Being better able to understand one's patients is a critical factor in becoming an effective practitioner.

The fourth aspect of the development of the therapist is taking responsibility for one's patients. Not only is the therapist responsible for acting as a role model, assessing and treating her patients, and suggesting certain nutritional changes or exercise, but the therapist is also responsible for following through with her patients even after the patient leaves the treatment room. This may mean calling the patient to see how he is feeling, studying the patient's problem and checking on the physiological interactions and side effects of medications, and contacting other health professionals for assistance or more information. When treating a patient, the Amma therapist must maintain a certain objectivity while at the same time reaching out to understand the difficulties experienced by the patient. There is no place in the therapist-patient relationship for disdain, judgment, or any other negative emotion. While the therapist cannot force patients to make certain efforts, he can suggest, encourage, and verbally urge the patient to make certain changes if the patient's condition necessitates such motivation and if the therapist can maintain the necessary objectivity. This is the therapist's responsibility to his patients. It is through the joint efforts of the Amma therapist-patient team that patients are educated to understand their condition and taught to value their health. Therapists must remember that another person's health, quality of life, and perhaps even duration of life has been entrusted to them, and this must be regarded with great respect.

The journey of becoming an Amma therapist is a remarkable experience, extending far beyond the art of bodywork technique. From the earliest levels, the sincere practitioner can begin sensitizing to his own energies, and then to the energies of others. Being able to help heal others through encouraging them to feel their inner physical and emotional experiences is to embark on a journey that helps to develop one's inner being. As an Amma therapist evolves, he comes more in touch with his spiritual existence and with that of his patients. Through consistent efforts to "know thyself," the therapist uncovers and nurtures the higher potential of all human beings and the ability to touch the deeper realities shared by and with the rest of nature.

Through this knowledge and experience, the ability to understand and feel the suffering of others and know how to best alleviate that suffering becomes possible. As the therapist travels this path of self-discovery with dedication to helping others, he gains not only sensitivity but health, strength, compassion, wisdom, freedom, and joy. He evolves from a practitioner into a true healer.

THE DEVELOPMENT OF SENSITIVITY, STRENGTH, AND PALPATORY SKILLS

Refined sensitivity, strength, and palpatory skills are crucial to the success of the Amma practitioner's treatments. The ability to assess and treat for imbalances in the bioenergy requires feeling beyond the gross material body—the skin, muscles, flesh, and bones—to the level of Qi, Blood, and Fluids. While kinesthetic awareness and physical development are necessary in the training of the Amma practitioner, more essential is the development of sensory awareness via the hands. The same techniques executed by different Amma practitioners will yield varying therapeutic effects because of the difference in sensory awareness and the ability of the hands to execute the appropriate movements.

SENSITIVITY

For the Amma practitioner the sense of touch is the most essential of all the senses. Developing sensitivity requires constant and focused attention in conjunction with relaxation of the hands. Although the hands are the least developed of our sensory organs, when used appropriately they can serve as primary information-gathering devices. The hands are the sensors through which important data relative to the patient's condition can be gathered. Through touch, important differentiations are made regarding variations in muscular tonus, temperature, and skin quality. For example, therapists must be able to differentiate between a tight muscle, a tendon, and a bone; a normal abdomen and a distended one; and changes in the tissue and swelling with edema. With long and serious practice and carefully channeled attention, the practitioner can receive increasingly subtle signals from the patient's body through the hands. Qualities of the vascular activities in the body and their disturbances, qualities of the respiratory rhythms and their anomalies, qualities of the cerebrospinal rhythmic pulsation and its disturbances, even the patterns of bioenergy flow and the disturbances in that field can be palpated and interpreted by the trained hands of an advanced Amma therapist.

The beginning practitioner who understands the importance of developing acute sensitivity must seek to develop a new relationship to her hands, regarding them as her eyes and ears. The desire to use the hands not to mechanically follow a prearranged series of motions but to sense the condition of the patient on more subtle and significant levels requires molding the hands into tools that will serve the practitioner's aim. The process of creating a new relationship to the hands as sensory tools does not require any special equipment. It is accomplished through constant attention to the practice of placing awareness into the hands and intentionally feeling whatever is touched—from the plasticity of a computer keyboard to the liquid energy of running water. Yet most of what is recognized as felt awareness—the feel of my pencil as I write, for example—goes unnoticed because there is no need for my attention to be more than superficially aware of the tactile sensations produced by the mass of objects and forces that are experienced in most daily activities.

Focused attention within oneself and toward the patient allows the hands to act as powerful and subtle sensors. Focused attention is the means by which a practitioner can learn to become delicately aware and capable of perceiving minute differences in the patient's physical and emotional condition. Physical sensitivity, the awareness of the condition of the physical body through the sense of touch, begins with a tactile awareness of the tone and texture of the skin and musculature. The sensations entering through all sense organs, including the hands, are monitored and filtered by the brain so that only those things requiring directed attention are allowed to enter beyond peripheral awareness; therefore, the novice practitioner must begin to be aware of all the information available through his hands about all the objects he touches. The difference in the qualities of objects in regard to their primary materials—that is, whether the object is made of metal as opposed to wood for example—can be assessed from the place of beginner's mind in the effort to develop awareness and sensitivity in the hands. Feeling for qualities of hardness or softness and roughness or smoothness is easy. The density of the material and the thinness or thickness of the substance are a bit more difficult to ascertain, but can certainly be felt with practice. The distinctions between hard plastics and bone or ivory can be clearly felt with well-sensitized hands. The hands are remarkable devices. With training they can become as keen as the clearest eyesight, and can provide information of the most subtle nature to the evolved practitioner. Thus the very first step in creating such sensory awareness in the hands is to pay attention to them. The evolving practitioner should acutely sense anything that is touched in order to develop awareness and sensitivity in the hands.

Relaxation of the hands is necessary for adequate development of this sensitivity. Once the hands are both strengthened and relaxed, they can begin to feel what is being touched. A hand that is stiff with tension and held almost like a claw cannot feel what is beneath the skin, even to the point of being unable to perform the basic skill of differentiating among the muscles that drape the body. When the physical strength is such that all that is necessary can be accomplished with ease during the course of a treatment, the practitioner can begin to make the more subtle efforts necessary to evolve hand sensitivity, resulting in deeper awareness. When the hand can mold to the contours of the body, and when areas and points can be manipulated with directed force while maintaining physical relaxation, then the mind can be directed to feeling more deeply the complex multiplicity of signals and indicators of the patient's body. Body temperature differences, subtle swellings or areas of fullness, areas of weakness or strain, and areas that feel "spongy" or "brittle" become gross and obvious facts next to the subtle yet powerful indicators available to truly sensitive hands regarding the patient's condition. The hands are sensors as well as tools.

Once developed, sensitivity allows the practitioner to become aware of the physical manifestation of a patient's emotional experience and to perceive emotional states as they are experienced by the patient. Ultimately it produces the ability to become aware of the bioenergy system. There is a world of experience available to the touch of a practitioner with developed sensitivity. Very few are born with the gift of extreme sensitivity. For those who are not, focused attention and relaxation is the means through which it can be developed.

STRENGTH

The effectiveness of Amma as a therapeutic modality is in great part dependent upon the strength and flexibility of the hands and body. Strength is defined as the ability to sustain a reasonable and intense level of effort for an extended time without tiring or allowing the techniques to deteriorate; it is the capacity for sustained exertion without deviation for many successive treatments. Inadequate strength or strength that manifests in spurts results in poking and jabbing at the patient, and may be the cause of unnecessary pain.

The hands must be sufficiently strong and flexible to be able to consistently manifest and control the degree of technical skill required in Amma therapy treatments. There must also be sufficient strength in the arms, shoulders, and back in order to deliver appropriate pressure and rhythm throughout the treatment.

Amma therapy requires sufficient strength in the upper body to guide, manage, and direct the hands and arms in both the broad strokes and the finely detailed hand and finger techniques described later in this chapter. Fine movements of the fingers are accomplished through actions of the intrinsic muscles of the hands, and the larger, gross movements of the hands are accomplished by actions of the muscles of the forearm. Since many of the forearm muscles originate on the humerus, actions of the forearm muscles on the hands involve some activation of the upper arm. Movement of the upper arms is a direct function of the muscles of the chest, shoulders, and back, again due to the origins and insertions of the muscles in these regions. The movement of the hands and arms, then, involves the total musculature of the upper body, and is directly affected by the strength of that muscle system.

An Amma therapy treatment lasts for approximately fifty to ninety minutes, with the therapist standing most of that time and directing pressure into the patient's body. The practitioner's back, legs, and abdomen must be fully developed to support the body in this upright and often forward-leaning position, the proper stance allowing the hands and arms to apply controlled pressure. Weakness of the torso muscles leads to fatigue, which invariably results in leaning on the table or on the patient. Basically the therapist must be capable of accomplishing fifty to ninety minutes of hard physical work without straining. The breath must remain even and controlled, and stamina and endurance must be evolved to the point that the last technique of each

treatment is applied with the same power and focus as the first, and that the last patient of the day is treated with the same power, degree, and level of skill as the first. The therapist must be able to concentrate fully on the patient without being distracted by the aches and pains that inevitably result from inadequate or incomplete physical development. The level of strength and consequent physical development of the Amma therapist is therefore equal to that required in the development of any serious athlete.

While strength is necessary throughout the body, the Amma therapist's primary strength must be manifest both in and through the hands. Strength of the hands is necessary for control of the hands. Control is the ability to guide the hands to the appropriate points and areas of the body, maintaining the sometimes difficult positions that the hands and fingers must hold, and properly maintaining the direction and the quantity of force. Great strength must be developed in the small muscles of the hand as well in the muscles of each finger. Each finger must move independently to hold points and control the direction of applied force without losing strength or allowing the force to dissipate into the palm or other fingers. Occasionally the hands are rotated and maintained in unusual and sometimes uncomfortable positions as specific areas of the body are treated. For example, the inner canthus of the eye is treated with the lateral aspect of the tip of the pad of the fifth finger. The point must be held and manipulated. Should the hand slip, it may cause injury to the eye of the patient. Development of the small muscles of the hand is required to accomplish this manipulation without danger to the patient. Strength is the root on which control grows. Both are essential to the development of the practitioner's hands.

Real force is manifested when the body is used correctly. Proper and consistent alignment of the musculoskeletal system provides a channel through which force can easily be developed and directed. If the alignment is maintained over a reasonable period of time, the consistent application of a powerful force can be easily accomplished with minimal amounts of tension and muscular contraction. Once the skeletal alignment of the body and hands as taught in t'ai chi chuan are properly maintained, the attention should be directed to relaxing the musculature, allowing only those muscles and tendons that are directly involved in maintaining alignment to remain in contraction. The hand is open—the fingers neither hyperextended nor curled toward the palm. Thus the musculature of the hand is relaxed and soft, and no joint is locked, although there must be sufficient tonus in the hand to maintain the alignment of the central metacarpal with the centerline of the forearm. Energy as force will move through a relaxed muscle but will be lost in the constriction of a muscle locked in unnecessary contraction. Therefore, when the body is aligned and the musculature is relaxed—a result of the release of tension in the legs, buttocks, torso, chest, neck, face, arms, and hands— authentic strength, strength that follows from the free flow of systemic energy, will be experienced. From that point the practitioner can direct force for various purposes throughout the course of the Amma treatment.

The Amma practitioner cultivates muscular strength, in order to develop and maintain proper musculoskeletal alignment. Through this alignment, the practitioner can direct force while relaxing his own musculature. Relaxation of the hands and body is necessary for adequate development of strength. Beginning practitioners often mistake tension for strength. People will tighten their muscles in order to feel their strength. But as t'ai chi students soon begin to learn, as long as they equate strength with muscular tension, whatever power they could develop is lost to the effort of the contraction. Their experience is only the power of the muscular contraction; the subjective "feeling" of strength is the very thing that opposes the attempt to manifest real strength. For a practitioner of Amma therapy, real strength lies in the ability to direct an appropriate force into another body. This force will be of greatest value when it is highly concentrated and directed. When force is contained in the maintenance of the muscle contraction, the force is lost within that muscle. Force developed through muscular contraction will not be expended at its intended location, that is, at the point of contact with the patient.

PALPATION

Palpation is exploration through touching the patient's body; it is examination of the superficial and deeper structures of the body through use of the hands. Through palpation the student of Amma therapy arrives at a broader understanding of the structure of the human body. Skin qualities, muscle shapes and qualities, tendon insertions, blood vessels and anastomoses, and lymph vessels and nodes are a few of the many aspects of the physical form that can be experienced through attentive and directed practice of palpation. This practice begins with formal study of the physical structure and its functions. Surface anatomy, general anatomy, and detailed myology must be studied carefully to produce a thorough understanding of the musculoskeletal system. The size, shape, and function of the structures within the skeletal system must be understood, as well as the structure and operation of the various joints. The aspiring Amma therapist must become equally familiar with the muscular system, learning the size, shape, and actions; fiber directions; innervations; and vascularization of each of the muscles of the body. This formal study must be enlivened by study of the therapist's own body.

The practitioner begins the actual practice of palpation by touching his or her own body, starting with gently stroking an area with the entire hand in order to sense its form and structure. Become aware of each part of the hand and what is felt in each part as the hand is moved over a limb or the torso. If you feel that one or another part of the hand is not in contact with the muscle, you must soften the hand and allow it to mold to the body's contours.

Since the contours of the body change, the form of the hand will change as it moves from one area of the body to another. Allow the hand to assume the contours of the surface over which it moves. The hand must be constantly corrected to retain maximum relaxation, using a very gentle touch to lightly contact the surface of the body. At first when practicing there is no need to apply pressure; rather, feel the texture of the skin and the configuration of the surface musculature, the interstices between the muscles, the tendons and the superficial blood vessels, and the form of the surface muscles. Start at the origin and follow each muscle to its insertion, attending to the size and shape of the muscle as well as its qualities such as fullness or emptiness, spasm or flaccidity. Feel for temperature variations and local spasms throughout the area being palpated. Look at what is being palpated and visualize the form of the muscle, as well as its placement and action. By combining cognitive awareness with sensory experience, you will broaden your understanding of the physical form.

When you can comfortably palpate the surface and sense the necessary configurations and differentiations, gradually increase the depth of palpation and try to feel the skeletal structure. This practice should encompass the face, skull, and posterior neck, and continue to the rib cage, shoulders, arms, hands, legs, and feet. The basic structure of the bones will be your first awareness. Try to become aware of the small hollows, ridges, and bony prominences on the surface of the bones. Various acupuncture points are located in these areas, so sensitivity to these small regions is essential for proper point location and manipulation. The same technique of combining cognitive awareness with sensory experience is required in this practice. As the mind is continually focused to attend to what is being felt, your experience of the body will change dramatically. Your level of skill in palpation will increase, and you will be on your way to developing your hands into the sensors and the tools that are needed to become a skilled practitioner of this art.

Since balance is an essential aspect of the development of an Amma therapist the student works with both hands so that they may be equal in strength and sensitivity. The imbalance between the dominant and nondominant hands can be corrected by using the nondominant hand in simple daily activities, such as brushing the teeth, using eating utensils, buttoning a shirt, closing a lid on a jar, or reaching for a glass of water. Learning to write with the nondominant hand develops the finer muscles of the hand and arm and cultivates fine coordination. By requiring the nondominant hand to do these tasks, daily activities become a major source of exercise toward balance.

The ever greater and finer development of the hands is necessary for acquiring the palpatory skills needed for assessment and treatment. Each level of the practitioner's evolving ability requires directed attention, persistent practice, and constant correction. This will result in the production of a pair of finely tuned instruments. As they are honed, these instruments will begin to produce wonderful experiences. They will be tools of great value, and unimagined sensitivity, and will serve the student well in his evolution as an Amma therapist.

HAND TECHNIQUES

CIRCULAR PRESSURE

Circular pressure, the most commonly used technique in Amma therapy,

involves the application of pressure and movement in small circles at a given point on the body. The technique is repeated in a smooth and rhythmic pattern that follows a channel pathway or the direction of muscular fibers. The novice practitioner, who has yet to develop fine coordination, will frequently execute large circles that cover a large surface area. The advanced Amma therapist creates minimal circles, the motion often looking as though it is going in an up-and-back direction.

Circular Thumb Pressure

In this technique the whole hand is in contact with the patient's body while the thumb performs circular pressure. The thumb is directly aligned with the radius of the practitioner's working arm and does not abduct or adduct unnaturally. This maintains a proper direction of force through the forearm and into the hand.

Depending on the area being treated, this technique can be executed with either the pad of the thumb, the arch of the thumb, or the thumb in combination with the thenar eminence. Minimal tension should be experienced in the working hand and arm, as the muscles of the upper back and shoulder initiate the movement. This technique is used in the manipulation of specific points on the body, the manipulation of channels, and in particular for deeper pressure on the Bladder Channel.

Circular Digital Pressure

In this technique the pads of the four fingers are used. However, depending on the size of the area being treated, you may use as much as the entire palmar aspect of the four fingers up to and including the metacarpophalangeal joint. Although the four fingers are used, the major direction of force comes through and from the middle finger.

In a more advanced technique the pad of the distal phalange of the index or the middle finger is used to provide directed circular pressure to a specific point. In this case the palm is held in contact with the body, with force being directed into the pad of the finger.

Circular Palmar Pressure

In this technique the entire hand is used in the manipulation. The palm focuses the movement while the fingers remain relaxed and in complete contact with the body. Pressure is disseminated evenly throughout the hand rather than being applied at the heel of the palm or the distal pads. The thumb is held beside the digits.

This technique is used in the manipulation of large muscle groups and at those places where more gentle treatment is required.

Circular Ulnar Pressure

In this technique the ulnar aspect of the hand, the so-called blade, is used to apply force. The direction of force is into the area of the hand from the pisiform to the metacarpophalangeal joint. Movement of the hand is in small circles. This technique is most frequently used in the area surrounding the scapulae to release the deeper muscles.

Circular Palm-Heel Pressure

In this technique circular pressure is applied with the heel of the palm.

Circular palm-heel pressure is frequently used in the release of larger muscle groups.

DIRECT PRESSURE

▼

Direct pressure refers to either steady direct thumb pressure or direct digital pressure to a specific area or point. The amount of pressure varies with the area of the body being manipulated and the patient's needs and sensitivities. This is a technique that is used in the direct stimulation of points and in the release of muscle spasms. It is generally followed by circular pressure to the area or point.

Direct Thumb Pressure/Direct Digital Pressure

This technique employs the use of the distal aspect of the pads of the five fingers. Typically used for the stimulation of specific points, either the whole pad or portions of the most distal aspect of the pad are used, depending on the area of the body being manipulated. Because this technique requires that the hand be perfectly controlled, the appropriate administration of this technique requires great strength in the completely relaxed hand.

STROKING

▼

The stroking technique involves a single uninterrupted movement repeated over an area of the body. The force is distributed equally throughout the whole hand or the aspect of the hand that is being used. Pressure remains constant and even throughout the movement.

Thumb Stroking

Thumb stroking involves the use of the entire palmar aspect of the thumb—the pad, the arch, and the proximal phalange. Pressure is distributed equally throughout the thumb. This technique is most commonly used in the treatment of the muscles of the forehead, the face, and the medial aspect of the foot.

Digital Stroking

This technique employs the use of the palmar aspect of the fingers. A large surface area may be covered with a gentle pushing movement. There is light contact between the hand and the patient, with little pressure applied. Digital stroking is frequently used to reduce edema in the extremities; the direction of movement is with the venous flow, that is, toward the trunk of the body, in order to facilitate lymphatic drainage.

Palmar Stroking

Palmar stroking involves the use of the entire palmar aspect of the hand in full contact with the body. A gentle gliding motion covers the surface of the area being manipulated. In the correct administration of this technique the relaxed hand molds to the contours of the body. This technique is often employed on the posterior surface of the body in long sweeping motions.

Loose-Fist Stroking

A very relaxed fist is formed with virtually no tension in the forearm. The fingers of the hand are flexed toward the palm, allowing the dorsal aspect of the middle phalange of the fingers to come in contact with the patient. The thumb is held in a relaxed fashion beside the index finger. Either a short up-and-back motion or circular pressure is used.

FOREKNUCKLE TECHNIQUE

This technique requires forming a relaxed fist by flexing the fingers of the hand toward the palm without flexing the metacarpophalangeal joints. Contact with the patient's body is made with the proximal interphalangeal joints of the fingers. The foreknuckle can be applied using circular pressure, direct pressure, or a stroking technique when deeper manipulation is appropriate.

EMBRACING

In this technique the hand is molded to the contours of the body and a drawing or suction motion is applied with the palm. Because this is a palmar technique, no fingertip pressure is applied.

Palmar Embrace

In this technique the thenar and the hypothenar areas of the hand are used in opposition to one another in a drawing motion that produces a vertical suction effect. The focus is in the palm of the hand, though some contact is made by the proximal phalange of the fingers. No fingertip pressure is applied.

The palmar embrace is effectively used in the release and relaxation of muscle groups.

Palmar/Thenar Embrace

In this technique the thenar and the hypothenar areas of the hand are again used to produce a vertical suction effect; however, in this manipulation the thumb is drawn toward the fingers at the end of the stroke. This technique is effectively used in the release and relaxation of larger muscle groups.

PERCUSSION

With percussion movements, a light tapping motion is applied in a rhythmic manner to the surface of the body, producing a stimulating effect. Care should be taken to produce a vibratory effect rather than producing pain from incorrectly applying the techniques. Percussion techniques should never be used directly over the spine.

Cupping

In cupping, the hand is held in a relaxed pyramid form. The four digits are held together with the fingers extended; the thumb is held beside the index finger. A slight bend at the metacarpophalangeal joint creates a hollow at the center of the palm. When executed properly, the palm never contacts the body. This technique is applied in a continuous rhythmic manner, with the two hands alternately striking the body. As a result it produces a highly stimulating yet relaxing effect.

This technique can be used on the back, buttocks, thighs, legs, and shoulders. When applied to the posterior aspect of the thorax, it stimulates the release of mucus and mucopurulent material from the lungs.

Chopping

The blade or ulnar aspect of the hand is used in chopping. The wrist is held in a relaxed manner, allowing the hand free movement at the joint. The fingers, while held together, are also relaxed. The striking area extends from the pisiform bone to the distal aspect of the fifth digit. The two hands strike in an alternating fashion in a continuous and rhythmic manner. This produces a stimulating yet relaxing effect when administered properly. Like cupping, this technique can be used on the back, buttocks, thighs, calves, and shoulders.

HAND EXERCISES

The following series of hand exercises should be practiced daily to develop strength, coordination, and sensitivity.

Exercises 1–4 and 11 are performed in a kneeling position; exercises 5–9 are performed in a seated position. Exercise 10 is performed standing.

1. FINGER STRETCH

This exercise will encourage the full extension of the fingers and palm, and helps to develop the fine muscles of the hand.

From a kneeling postion, place your palms flat on the floor. Elongate your fingers, stretching each finger out so that it is as long and as flat as possible. Relax your fingers and the center of the palm to maintain full palmar contact with the floor. Do not allow the fingers to bend. Hold this position for 10–15 seconds. Slowly withdraw your hands from the floor and shake them out. Repeat this exercise four or five times.

2. PALMAR EMBRACE

▼

This is an exercise for the very fine muscles of the hand. Practically no movement will occur in the gross muscles.

Place your palms on the floor as in exercise 1. Focusing on the center of the palm, draw the palm directly upward away from the floor, keeping the weight evenly distributed throughout the hand. You should see only a slight movement of the muscles along the entire perimeter of the hand. After the palm is drawn upward, relax it again so that the centermost part is touching the floor. This is similar to the action of a suction cup.

Repeat this motion ten to fifteen times, taking care to maintain straight, relaxed fingers. Slowly withdraw your hands from the floor and shake them out.

3. WRIST STRETCH

▼

This exercise is instrumental in developing stretch and flexibility in the palmar surface of the hands, in the wrists, and in the forearms.

Place your palms on the floor so that the anterior aspects of the wrists are touching and the fingertips are pointed in opposite directions. Elongate your fingers and keep the hand as flat as possible. The cubital crease of the elbow should be facing forward. Keeping your fingers elongated and without allowing the knuckles to bend, slowly rotate your forearms so that the elbow folds are facing each other. Do not allow the heels of the palms to lift up off the floor, and do not allow your shoulders to roll forward as you rotate your forearms. Hold this position for 5 counts and then slowly rotate your forearms back to the initial position. Repeat four or five times.

4. FINGERTIP STRENGTHENING

▼

This exercise develops proper alignment of the fingers and the strength necessary for adequate hand control in the implementation of digital pressure techniques.

Place your fingertips on the floor so that your fingers are relaxed but extended. The palm of your hand should be well up off the floor. The joints in your fingers and hands are neither flexed nor hyperextended. Keep your hands and fingers relaxed but straight, without bending the knuckles. Your hands take on the appearance of a smooth, curved line that extends from your fingertips to your wrist. Gradually shift your weight onto your fingertips, repeatedly checking to make sure that your fingers remain straight. The most distal aspect of the palmar surface of each finger, not the pads of the distal phalanges, are in contact with the floor. Hold this position for 5 counts and release. Repeat this four or five times. Withdraw your hands and shake them out.

When you are able to maintain this position without locking or bending any of the joints in your fingers or hands, slowly lift your knees off the floor approximately 2 to 3 inches. Hold this position for 5 counts and release. Repeat four or five times.

5. CROSSING FINGERS

▼

The children's game of crossing the fingers is a good exercise for stretching the fingers and developing flexibility.

Starting from a seated position, place the fifth digit over the fourth, the fourth over the third, and the third over the second. Hold this position for 5–10 counts and then slowly relax the fingers and shake out your hands. Cross the fingers in reverse order and repeat.

6. ROLLING STONES
▼

A good, accessible method of exercising the hands is with the use of two large walnuts or two stones; both should fit comfortably in the palm of one hand. Exercise the fingers and hands by rolling the walnuts or stones around in the palm of the hand. A variation on this exercise is to roll and squeeze a hard rubber ball in the palm of the hand. The rolling and squeezing motion develops strength and coordination of the fine muscles of the hands and fingers.

7. FIST—STRETCH REPETITIONS
▼

The following exercise is recommended for building strength and endurance.

Make a tight fist by slowly flexing the fingers into the palm and wrapping the thumb around the fingers. From the fist position, fan your hands out, stretching the palms and fingers as widely as possible. Alternate the fist position with the stretch position, beginning with fifteen to twenty-five rounds and working up to two hundred rounds. An advanced Amma therapist can perform upward of five hundred rounds. Build your endurance slowly. It is important that you not sacrifice the detail of correct positions simply to accomplish more rounds.

8. ROTATING THUMBS
▼

This exercise is used to relax the hands and develop muscle isolation and strength of the individual muscles in the thenar region.

Abduct and extend the thumbs keeping them straight at the interphalangeal joints. Rotate the thumbs first in a clockwise direction and then counterclockwise. You must make certain that the rotation takes place from the carpometacarpal joint, and not the metacarpophalangeal joint. Begin with twenty-five rounds and work up slowly to one hundred rounds.

9. FINGER-PAD PRESS
▼

This isometric exercise builds finger strength.

Oppose the center of the pad of each finger in sequence with the center of the pad of the thumb. Apply maximum pressure with each press. Begin with twenty-five rounds and slowly increase.

10. STRENGTHENING THE WRISTS
▼

This exercise strengthens the wrists by building up the forearm flexors and extensor muscles.

Tie one end of a cord to a one- or two-pound weight and the other end to the center of a wooden dowel. Stand with the arms extended at shoulder height. Elbows must remain straight but not locked. Hold the dowel in both hands with palms facing downward, allowing the weight to hang freely. Using only the muscles of the hand, wind the cord around the dowel drawing the weight up to it. Once the weight is raised, reverse the winding movement so that the weight is lowered toward the ground, making sure to control the descent carefully.

Repeat this exercise two or three times. The same exercise may be repeated with the palms turned upward.

11. FINGER RAISES

This exercise will increase strength and agility of the hands and improve coordination.

From a kneeling position, place your palms flat on the floor and elongate your fingers as in exercise 1. Keeping the weight evenly distributed throughout the hand, and with the palm "glued" to the floor, raise and stretch the index fingers of both hands while keeping the remaining fingers and the palm on the floor. Relax the index fingers, drawing them back down to the floor. Repeat with the third fingers, then the fourth and fifth fingers and thumbs successively, each time keeping the rest of the hand completely in contact with the floor. Once this is mastered, combinations of fingers may be practiced, such as raising the second and fourth fingers together, or the third and fourth fingers, and so forth.

This exercise may also be done off the floor, with the arms slightly extended and bent at the elbow and palms facing the practitioner. Close the second and fifth fingers into a loose fist. Raise the index fingers of both hands while the other fingers remain in a loose fist, then relax them and bring them down. Repeat with the third, fourth, and fifth fingers successively, each time extending and stretching the fingers as they are raised. Now try combinations—raise the index and third fingers while the fourth and fifth fingers remain closed, then raise the second and fourth while the third and fifth fingers remain closed, and so forth.

THE IMPORTANCE OF T'AI CHI CHUAN TO AMMA THERAPY

The evolution of a therapist begins with self-development. Critical to this self-development is self-awareness. The process of developing self-awareness requires training in each of three arenas: physical, intellectual, and emotional. Of the three, the physical center should be trained and developed first. One practice by which to facilitate this goal is the study of t'ai chi chuan, an ancient Chinese system of exercise that is sometimes called "meditation in motion." The study of t'ai chi is important for prospective therapists, because strength, physical and emotional control, and heightened self-awareness are critical to the practice of bodywork therapy. At the New York College for Wholistic Health Education and Research, t'ai chi is a mandatory part of the curriculum for all students. Traditionally a martial art form, t'ai chi chuan has tremendous value to offer anyone seeking to develop awareness of the body, the emotions, and the energy system. It also produces great physical strength and endurance when practiced seriously. Because of its graceful appearance and many healthful effects resulting from its practice, t'ai chi has also often been referred to as the "grand dance for health."

The phrase *t'ai chi chuan* means "boxing with application of the principles of energy balance and harmony with the energy of the planet." The t'ai chi form is a series of slow, continuous movements performed with great attention. Movements are done without strain, although in the early stages a certain amount of strength must be developed. The practice is therefore initially not as soft and easy as it becomes when the proper strength is developed. These movements provide exercise and toning for every part of the body, including the internal viscera. The t'ai chi form usually takes fifteen to twenty minutes to complete, and should be practiced twice daily, in the morning and before retiring at night. Through regular practice, this beautiful series of movements helps to develop and coordinate the body.

A primary purpose of t'ai chi is to develop control of Qi. The word Qi is usually translated as "intrinsic energy" or "vital energy," considered the basic life force of the individual. T'ai chi chuan is concerned with the development and control of this energy. The practice of t'ai chi chuan has been associated with many positive changes. Among these are:

- Greater physical power resulting from increased flow of Qi through the muscles, increased strength in the legs and lower torso, and decreased oxygen needs.
- Greater physical endurance resulting from more effective use of oxygen.
- Increased efficiency of movement as the t'ai chi practitioner learns not to use muscles that are not necessary for the accomplishment of her intended movement. Such unnecessary expenditure is a big part of energy waste in most activities.
- Greater control of emotional expression resulting from proper control and utilization of energy in the body.
- Greater control and stamina in sexual activity resulting from an increased awareness of the pelvic area and increased energy available for sexual activity.
- Less need for sleep, with deeper and more restful sleep resulting from more efficient and appropriate energy use, decreased aerobic needs, and a general decrease in disturbing emotions.
- Less need for oxygen and less cardiovascular strain resulting from the very basic practice of relaxed and efficient movement.
- Less need for food intake resulting from the decrease in oxygen usage and decrease in fuel burned—a general basic reduction in stress and tension.
- Less negative emotionality resulting from the practice of efficient posturing and the t'ai chi form.
- Greater calm and inner peace resulting from many of the above.
- Greater stamina and energy resulting from all of the above.

T'ai chi is a vehicle for the therapist to attain a new kind of strength, encouraging proper positioning and use of the arms and shoulders for the efficient and correct use of force while discouraging back pain and fatigue. This physical component is of vital importance to the practice of healing others. Beyond physical strength, t'ai chi is also a powerful medium for developing self-awareness. In order to heal others, it is critical to have control over one's own body and emotions. The first step toward this level of control is self-awareness.

The practice of t'ai chi begins with learning the t'ai chi posture. Good posture is fundamental to physical, emotional, and intellectual balance. This balance has its roots in the mind as well as in the body. The principles of t'ai chi assert that realignment of the spine will provide for the natural balance and free flow of energy in the body, especially in the spine. Realignment of the spine is accomplished through relaxing and placing the attention of the mind on the *tan tien*—the area of the lower belly, below the navel—while practicing the t'ai chi form.

The word *tan tien* literally means "field of elixir" (or "medicine"), implying an area that is a source of healing. This is the center in which the psychic energies are conserved and transformed. The primary goal of t'ai chi is the opening of the tan tien. When it opens, physical health improves dramatically, and the use of awkward muscle strength becomes obsolete in light of the new powers of relatively free-flowing Qi. This in turn results in better physical, emotional, mental, and spiritual health.

Opening the tan tien begins with practicing a posture wherein the shoulders are drawn back and dropped and the lower belly is fully released. This posture drops the center of gravity into the lower body. Standing in his usual posture, a person who does not practice t'ai chi will fall over from an effortless push because his center of gravity is up in the chest and head. A person who is relaxed will feel surprisingly stable and can withstand even a hard, quick thrust. Long practice is necessary to effect a change in the body's center of gravity so that such a posture can be held naturally.

Understanding the proper t'ai chi posture is often difficult for novices. It may seem like a contradiction that instructors describe the posture as one to both approach with and engender relaxation, yet getting into the correct posture—simultaneously bending at the knees, drawing the shoulders back and down, hollowing beneath the solar plexus, filling in the lower back, releasing the lower abdomen below the navel, straightening out the neck—requires great effort. Holding this posture is even more difficult. It feels tense and seems to be a contradiction to what the student has been told—that the purpose of the posture is to enhance one's ability to relax. However, what seems like a contradiction is not. The skill of correctly holding the t'ai chi posture will enable students to let go of their tensions and finally begin to relax their bodies. By making a conscious effort to hold the posture, one must also put himself in a properly directed frame of mind that can ultimately lead to a powerful learning experience—an experience of a balanced state of body, intellect, and emotions.

When one works on being centered in himself in light of the principles of the t'ai chi philosophy, he begins to evolve toward a balanced physical, intellectual, and emotional state. The Taoists say this takes three years for a minor success and ten years for a major success. Once accomplished, the practitioner can then begin to shift into a much larger view and understanding of life and of himself.

For the therapist, this will radically effect the way he sees and experiences the world and his own state. Only when someone is aware of his emotions does he have the possibility of controlling them and using them appropriately. If the therapist has uncontrolled emotions within him or is unaware of a negative emotional state, the potential is greater for those emotions to manifest in his voice and body language and through his hands during treatment, which is antithetical to his purpose of healing the patient.

As well, if the therapist is in a negative psychological state, his body will reflect that in the form of physical tensions that restrict the flow of energy. If his energy is blocked, there is no way that he can feel the energy of others. As soon as the open and aware therapist puts his hands on a patient, he can experience both his own energy and that of his patient. However, if he is not rooted in the t'ai chi posture with his tan tien open—if he is not aware of himself—then he will not treat very effectively.

By applying the principles of t'ai chi chuan, one learns to pay attention to his inner world and to act and respond appropriately. As one becomes rooted in this new way of thinking and seeing, the tan tien begins to open. The practitioner then begins to perceive reality through a new set of eyes, and develops the ability to observe emotions that arise within himself, particularly while in the treatment room with a patient, without allowing them to gain control of his body, mind, or facial expressions. As a therapist, one is in a position of great responsibility—not only having to cope with the emotions of the patient as they arise during the treatment, but with his own emotions as well. It is vital for him to put himself into an appropriate relationship with these emotions, so that they do not interfere with or disturb his work.

Even when a therapist experiences negative emotions, he can protect his patients by staying in that place where nothing gets passed to the patient either psychologically or energetically. The key is being aware that while he may be feeling upset, he will not pass on large amounts of his own life force, in the form of negativity, to the patient. This is also self-protection for the therapist, to avoid draining his own energy and/or absorbing the negative Qi of his patient.

By maintaining the t'ai chi posture, remaining in a state that is relaxed and centered, and staying fully aware of the dynamics of the emotional conditions going on within, the therapist can carry on with his responsibilities without being affected by negativity. Learning to remain immune to negative emotions will help the developing bodywork therapist to become more effective at what he does. An awareness of the tan tien and one's own body should always be part of the therapist's attention and consciousness, not only when treating another but as a constant throughout life.

The process of becoming self-aware begins to put one on the path toward healing oneself and becoming more balanced in the three centers: physical, emotional, and intellectual. As one heals himself and becomes more self-aware, he becomes better as a therapist. As he becomes a role model, his effect on patients will be better and stronger. Following his guidance, patients will become educated about their bodies and their states of health, and will become more aware of how they are feeling. A good therapist stimulates his patients' growth and development while his own development is also taking place, offering his patients the results of his own acceptance of both his emotions and their emotions. As one becomes more aware and in control of his internal world through the practice and application of the principles of t'ai chi chuan, he is able to expand and increase his awareness to encompass that of his patients. The principle is this: the more self-aware the beginning Amma therapist becomes, the greater the potential for him to be more aware and sensitive to the emotional states and needs of his patients. He can then treat them most effectively and make the most appropriate recommendations for their development and well-being.

CHAPTER

12

ETHICS AND THE
AMMA THERAPIST

Broadly defined, the word *ethics* refers to a set of values, codes, or principles that a profession embraces in its efforts to define itself, both to itself and to the public. Ethics implies a way of acting and behaving as well as feeling and believing. Ethics are therefore a vital underpinning of what we do, and of who we are as healing practitioners.

Every evolved profession has an articulated code of ethical conduct set down in a series of individual principles. These principles encompass both the highest ideals of the profession and the minimum standards of acceptable behavior; in this way, ethics codes contain both the "shoulds" and the "musts" of professional behavior. Why is it important for a practitioner of Amma therapy to identify and implement a code of ethical behavior? Because ethics codes, above all, invoke the primary rule of the healer set forth by Hippocrates, which is to do no harm. At its most basic level, a code of behavior protects the patient. By being recognizable as setting a high standard of acceptable practice, an ethics code also serves to protect the profession. An identified code of ethics that all practitioners agree upon sends a message to the public that the profession has evolved, and is dedicated to serving in the public's best interest.

What ethical principles does the Amma therapist embrace? The first, and perhaps most important, is *respect for the patient*. Respect for the patient means understanding that the patient is a unique individual with a history of likes and dislikes, strengths and challenges, and reactions to touching and being touched. Respect implies treating the patient as an equal in the healing relationship without losing sight of the ultimate responsibility for the healing process. This principle encompasses respect for the person's physical, emotional, and energy bodies, understanding that all play an equally important role in the healing process. And respect for the patient demands that no person is discriminated against in the treatment relationship by virtue of personal characteristics unfamiliar or discomforting to the healing professional.

The principle of respect requires a high level of self-awareness in the Amma practitioner. It is normal human behavior to have biases or stereotypes about people who are different from ourselves. However, as stated earlier, a true health professional is one who demonstrates a concern and a compassion for others that is beyond what might be expected from everyday human concern. Therefore, the Amma therapist must explore his own biases, beliefs, and discomforts with different types of people and personalities in order to neutralize their potential negative impact on the treatment relationship.

The next ethical principle of the Amma therapist is that of *professional integrity*. This principle implies that the Amma therapist conducts him- or herself in a manner demonstrating the utmost honesty and professionalism. Amma therapists must understand the limits of their training, knowledge, and experience, and treat patients accordingly. What can be attempted by a healing sensitive must not be tried by the novice. Similarly, a novice of Oriental bodywork must not present himself to the public as an Amma therapist until that portion of the advanced training has been satisfactorily completed.

Professional integrity demands a commitment to excellence, both personal and professional, that should be regularly assessed and strengthened through ongoing participation in continuing education and training. This attitude toward self-development acknowledges that the acquisition of skills, knowledge, and abilities in the healing arts is a lifelong process.

Integrity and a commitment to excellence are evident in both the personal and professional behaviors of the Amma therapist. Mode of dress, manner of speaking, personal hygiene and health behaviors, and public conduct are all evidence of a person's commitment to the highest standards of behavior. All are also evidence of the self-discipline that is essential in developing the kind of sensitivity, awareness, and technical ability of the advanced Amma practitioner.

Finally, professional integrity implies having a thorough knowledge of what the practitioner is and is not capable of. This means understanding the limits of Amma therapy and individual limitations, developing a good working relationship with other health practitioners, and knowing when and how to refer a patient to another health professional.

A final yet critically important ethical principle is that of *intention and trust*. Intention is the aim, the course of action the therapist plans to follow. It is something that takes place within the therapist, in her personal commitment to healing—and not harming—the patients with whom she works. Trust is something that takes place between therapist and patient, and has to do with establishing and maintaining safety and appropriate boundaries in the therapist–patient relationship. Establishing an atmosphere of safety and trust is essential in creating the conditions in which healing can occur. Patients come for treatment in a vulnerable state. They are vulnerable because they are sick or injured, they possess less knowledge than the therapist, and they have to lie down and may have to undress in order to be treated. These add up to a situation in which the balance of power between the patient and the therapist can be clearly weighted toward the therapist. Patients are also vulnerable because, in order to cooperate with the healing process, they will have to give up ways of behaving in the world that, although maladaptive, have until now provided a certain amount of comfort and security.

All of this adds up to a potentially frightening situation, and patients' defenses must be respected as they are slowly encouraged to change. Providing a safe atmosphere in the therapeutic setting means allowing patients to progress at their own rate, without judgment. It means allowing patients to speak confidentially and to protect their privacy at all costs. It means setting and maintaining clear boundaries: patients are not coming to the Amma therapist because they want to be friends, nor are they coming because they want psychotherapy or advice about how to conduct their lives beyond the confines of their health behaviors. Although all of these things might be discussed in an Amma therapy session, and although Amma therapists certainly care about their patients, appropriate boundaries must be maintained.

Nowhere is the issue of boundaries more important than in the realm of sexuality. Because Amma therapy involves touch, often of an intimate nature, it is normal that sensual feelings can arise in both therapist and patient. Human contact is sensual contact, and contains the seeds of the healing relationship. It is only where the sensual aspect becomes sexualized that there is a violation of the boundaries of the therapist–patient relationship. Sexualization of the relationship occurs when one or both parties extends the realm of contact to include that of a sexual nature. This could include sexual comments, such as "You have a great body," types of touch, parts of the body worked on, and even entering into a consensual sexual relationship outside of the treatment relationship. For an Amma practitioner, indeed for any health professional, sexual contact between therapist and patient is a violation of appropriate boundaries and is *never acceptable,* even if the patient initiates it. Furthermore, sexual contact in the therapeutic relationship *always* leads to harm—for the patient, and possibly for the practitioner. Sexual contact in the treatment relationship is against the ethical standards of every profession, and in most instances is also against the law. Refraining from sexual intimacy with a patient, even when the patient consents, is an ultimate "must" for the Amma therapist.

In addition to these principles, what else must a therapist understand in order to act ethically? The Amma therapist must be aware that he is in a relationship with his patients in which there is a power differential, as is always the case in a therapist–patient relationship. One of the reasons that this is true has been already mentioned: the patient is less powerful because he is more vulnerable when presenting for treatment. The patient is also less powerful because we live in a culture wherein the person in authority—in this case the Amma therapist—holds more power. That is why professional organizations and the law always recognize the therapist as holding ultimate responsibility for the treatment, even if it is the patient who tries to alter the treatment boundaries. Because of the inherent power differential, the Amma therapist has an obligation to protect the patient's welfare. This includes understanding the impact that the relationship has upon the patient, which will be determined in part by the patient's previous relationships with authority figures. If, for example, the patient has had previously positive relationships with teachers, parents, and other people in authority, then the chances are much greater that the patient will experience the Amma therapist as helpful and having a positive impact. If, however, the patient has had negative or traumatic experiences with people in power over him, then the chances are much greater that the Amma therapy treatment might also be perceived as harmful. This might be so in spite of the therapist's intention to do no harm. That is why an understanding of the patient's positive and negative reactions to the therapeutic situation is so important. It minimizes the potential for harm, the seedbed for which is based upon the patient's previous life experiences.

It is also crucial that the Amma therapist understands the power differential that exists in the Amma therapy setting in order to minimize the risk that the patient will be coerced or exploited, again without the intention of the therapist to do so. This is due to the tendency for people in the less powerful position to be compliant with authority, even if they do not understand the reason or if it is not in their best interest. This tendency toward compliance means that patients will often tolerate painful treatments or uncomfortable recommendations without complaining or asking the reason why something has been recommended. It also means that patients may not communicate when something about the treatment setting does not feel safe to them, as might happen when the therapist asks too many questions of a probing or personal nature or makes judgments about the patient's lifestyle or behaviors. By developing an ever-increasing awareness of the effect of the power differential on her patients, the Amma therapist minimizes the risk of harm through sensitizing her communications and continually assessing her impact upon the patient. Additionally, the Amma therapist must develop an awareness of her own reactions to the effect of the power differential, which will also be determined by her history and personal experiences of having more and less power.

How can the Amma therapist maximize the possibility that the treatment relationship will be safe, effective, and positive for the patient? First, by upholding the ethical principles of the profession, as stated above. Second, by understanding the impact of the power differential on herself and the patient. Third, by continually seeking supervision and support from appropriate advisors, including advanced Amma practitioners and experts in the fields of human relationships and ethical conduct, such as clinical psychologists. Fourth, and finally, by keeping the lines of communication open between herself and the patient.

Good communication is an essential element that makes safety and treatment effectiveness possible. Good communication begins at the first moment of contact with a person who is a potential patient. Good communication entails helping the patient to articulate why he is coming for treatment and how the therapist's skills and the treatment itself may be helpful. Good communication means relating important clinical information to the patient in a way that is understandable and with a sense of timing that takes into consideration the patient's particular sensitivities, expectations, and resistances or defenses against the healing process.

As with good boundaries, good communication is ultimately the therapist's responsibility. Good communication starts with articulating the basic therapeutic contract, naming what it is that the patient can expect from the therapist and from the treatment as well as what will be expected of the patient. The therapeutic contract is essential in order for healing to occur, and includes the important ethical—and legal—consideration of informed consent.

Informed consent is what the patient gives when he understands the treatment process and consents to participate in it. As such, he must understand what to expect from the treatment—in what way touch is involved; how much clothing he will have to take off; how the treatment effects healing; and what will be expected of him from financial, behavioral, and psychological perspectives. If a patient is not adequately informed, true consent cannot be given. When this is the case, the law recognizes that a therapeutic contract was never truly in effect, and in such cases there may be negative conse-

quences for the therapist and patient alike. Informed consent is therefore a protection for the patient as well as the therapist, who will gain an understanding of the patient's willingness and ability to participate in a depth-oriented treatment such as Amma therapy, a treatment that requires time, energy, and commitment on the part of both participants.

In summary, upholding the ethical standards of Amma therapy serves as a protection for both the public and the practitioner. By incorporating the principles of respect, integrity, and intention and trust, the Amma practitioner demonstrates his commitment to the patient's welfare and to his own evolution toward the highest plateau of the profession, that of healing sensitive. By understanding the role of the power differential, the therapist avoids harming the patient by inadvertently exploiting or coercing the patient, either through his own or the patient's response to power and authority. And by understanding the concepts of the therapeutic contract and informed consent, the therapist sets the stage for good communication and appropriate expectations throughout the course of treatment.

Ethical behavior and the making of decisions based on ethics are not practices that develop overnight. Similarly, they are not something that you either have or do not have. A sense of ethics and the rightness or wrongness of particular behaviors develop over time, with experience, training, and introspection. There are some rules to follow and, when in doubt, a true healing professional errs on the side of caution in order to uphold the ultimate ethical code stated by Hippocrates so long ago: *"Above all, do no harm."*

THE BASIC AMMA THERAPY TREATMENT

This chapter describes in detail the sequence of movements and techniques that comprise the basic Amma therapy treatment. In the beginning a student must devote many hours of concentrated attention to learning these techniques, utilizing them in the proper sequence and evolving his coordination and skill. While a typical session given by an advanced Amma therapist can last anywhere from forty-five minutes to one and one-half hours, the beginning student may find it takes him an hour simply to perform the techniques for the head. This pace during the learning process must be accepted, and viewed in the context of Amma therapy as a healing art. In the same way that a beginning karate student must master basic *katas* before advancing to more difficult forms, the novice student must master the basic treatment before learning the more advanced techniques discussed in part IV.

For those readers who have a background in other bodywork techniques, this chapter will provide the groundwork for learning some basic Amma manipulations. However, like any other true art, mastering Amma therapy requires a teacher who can guide, correct, and impart in-depth understanding. I encourage those who are interested in learning Amma therapy to its fullest extent to enroll in a school of Amma therapy, where they can study under the tutelage of certified instructors.

It should be noted that there are no specific contraindications for Amma therapy. The therapist may be limited by the patient's condition but can still utilize a variety of techniques, and can adapt the treatment to the patient's individual needs. For example, if a patient suffers from varicosities or edema, the treatment of the affected areas will be tempered with appropriate pressure and herbal liniments. Even in hospitals where patients are confined with medical equipment, such as ventilators, IVs, and cardiac monitors, Amma therapists can adjust their treatments to accommodate these limitations. Infants and children respond exceptionally well to Amma therapy.

The proper execution of Amma therapy techniques applied directly to the physical body, along with specific manipulation of the energies in the twelve Primary and Tendino-Muscle channels, the Conception and Governing Vessels, and the Cutaneous Regions, affect both the superficial and deep tissues as well as the energy system. These include the myofascia, all the major systems of the body (that is, the circulatory, lymphatic, respiratory, digestive, nervous, and endocrine systems), and the craniosacral system. The specific benefits of a basic treatment are discussed in detail in chapter 15, "General Treatment for Revitalizing and Balancing the Body."

Because it works on both the Primary and Tendino-Muscle energy pathways of the body, Amma therapy affects all the systems of the mindbody complex and therefore can treat most any illness. However, the decision of what to treat, when to treat, and how to treat will depend on the assessment of the therapist, the purpose for the patient's visit, and the severity of the symptoms and signs. Part IV gives detailed guidelines for treatment protocol for various conditions. While I encourage readers to use the information in part IV to the best of their abilities, it is important to realize that finely tuned assessment capacities and the skillful employment of technical

information and intuitive understanding that make healing a true art form, can only be gained through diligent study with respected teachers.

In the course of an Amma therapy treatment the practitioner works from both seated and standing positions. Whether seated or standing, the therapist must always strive for proper postural alignment. This is where the practice of t'ai chi chuan proves invaluable—through t'ai chi the student learns how to maintain alignment while in motion. At the beginning of the treatment the spine should be in alignment so that energy is free-flowing and strength is not lost. In the standing position, weight is distributed evenly on both feet, with the knees slightly bent. The shoulders and scapulae are held back and down; the rib cage is dropped; the perineum, buttocks, and anus are relaxed; and the tan tien is opened and filled. The practitioner is relaxed, with her weight dropping into her legs and feet; this stance is referred to as "sinking." The aligned neck is straight and relaxed. In the seated position the feet are placed comfortably on the floor without crossing the legs or ankles, and alignment through the spine is maintained, as is the holding of the tan tien. The head is held erect and the entire body is relaxed.

The treatment begins with the patient lying comfortably on the table in the supine position. Patients may wear gowns or loose, comfortable clothing. The practitioner is seated behind the patient's head. In the course of executing each technique, the area being worked on should be palpated as the movement is made, noting any surface changes and/or skeletal contours.

STEP 1

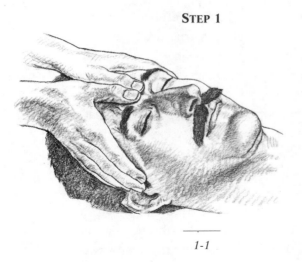

1-1

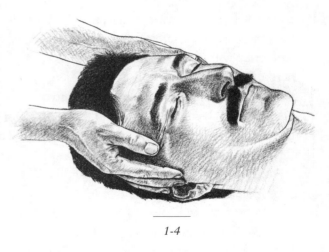

1-4

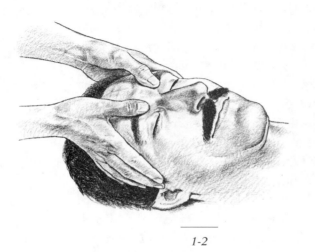

1-2

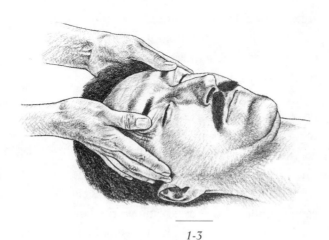

1-3

Step 1: Gently center the patient's head. Place the hands on the patient's forehead with the pads of the thumbs lying midway between the eyebrows. The radial edges of both thumbs, from the thumbnails to the thenar eminences, are aligned and touching at the center of the forehead, pads of the thumbs on the eyebrows. The palms are resting on the forehead, with the fingers resting on the lateral aspects of the head and face.

Using thumb stroking with the pads of the thumbs, gently stroke over the eyebrows, starting at the midpoint of the eyebrows and moving horizontally across the forehead toward the temples to end just inside the lateral hairline. Thumbs should remain in a vertical position during thumb stroking; the hand moves laterally as a unit with the thumbs. Repeat this movement five times.

Step 2: Place the hands on the patient's forehead with the pads of the thumbs in contact with the midpoint between the eyebrows. Hyperextend the thumbs at the distal phalange and stroke above the eyebrows, in the superciliary arch, moving across the forehead to the lateral hairline. Repeat five times.

Note that, in this stroke, pressure is shifted from the pads of the thumbs to the arch of the thumbs. This allows stroking of the area just above the eyebrow rather than directly on the eyebrow.

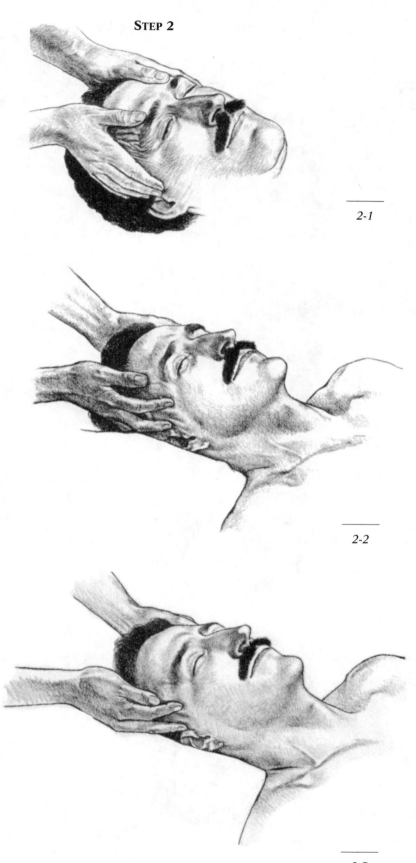

STEP 2

2-1

2-2

2-3

Step 3: Return the hands to the midpoint between the eyebrows. Using thumb stroking with the pads of the thumbs, stroke up the midsagittal line of

STEP 3

the forehead approximately one inch, and then stroke across the forehead to the lateral hairline. Repeat this movement, moving up the forehead in half-inch increments until the superior hairline is reached. End this group of strokes with thumb stroking at the level of the superior hairline. All strokes should begin with an upward movement along the midsagittal line of the forehead. Repeat each increment five times.

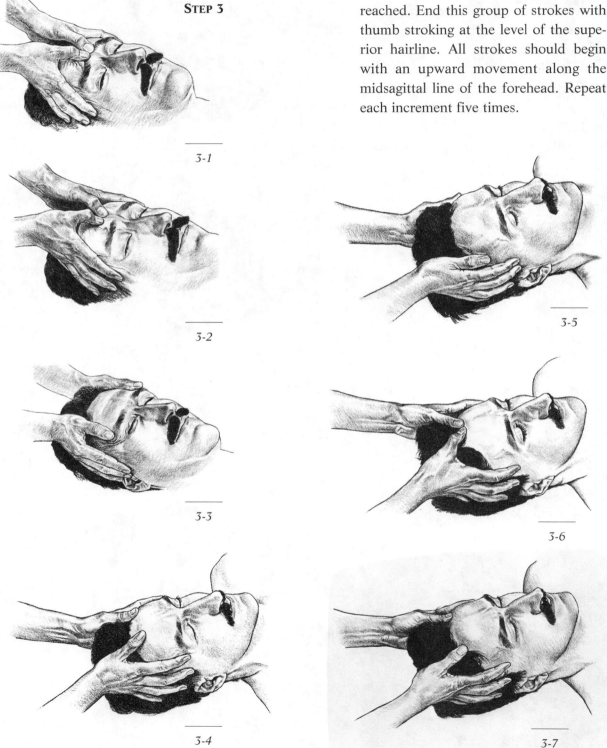

3-1

3-2

3-3

3-4

3-5

3-6

3-7

STEP 4

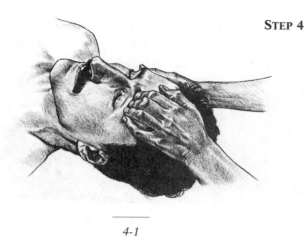

4-1

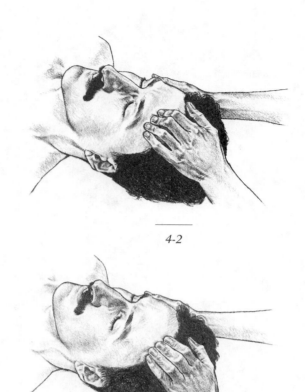

4-2

4-3

Step 4: Place the second, third, and fourth fingers on the superior border of the eyebrow, with the second finger in line with the medial end of the eyebrow and the thumb and fifth finger resting comfortably on the forehead. Begin circling with the pads of the fingers, using even, circular digital pressure and moving toward the superior hairline in half-inch increments, stopping just superior to the hairline. Focus is on the pads of the three central digits. One hand works while the other hand is used to support the opposite side of the patient's head. The supporting hand can either gently cup the ear or lay flat over the temple. Repeat the manipulation of each side of the forehead five times.

STEP 5

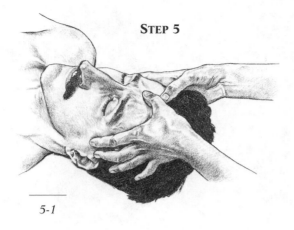

5-1

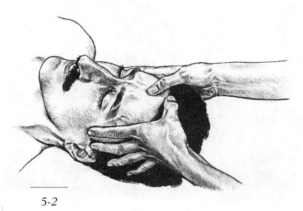

5-2

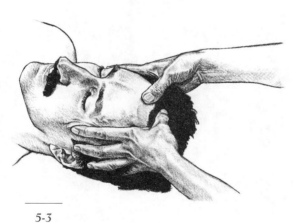

5-3

Step 5: Place the hands on the patient's head with the pads of the thumbs in contact with the midpoint between the eyebrows. Using the thumb-stroking technique, stroke up the mid-sagittal line to the superior hairline, alternating thumbs as you stroke. As soon as the thumb of one hand reaches the hairline, the other thumb begins its vertical stroke. The hands rest on the patient's head as much as possible. Repeat five times.

STEP 6

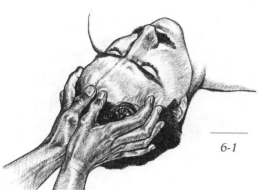

6-1

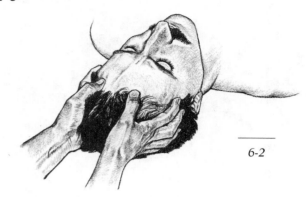

6-2

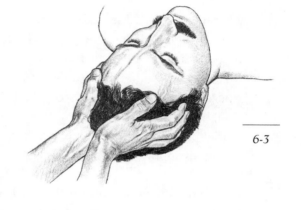

6-3

Step 6: Place the thumbs on the mid-sagittal line of the forehead at the superior hairline. The hands are relaxed and resting on the head. Using the thumb-stroking technique, stroke laterally from the midpoint of the forehead at the superior hairline to the lateral hairline. Both hands work simultaneously. Care should be taken to avoid stroking in an inferior direction (toward the ears). Repeat five times.

The manipulation of the forehead relaxes the temporalis and frontalis portion of the epicranius. This promotes relaxation of both the galea-aponeurotica and the occipital muscles at the base of the occiput, thus encouraging upper body relaxation. The forehead often reflects a patient's emotional state; in biofeedback therapy, the tension of the frontalis muscle is used to gauge a person's overall stress level. The techniques of thumb stroking and circular digital pressure to the forehead helps to relax the patient by releasing muscle strain and tension.

In addition to providing muscular relaxation, these techniques also help to treat the frontal sinus cavities, providing relief for those who suffer from acute, chronic, and allergic sinusitis and rhinitis. Various types of headaches as well as eyestrain are also successfully treated with this technique. Portions of the pathways of the Bladder, Gall Bladder, and Stomach Primary channels are stimulated, as are portions of the Bladder, San Jiao, and Small Intestine Tendino-Muscle channels, thus helping to remove energetic obstructions in these pathways that can manifest as problems locally or at other areas along the channel.

STEP 7

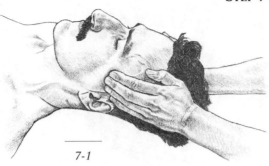

7-1

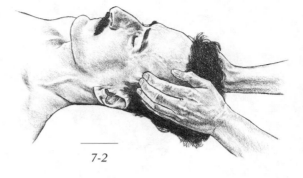

7-2

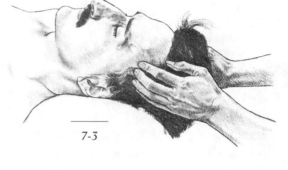

7-3

Step 7: Place the pads of the three central digits at the temples, with the index finger in line with the outer canthus of the eye and the third finger superior to the tragus of the ear. You will feel a slight indentation just above the zygomatic process of the temporal bone. Using even circular digital pressure manipulate the temple area, moving in half-inch increments toward the level of the superior hairline and stopping just superior to the hairline. One hand works while the other hand supports the opposite side of the head. Repeat the manipulation of each temple five times.

Manipulation of this area relaxes the temporalis muscle and can have a profound effect in promoting overall relaxation. A simple but very effective technique is to hold the temple area with the hands for 15–40 seconds. This produces a calming effect on the entire body and may be used at the beginning of the treatment to relax patients who are quite stressed. Manipulation of this area should be emphasized with patients suffering from headaches in the temporal region, patients who suffer from bruxism and temporomandibular joint syndrome, and those who are suffering from stress and tension.

This technique affects portions of the superficial pathways of the Stomach, San Jiao, and Gall Bladder Primary channels and portions of the Colon, Stomach, San Jiao, and Gall Bladder Tendino-Muscle channels.

Step 8: Turn the head to one side, making sure that the head is supported with your hands and that the patient is comfortable. This movement should be done with particular care and attention; overturning should be avoided. Observe and feel any muscular tension of the neck and any limitations of the patient's range of motion. When turning the patient's head, cup the ears gently but firmly with both hands to provide sufficient stability. Overturning the head produces tension in the soft tissues of the neck and makes manipulation of the sternocleidomastoid muscle more difficult.

Using circular digital pressure, manipulate from the top of the sternocleidomastoid muscle, moving from the mastoid process at the area of the occiput down to the clavicle. The third finger rests on top of the muscle while the index and fourth fingers rest alongside the muscle. Focus is on the third finger; however, the other two fingers are also applying pressure. The hand moves in small increments, approximately one finger space or one vertebral space at a time. Begin with the distal and middle phalanges; as the movement proceeds toward the clavicle, extend the contact to include the proximal phalanges and metacarpophalangeal joint area of the hand.

In this technique, circular digital pressure of the right hand is performed in a clockwise direction while movement of the left hand is performed in a counterclockwise direction. This assists in the drainage of the cervical lymph nodes. Repeat the manipulation five times before gently turning the patient's head to treat the other side of the neck.

Do not attempt to turn the head of patients who have a very limited range of motion. As an alternate technique, both hands may work simultaneously with circular digital pressure down the sternocleidomastoid, from the mastoid process to the clavicle; move in very small increments, approximately one finger space or one vertebral space at a time. During this manipulation the head is cupped and supported by both palms as the fingers manipulate down the muscle.

The manipulation of this area has multiple benefits. Tension in the sternocleidomastoid muscle and the platysma is relieved; this serves to relax the neck, upper chest, jaw, chin, and throat—all common areas of tension. For those suffering with shoulder tension, neck tension, bruxism, and temporomandibular joint

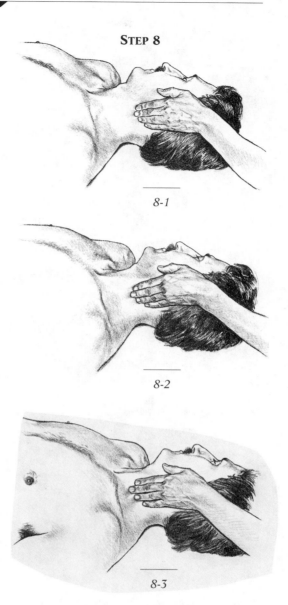

STEP 8

8-1

8-2

8-3

dysfunction, this is a particularly effective technique. Manipulation here also promotes drainage of the cervical lymph nodes, which may become swollen due to allergies or infection.

This manipulation stimulates portions of the Colon, Stomach, Small Intestine, Bladder, Gall Bladder, and San Jiao Tendino-Muscle channels. In addition, the superficial pathways of the Gall Bladder, San Jiao, Small Intestine, Stomach, and Colon channels all intersect with the sternocleidomastoid muscle.

STEP 9

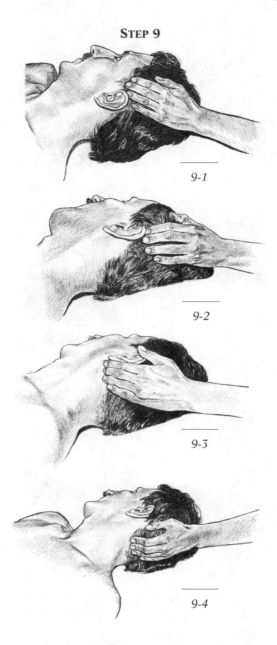

9-1

9-2

9-3

9-4

Step 9: Beginning at the temples, treat the area around the ear using circular digital pressure on a line that approximates the path of the squamosal suture, approximately one inch above the ear. With careful palpation of this area you will feel a shallow indentation at the suture line. The middle finger of your working hand remains in contact with this indentation. Work around the ear and down to the base of the occiput following the superficial pathway of the Gall Bladder Channel. Repeat five times, then turn the head and repeat this manipulation on the opposite side. Work only one side at a time, supporting the patient's head with the opposite hand.

After completing the second side, turn the head back to the original side. Using circular digital pressure, work medially from the mastoid process, along the occiput to the midline. Repeat five times. Turn the head and repeat five times on the opposite side. Care must be taken not to overturn the head. The patient's range of motion can be ascertained through observation and palpation of muscular tension while gently turning the head.

With practice this sequence can be done one complete side at a time, so that the last repetition following the Gall Bladder Channel around the ear to the mastoid process moves smoothly into the manipulation at the base of the occiput to its midline.

This technique stimulates portions of the Gall Bladder Tendino-Muscle pathway and the superficial pathway of the Primary Channel. The Gall Bladder Channel reflects and affects emotional energy. Manipulation here produces emotional calm and physical relaxation. The manipulation at the base of the occiput releases the splenius capitis, the origin of the upper trapezius, and the smaller deep muscles that connect the skull to the cervical vertebrae (longissimus capitis, spinalis capitis, semispinalis capitis, rectus capitis posterior major and minor, obliquus capitis superior). The combined manipulation releases muscular tension in the neck and shoulders and can also be used with patients suffering from stress, headache, arthralgia, upper back pain and spasms, and temporomandibular joint dysfunction. This technique also helps to remove obstructions from the Primary and Tendino-Muscle Bladder channels, which energize the occipital area, and therefore can have a positive effect on genitourinary disorders. It also

STEP 10

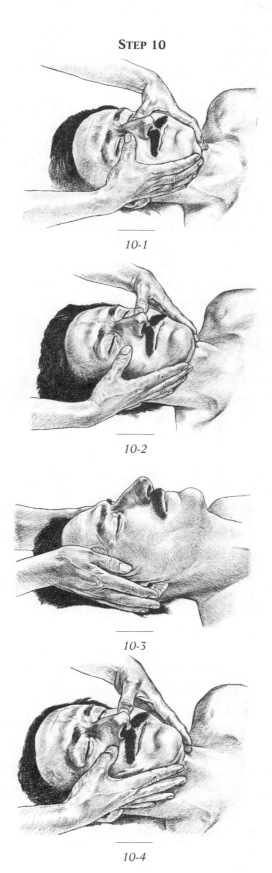

10-1

10-2

10-3

10-4

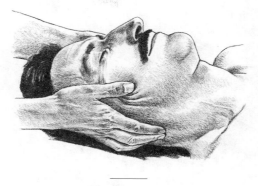

10-5

affects the Kidney, Small Intestine, and Gall Bladder Tendino-Muscle channels.

Step 10: Using the thumb-stroking technique, stroke laterally over the nose and cheekbones toward the temples. Begin with the pad of each thumb in contact with the nasal bones, with the thumbs molding to the contours of the superior aspect of the maxilla and zygomatic arch, stroking along the bony structure of the cheeks. End the stroke at the temple, using the hairline as a guide.

After repeating this stroke five times, repeat the stroke again, this time following the inferior aspect of the maxilla and the zygomatic arch. Repeat five times.

This manipulation helps to drain the maxillary sinuses and reduce swelling. It is beneficial to those suffering with chronic or acute sinusitis and rhinitis, and treats sinus headaches. In addition, manipulation of this area relaxes the facial muscles and promotes general relaxation.

This technique stimulates portions of the superficial pathways of the Primary channels of the Stomach and Small Intestine. Deep portions of the Conception Vessel, Heart, Small Intestine, San Jiao, Liver, and Gall Bladder Primary channels all move through this area. Also portions of the Colon, Stomach, Small Intestine, Bladder, San Jiao, and Gall Bladder Tendino-Muscle channels are stimulated.

STEP 11

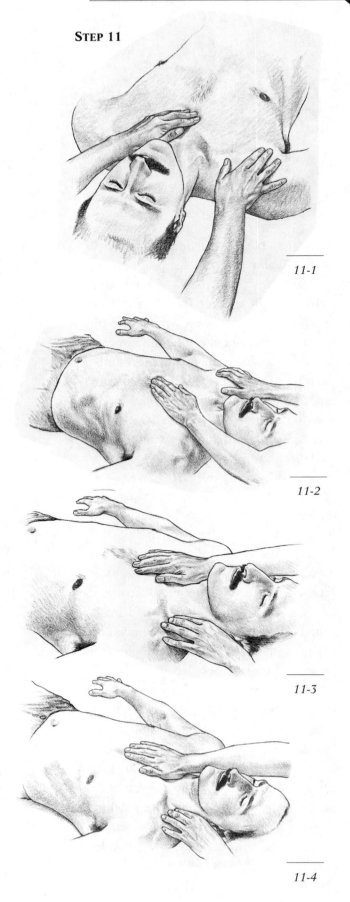

11-1

11-2

11-3

11-4

Step 11: Beginning with the left hand and using circular digital pressure, manipulate the sternum. Movement proceeds downward from the interclavicular notch to the xiphoid process. As you move inferiorly along the Conception Vessel, the movement includes both circular digital pressure and circular palmar pressure. This manipulation also affects portions of the Lung, Heart, and Heart Envelope Tendino-Muscle channels. Repeat with each hand three times, alternating hands.

As an alternate technique, begin with either the right or left hand and then, alternating hands, move down the sternum in small increments from the area directly below the interclavicular notch to the xiphoid process. Move with attention on the pads of the second, third, and fourth digits. The hands remain relaxed, moving one directly after another as the fingers execute the technique.

In both the classical Chinese and Hindu medical and philosophical systems, the emotional center resides in the chest. Oriental medicine traditionally regards the emotions as a primary cause of disease. In recent years Western medicine has begun to recognize that there is a strong emotional component in illness. This technique helps to move the energy down, moving it out of the emotional center, and thereby promotes emotional calming. Since manipulation of this area helps to release emotional tension, it may be repeated several times during the course of the treatment.

Step 12: Using circular digital pressure, treat the upper chest, beginning beside the sternum and working laterally to the shoulders in the intercostal spaces. Begin in the first space at the interclavicular notch. Work one side at a time, with the left hand manipulating the patient's left side and the right hand manipulating

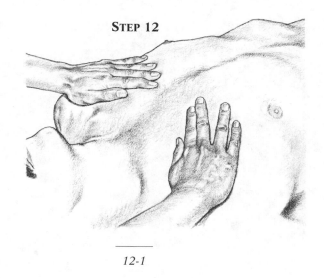

12-1

the patient's right side. Manipulation begins with one intercostal space at a time. The focus is on the pads of the digits, with as much of the palmar aspect of the fingers as possible resting in the intercostal spaces. The first move begins with the thumb resting on top of the clavicle and the index finger lying in the costoclavicular space. The two fingers gently grasp the clavicle. The focus is on the index finger while the thumb lightly assists along the top of the clavicle. (Be careful not to dig the thumb into the supraclavicular fossa).

A variation on this movement is to let the thumb rest on the clavicle and apply pressure only with the index finger. After this manipulation is repeated several times, the next intercostal space is manipulated with the focus on the second and third fingers together (depending, of course, on the size of the therapist's fingers and the width of the patient's intercostal spaces), and then is followed with manipulation between the third and fourth ribs. This sequence is repeated several times.

As an alternate technique, depending on the skill of the therapist and the structure and condition of the patient, the practitioner can treat all three intercostal spaces simultaneously, spreading the fingers so that the second, third, and fourth fingers rest within the respective intercostal spaces. In both cases the palmar aspect of all the fingers remains in contact with the chest. Care must be taken not to manipulate the breast tissue in female patients. In some women, this may mean that only the first or first and second intercostal spaces may be accessible. In that case, the technique first described is the preferable one to use.

The practitioner should be attentive to the patient's shoulders, which may be elevated. If one or both shoulders are elevated,

the therapist can slowly depress the shoulder with the heel of the palm of his or her opposite hand. Advanced therapists may use circular thumb pressure to relax the shoulder joint if the shoulder is raised. The Lung, Kidney, Stomach, and Spleen Primary channels are affected by this manipulation, as is the Conception Vessel. All of the Arm Yin Tendino-Muscle channels—the Lung, Heart, and Heart Envelope— enter into the upper chest, as do portions of the Stomach, Bladder, and Gall Bladder Tendino-Muscle channels. Manipulation of the sternum and chest is used clinically in the treatment of respiratory problems, such as coughs due to colds, allergies, asthma, bronchitis, and pneumonia. Cardiovascular problems, high and low blood pressure, and poor circulation can be treated through the Heart and Heart Envelope Tendino-Muscle channels. Stress-related digestive disorders can also be affected through release of muscle tension and emotions from the chest and by affecting portions of the Stomach and Gall Bladder Tendino-Muscle channels. These include sluggish digestion, irritable bowel syndrome, constipation, diarrhea, and colitis. In addition, relaxing the chest muscles is very helpful in correcting and restoring proper posture.

STEP 13

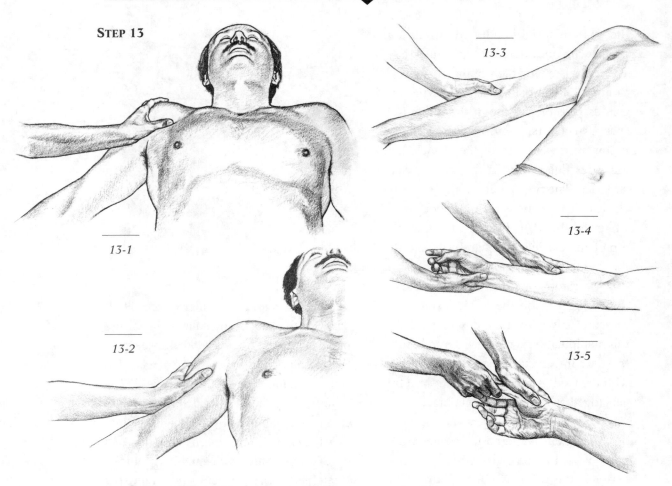

13-1

13-2

13-3

13-4

13-5

Step 13: Upon finishing the last manipulation of the intercostal spaces, move to a standing position at the patient's right side. Both hands must never leave the patient's body at the same time—one hand must always remain in contact with the patient's body. Therefore, a quick transition is made from the right hand to the left. Using circular digital pressure, the left hand moves in a counterclockwise direction, beginning in the Lung area of the pectoralis muscle distal to the clavicle and moving laterally to the shoulder. (This is an exception to the general rule of circular movement, in which the left hand moves in a clockwise direction.) When the fingers reach the deltopectoral groove, a switch is made to circular thumb pressure. The hand will naturally grasp the shoulder and arm in a palmar embrace. On the patient's left side, the therapist's right hand will move in a clockwise direction from the pectoralis to the shoulder, and then switch to circular thumb pressure.

With the patient's forearm supinated, gently support the patient's right wrist and hand with the palm of your right hand, and move down the arm between the anterior and the lateral middle deltoid. Work down the anterolateral aspect of the arm, securing the arm in a palmar embrace. Move down to and over the thenar eminence and over the thumb. Use circular thumb pressure with the focus on the pad of the left thumb. Repeat this manipulation five times.

An alternate technique is to manipulate a portion of the Lung Channel down to approximately the cubital crease and then return to the top of the shoulder. Manipulate the top of the shoulder from

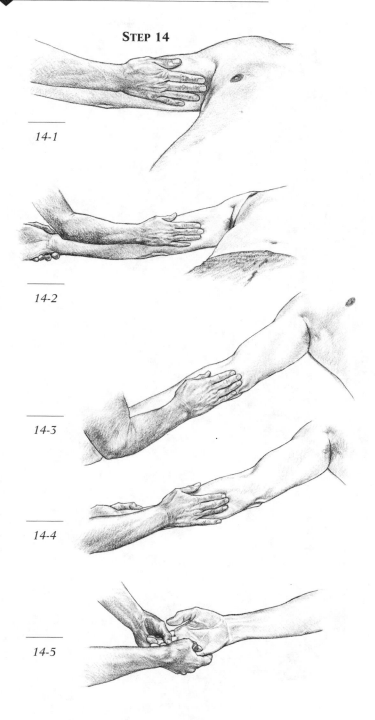

STEP 14

14-1

14-2

14-3

14-4

14-5

the neck to the acromion using circular digital pressure with the four fingers of the left hand. The right hand gently holds the patient's arm or wrist. After repeating this movement several times, the full length of the Lung Channel may also be manipulated several times. This is especially helpful for neck and shoulder problems. Manipulation to the top of the shoulder affects portions of all the Yang channels.

Treatment of the lateral chest and arm follows the pathways of the superficial and Tendino-Muscle Lung Channels and portions of the Spleen Primary Channel. Manipulation of these areas benefits the lungs and will treat respiratory problems, such as coughs due to colds or smoking, asthma, bronchitis, upper respiratory tract infections, and pneumonia. These manipulations are also beneficial for pinched nerve problems, arthritis, bursitis, and frozen shoulder.

Step 14: Gently support the patient's right hand in the palm of your left hand while slowly abducting the arm to open up the axilla region. Place your right palm on the medial surface of the supinated arm with the fingertips pointing into the axilla. Using circular palmar pressure in a clockwise direction, continue down the anteromedial portion of the arm to the wrist. The purpose of moving the palm toward the patient's body is to contain the energy of the Heart. As the patient's wrist area is approached, the gradual reduction in forearm width may necessitate the use of only three or two fingers, along with a change to using pressure from the palmar aspect of the fingers. Finally, change to circular thumb pressure at the pisiform bone and continue down the hypothenar eminence, moving between the fourth and fifth metacarpals and continuing to the radial side of the fifth digit.

This manipulation follows the superficial and Tendino-Muscle pathways of the Heart Channel. This technique will help to balance and strengthen the energies of the Heart. It is beneficial for relaxing patients who suffer from anxiety or depression and is also used in the treatment of cardiovascular problems, such as hypertension, poor circulation, palpitations, and insomnia.

STEP 15

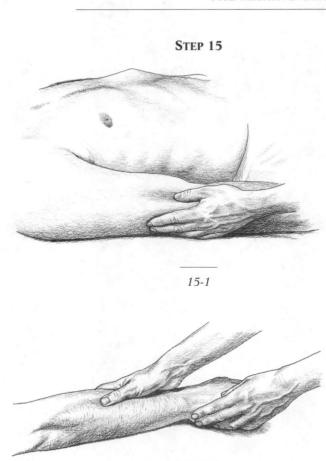

15-1

15-2

STEP 16

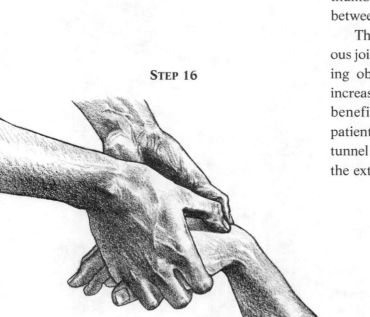

16-1

Step 15: Upon completion of the manipulation of the Heart Channel, gently pronate the patient's forearm. Using circular thumb pressure of the left hand, descend along the lateral arm from the shoulder to the elbow and then from the elbow to the wrist, manipulating between the brachioradialis and the wrist extensors. Repeat this manipulation five times.

This technique affects portions of the superficial pathway of the Primary Colon and San Jiao channels and portions of their Tendino-Muscle channels as well. It is effective in treating neck, shoulder, and elbow problems as well as removing energy obstructions from these channels. (Circular palmar pressure may be substituted from the shoulder to the elbow, switching to circular thumb pressure from the elbow to the wrist.)

Step 16: Use both hands to support the patient's hand; allow the patient's elbow to rest on the table. Using circular thumb pressure, manipulate the spaces between the carpal bones of the wrist.

This manipulation opens the numerous joint spaces of the hand, thereby freeing obstructions of Qi and Blood and increasing circulation, both of which are beneficial for all patients. This aids patients who suffer from arthritis, carpal tunnel syndrome, or poor circulation to the extremities, as in Raynaud's disease.

STEP 17

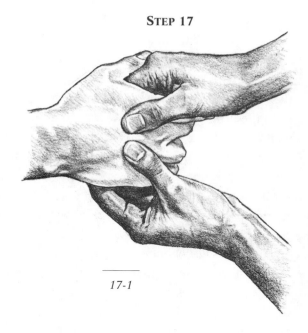

17-1

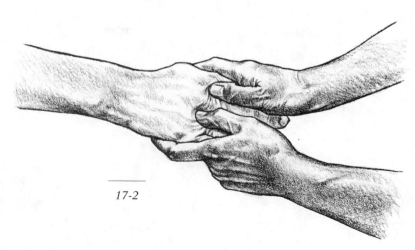

17-2

Step 17: Using circular thumb pressure, manipulate between the metacarpal bones of the hand, moving from the wrist to the metacarpophalangeal joints. Treat each space two or three times.

Step 18: Treatment of the hand ends with a manipulation of the anterior, posterior, medial, and lateral surfaces of each finger. The fingers are treated in the following order: third, fourth, second, fifth, and first digit.

The beginning and ending points of many channels are located in the fingers and toes. These are the areas where the energies of the Nutrient Cycle pass from Yin to Yang and from Yang to Yin. Manipulation of the fingers is important because it stimulates the circulation of Qi, Blood, and Fluids from channel to channel. Points in the fingers and toes can be used to affect areas that are located at opposite ends of the channels. This technique also serves to reduce swelling in the joints and is helpful for treating arthritis of the hands.

STEP 18

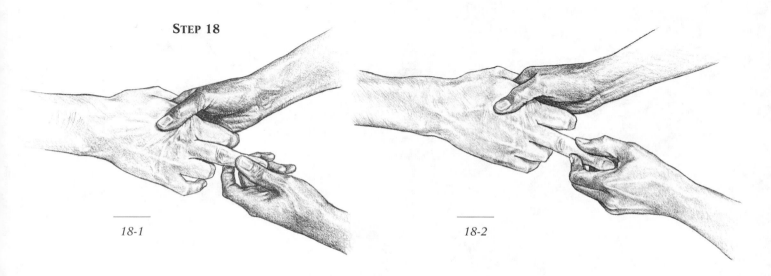

18-1

18-2

STEP 19

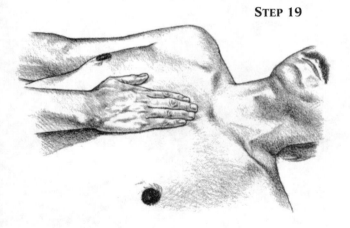

19-1

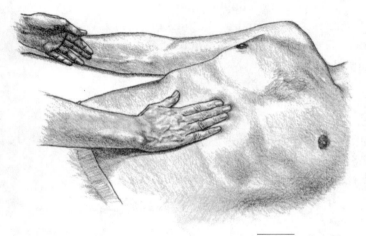
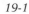

19-2

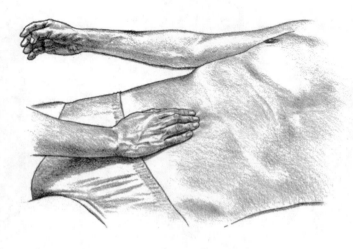

19-3

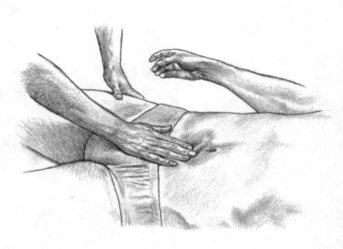

19-4

Step 19: Beginning with the fingertips at the interclavicular notch and using circular palmar pressure with the right hand, manipulate down the midline of the chest, lifting the heel of the palm so that the fingertips terminate approximately at the level of CV5 (2 tsun below the umbilicus). Repeat this technique five times.

This movement manipulates the energy of the Conception Vessel as well as the Heart, Heart Envelope, and Lung Tendino-Muscle channels and portions of the Stomach, Spleen, Liver, and Kidney Tendino-Muscle pathways. The Conception Vessel is considered to be the storehouse of all Yin energies; all the Yin channels flow along the anterior of the body, as does the Stomach Channel, considered to be the most Yin of all the Yang channels. This technique helps to release tension in the chest and calm the emotions by stimulating the flow of Qi, Blood, and Fluids toward the tan tien.

Step 20: Place both thumbs on either side of the sterno-xiphoid junction. Using circular thumb pressure, manipulate bilaterally down and along the edges of the rib cage, stopping at the eleventh floating ribs.

This manipulation stimulates the energies of the Stomach, Spleen, Kidney, Liver, and Gall Bladder Primary channels, as well as the Tendino-Muscle channels of the Stomach, Spleen, and Gall Bladder. This technique also helps to relax and release the abdominal muscles and assists in the process of digestion.

Step 21: Returning to the chest, place both hands down with the fingers at the level of the sterno-xiphoid junction. Beginning with the right hand and using a combination of circular palmar and circular digital pressure, move laterally across the lower rib cage with the pads of the fingers in the intercostal spaces. The technique ends at the midaxillary line in the area of Sp21. Alternate hands and repeat five times.

An alternate technique is to place the palm of the left hand across the patient's right lower rib cage, with the lateral edge of the hand resting on the tenth rib. The right hand supports the right side of the body. Move laterally using circular palmar pressure. When the practitioner treats the left side of the body, the right palm is used across the left lower rib cage and the left hand supports the body.

This manipulation stimulates the energies of the Stomach, Spleen, Kidney, Liver, and Gall Bladder Primary channels, as well as the Tendino-Muscle pathways of the Stomach, Spleen, and Gall Bladder. Liver Qi is often obstructed in the Middle Burner, and this interferes with proper assimilation of foods and

STEP 20

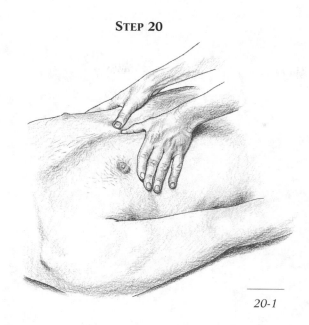

20-1

digestion. Manipulation of this area assists in digestion, the elimination of toxins, and the smooth flow of nutritive substances. In addition, Stagnant Liver Qi is a primary cause of increased emotionality and illness. Smooth and free-flowing Liver Qi is essential for emotional well-being.

STEP 21

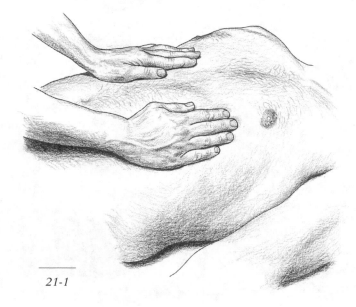

21-1

STEP 22

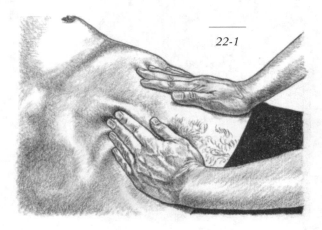

22-1

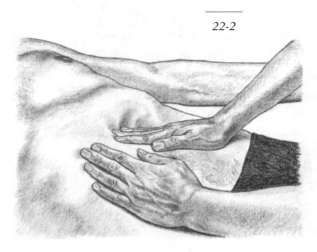

22-2

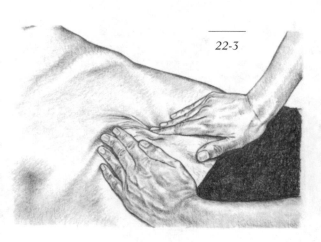

22-3

Step 22: Place both hands on the abdomen, with the fingertips inferior to the lower ribs and the whole hand maintaining contact. Using palmar embrace and alternating hands, manipulate the abdomen. Movement begins with the heel of the palm of the left hand performing a rolling motion from the palm to the fingers. The motion is then transferred to the right fingers and then to the right palm-heel. This technique imitates the movement of the colonic contents from the ascending colon on the patient's right side to the transverse colon and finally to the descending colon on the left side. It is useful for treating abdominal pain and distention, digestive stagnation, and other dysfunctions of the Colon, Spleen, and Stomach, such as flatulence, indigestion, constipation, irritable bowel syndrome, and diarrhea.

An alternate technique is to massage the colon with circular palmar and circular digital pressure, up the ascending colon, across the transverse colon, and then down the descending colon. The movement begins with the left hand and transfers to the right hand at approximately the midline of the abdomen. This manipulation is beneficial for stimulating peristaltic activity in patients who can tolerate deeper manipulation and who suffer from constipation. If the patient suffers from diarrhea, the manipulation can be done in reverse, going up the descending colon, across the transverse colon, and down the ascending colon. This facilitates reabsorption of fluids by slowing down peristaltic activity.

Step 23: Placing the hands with the fingertips at both axillas, manipulate down the coronal plane to the hips. As the movement proceeds, the pads of the fingers should be emphasized more than the palm.

This manipulation stimulates the Sp21 area and portions of the Spleen,

Bladder, and Gall Bladder Tendino-Muscle channels. Sp21 is a special point that influences all of the Blood Connecting Channels and helps to facilitate Qi and Blood flow. Manipulation of this area also helps to open up and relax the chest.

Step 24: Upon completion of the manipulation of the coronal plane, place your left hand on the anterolateral portion of the patient's right thigh. Support the medial thigh or the lower leg with the right hand. Beginning with the fingers of the left hand at the level of the anterior superior iliac spine, use circular palmar pressure to manipulate the thigh, moving distally from the hip to the knee. Repeat five times.

Manipulation of this area relaxes the large muscles of the anterolateral thigh, which includes portions of the sartorius, rectus femoris, vastus intermedius, and vastus lateralis. This stimulates the circulation of Blood, Qi, and Fluids to the thigh and lower leg. This technique is helpful for hip and knee dysfunctions due to injury or arthritis, as well as poor circulation to the lower extremities. Since the Gall Bladder and Stomach Tendino-Muscle channels and the superficial aspects of the Stomach Channel move through this portion of the thigh, manipulation of these pathways helps to remove obstructions and stagnations of Qi, Blood, and Fluids and can improve and benefit digestion. It can also help in a wide range of gastrointestinal disturbances.

STEP 23

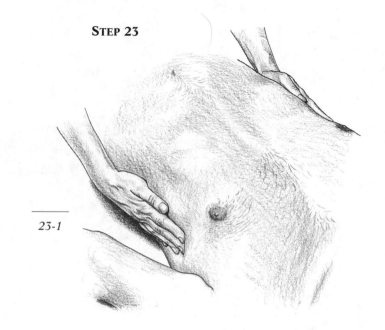

23-1

STEP 24

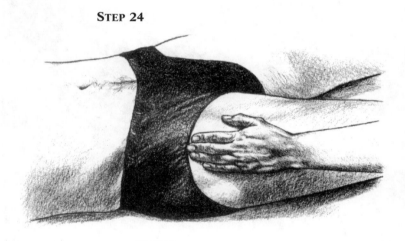

24-1

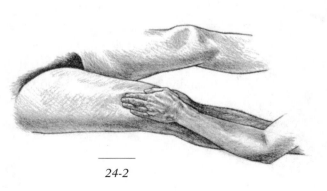

24-2

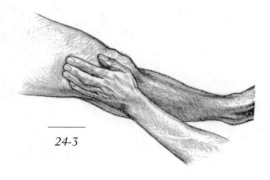

24-3

STEP 25

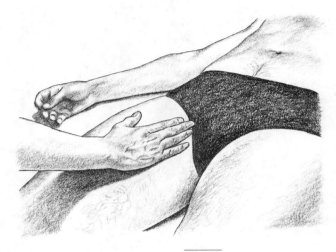

25-1

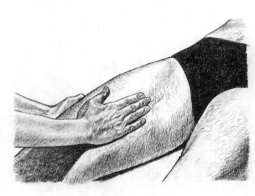

25-2

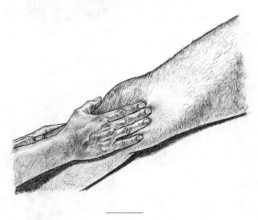

25-3

Step 25: Support the lateral aspect of the thigh with the left hand. Using circular palmar pressure with the right hand, manipulate the medial aspect of the thigh from the groin to the medial knee. This manipulation begins with the finger pads at the area of Liv10–Liv11, with the middle finger resting on the tendon of the gracilis muscle. If the tendon feels unusually tight, the edge of the hand may be used in a back and forth rocking motion to release the tension and relax the tendon.

Manipulation here affects portions of the adductor longus and adductor magnus, gracilis, vastus medialis, and the distal portion of the sartorius. Treatment in this area facilitates the drainage of lymphatic fluid through the inguinal lymph nodes. This is important for cleansing and circulating tissue fluids and blood and therefore is helpful to patients suffering with systemic acute and chronic infections, genitourinary tract infections, menstrual problems, and circulatory problems related to the lower limbs.

This technique treats the Tendino-Muscle and superficial aspects of the Liver and Spleen channels and therefore helps to unblock stagnated Liver and Spleen Qi. The Liver is responsible for the free flow of Qi, Blood, and Fluids throughout the body. The Spleen is called the Source of Blood because it provides the vital components that make up the Blood. In addition, it helps to transform and transport the Qi, Blood, and Fluids throughout the body. Stimulating and balancing the energies of both the Liver and Spleen channels is essential for encouraging a state of health and vitality.

STEP 26

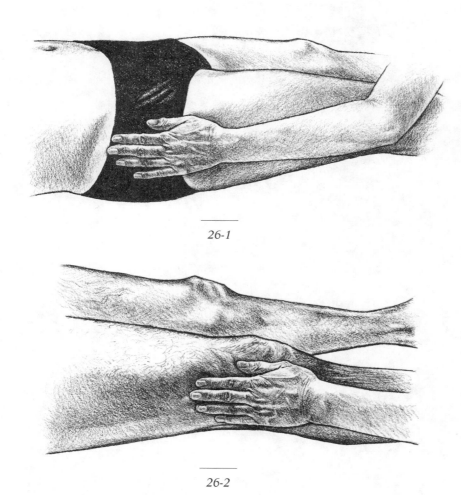

26-1

26-2

Step 26: Using circular palmar pressure with the left hand, manipulate the lateral portion of the hip and thigh down to the knee. Begin lateral to the anterior superior iliac spine, on the coronal plane of the body. Support the medial leg with the right hand. Repeat five times.

Manipulation of this area relaxes the tensor fascia latae, the iliotibial tract, and the vastus lateralis. Portions of the Tendino-Muscle and superficial aspects of the Gall Bladder Channel as well as portions of the Stomach and Bladder Tendino-Muscle channels lie in this area. This technique will treat arthritic problems of the hip, knee, and lower leg, as well as digestive dysfunctions.

STEP 27

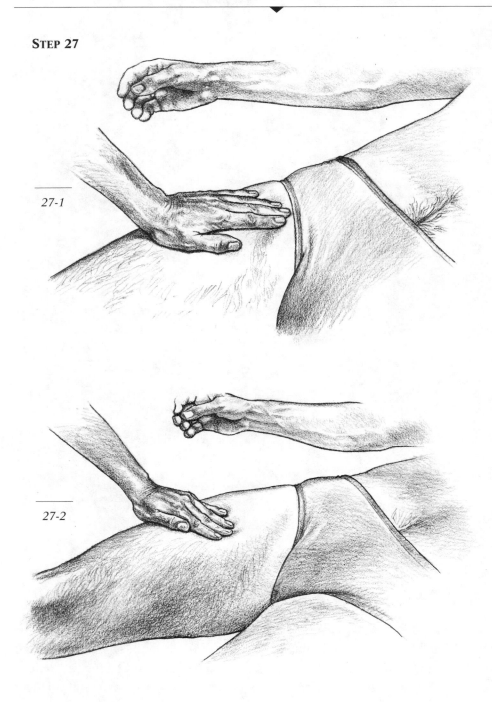

27-1

27-2

Step 27: Support the medial leg with the right hand. Beginning with the left hand at the ASIS and using circular palmar pressure, follow the course of the sartorius muscle down to its insertion at the medial aspect of the tibia. The hand begins at the hip on the anterolateral aspect of the body with the fingers facing superiorly. Manipulation of this muscle ends at the medial knee with the fingers directed inferiorly. As the hand moves down the thigh following the course of the sartorius muscle, it rotates at mid-thigh, using the heel of the palm as its point of rotation. The

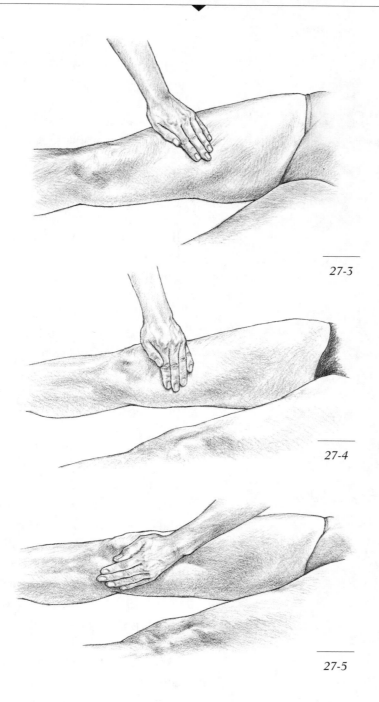

27-3

27-4

27-5

practitioner will need to turn his body toward the patient's feet in order to complete this manipulation.

The sartorius, the longest muscle of the body, crosses both the hip and the knee, two major joints of the lower extremities. The manipulation and relax- ation of this muscle affects the Tendino-Muscle channels of the Stomach, Spleen, Liver, and Kidney. This technique helps to circulate obstructed or stagnated Qi, Blood, and Fluids and is beneficial in the treatment of joint dysfunctions and problems affecting the lower extremities.

STEP 28

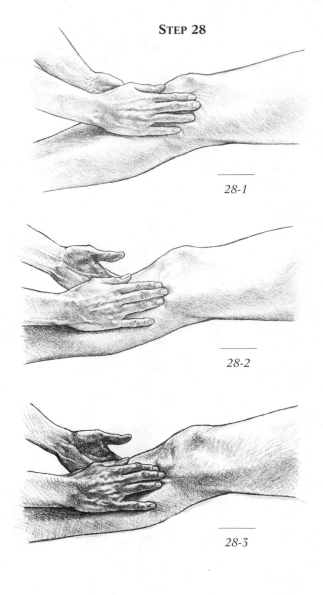

28-1

28-2

28-3

STEP 29

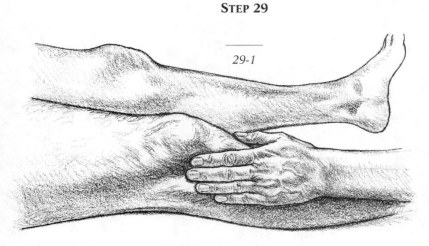

29-1

Step 28: Using circular digital pressure with the right hand, manipulate the medial knee, moving from the area superior to the medial epicondyle of the femur to the area just distal to the medial condyle of the tibia. The insertions of the sartorius, gracilis, semimembranosus, and semitendinosus muscles are manipulated. Repeat five times.

The treatment of this area promotes the free flow of synovial fluid within the knee joint. Because of its weight-bearing function, the knee is one of the most easily injured joints and often the site of arthritic changes. Therefore the circulation of Qi, Blood, and Fluids at this joint is extremely important. This technique primarily affects the Liver, Spleen, and Kidney Tendino-Muscle channels.

Step 29: This motion is now repeated on the lateral side of the knee. Supporting the medial leg with the right hand, use circular digital pressure with the left hand to manipulate the lateral aspect of the knee joint. Manipulation of the lateral knee relaxes and stimulates portions of the vastus lateralis and tensor fascia latae, and portions of the patellar ligament. This technique also affects the Stomach, Gall Bladder, and Bladder Tendino-Muscle channels. Repeat five times.

As an alternate technique, the area surrounding the patella can also be manipulated with the thumbs, using them to reach gently but firmly into the joint spaces. In addition, the practitioner can support the knee with the right hand and use the right thumb to manipulate the lateral side of the knee. Support the knee with the left hand and use the left thumb to treat the medial side.

Step 30: Supporting the leg with the right hand and using circular digital or circular palmar pressure with the left, manipulate the lower leg beginning at the lateral condyle of the tibia and following the lateral aspect of the tibia down to the lateral malleolus. Repeat five times.

The manipulation of this area follows the tibialis anterior and the extensor digitorum longus muscles. This improves the circulation of Qi, Blood, and Fluids to the foot and ankle. The ankle is an area that is easily injured and where Qi can be easily obstructed. This manipulation affects the Stomach Primary Channel and the Stomach, Gall Bladder, and Bladder Tendino-Muscle channels.

STEP 30

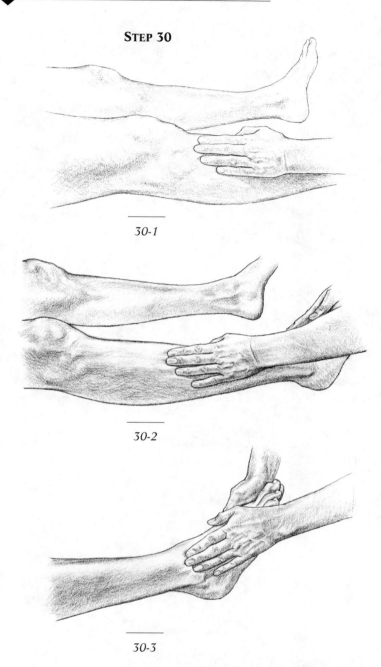

30-1

30-2

30-3

STEP 31

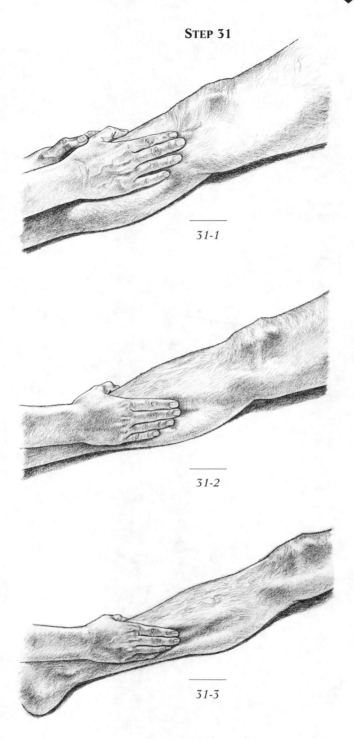

31-1

31-2

31-3

Step 31: Manipulate the medial aspect of the lower leg from the head of the tibia to the medial malleolus, using circular digital pressure with the right hand. Support the leg with the left hand. This affects the energies of the Spleen, Kidney, and Liver Primary and Tendino-Muscle channels. Points along these pathways are used to treat a wide range of digestive, menstrual, and genitourinary disorders. Repeat five times.

An alternate technique is to start with the left hand on the medial knee, with fingers pointing toward the table. Using circular digital pressure, rotate down to the ankle. The foot is held gently but firmly with the right hand to keep it stabilized.

Step 32: Using circular digital pressure with the left hand while supporting the foot with the right, manipulate around the lateral malleolus. Begin at the calcaneus and move distally toward the toes. Rotate around the medial malleolus in the same way, using the right hand while supporting the foot with the left hand. Repeat the manipulation of each side five times.

Portions of the superficial pathway and Tendino-Muscle channels of the Bladder and Gall Bladder surround the outer ankle, while portions of the superficial pathway and Tendino-Muscle Channel of the Kidney surround the medial aspect of the ankle. Manipulation of these areas is useful in the treatment of genitourinary dysfunctions, lower back pain, and local problems of the foot and ankle.

Step 33: Support the plantar surface of the foot with the palm of the right hand. Using circular digital pressure with the left hand, manipulate the dorsal surface of the foot from the ankle to the toes. The hands may be switched if that is more confortable. Work between the tarsal bones and between the metatarsals. Complete the movement with a manipulation of each toe, following the third-fourth-second-fifth-first pattern used with the treatment of the fingers in step 18.

STEP 32

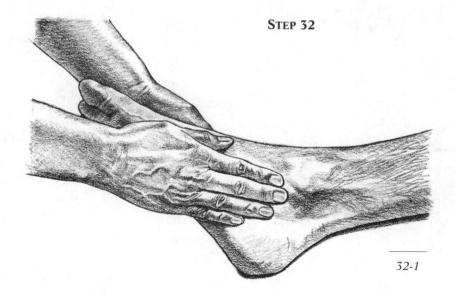

32-1

An alternate technique is to place the two thumbs together at the dorsum of the ankle joint while gently grasping the foot on both sides with the remainder of the hands. Use a stroking motion with the two thumbs, stroking down the top of the foot to the toes.

Portions of the superficial and Tendino-Muscle pathways of the Bladder, Gall Bladder, Stomach, Liver, and Spleen channels flow through the dorsum of the foot. Energy pathways transform from Yin to Yang and from Yang to Yin at the toes, providing for the continuous flow of energy in the Nutrient Cycle.

Manipulation of the feet and toes is beneficial for a wide range of disorders, including digestive dysfunctions; genitourinary problems; headaches; neck and shoulder problems; eye, ear, nose, and throat problems; vertigo; hypertension; anxiety; depression; seizures; and local problems of the feet.

STEP 33

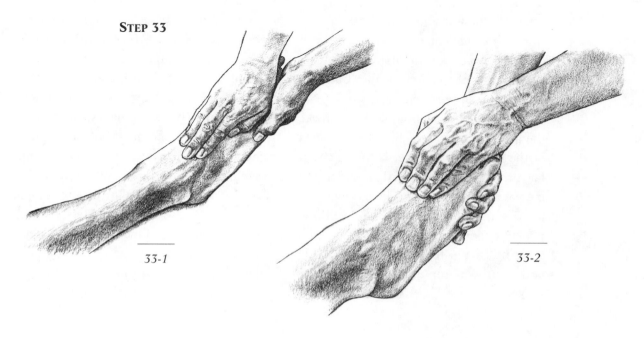

33-1

33-2

STEP 34

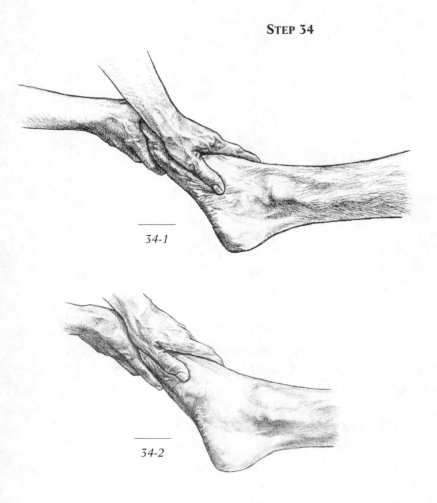

34-1

34-2

Step 34: Using thumb stroking with the left hand, stroke over the medial aspect of the foot. Begin at the area inferior to the medial malleolus and work distally toward the great toe, following the contour of the arch of the foot. The right hand supports the foot.

An alternate technique is to stroke the arch of the foot using all the fingers of the left hand. Another is to use circular thumb pressure starting under the medial malleolus and working down past the first metatarsophalangeal joint. If the patient's foot should begin to spasm, go underneath the foot to the soft muscle and gently manipulate to release the spasm. If the calf muscle is in spasm,

raise the foot and gently press with your thumb along the tibialis anterior.

This movement follows portions of the superficial pathways of the Spleen and Kidney channels and is used to treat gastrointestinal problems, blood sugar imbalances, genitourinary conditions, and back pain.

Step 35: This completes the treatment of the right side of the body. Step to the left side of the patient to begin manipulation of the Lung Channel. Perform steps 13 through 34 on the patient's left side, reversing hand directions when necessary.

Step 36: Return to the head of the table and repeat steps 1 through 10 in an abbreviated fashion, using less repetitions of each stroke.

This completes the treatment of the supine patient. The patient then turns over to a prone position and the treatment continues with the manipulation of the upper back. The practitioner begins from a seated position at the head of the patient.

Step 37: Begin with the hands resting upon the shoulders, the thumbs lying on both sides of the C7/T1 area. Starting with the right thumb and using circular thumb pressure, manipulate from the C7/T1 area laterally to the acromioclavicular joint. The manipulation is directed across the top of the shoulders in the belly of the upper trapezius. Repeat this manipulation five times. While the right hand rests, the manipulation is repeated on the opposite side with the left thumb.

A second line of manipulation begins also at the C7/T1 area and moves laterally along the superior border of the spine of the scapula, ending again at the acromio-

STEP 37

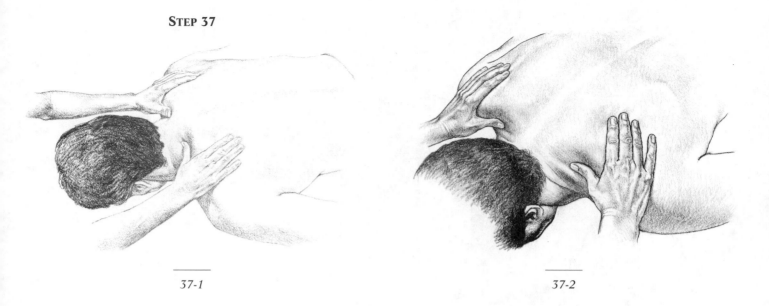

37-1   *37-2*

clavicular joint. In both techniques the focus is on the thumb, which is supported (but not dominated) by arm motion and strength. An alternate technique is to use the palmar embrace across the top of the shoulders. Repeat five times.

Manipulation of this area relaxes and facilitates the release of the upper trapezius muscle and helps to treat shoulder and neck tension, upper back pain, headaches, arthralgia, and bursitis. All the Yang Primary channels, either deep or superficially, pass through the shoulder area and are stimulated by this technique. The area is also energized by portions of the Colon, Small Intestine, Bladder, San Jiao, and Gall Bladder Tendino-Muscle pathways.

Step 38: Manipulate from C7/T1 down to the level of T3 at the root of the spine of the scapula, using circular thumb pressure and alternating thumbs. Repeat five times.

A very important Governing Vessel point, GV14, is located between C7 and T1. All of the Yang channels converge at this point. Manipulation of this area will

help to stimulate and remove energetic obstructions in these pathways. These obstructions are often reflected in people who suffer with dowager's hump. Treatment of this area helps to relieve neck and shoulder tension and pain, upper back pain, headaches, cervical arthritis, and neuralgia.

STEP 38

38-1

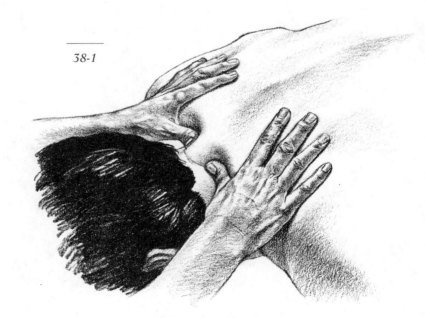

STEP 39

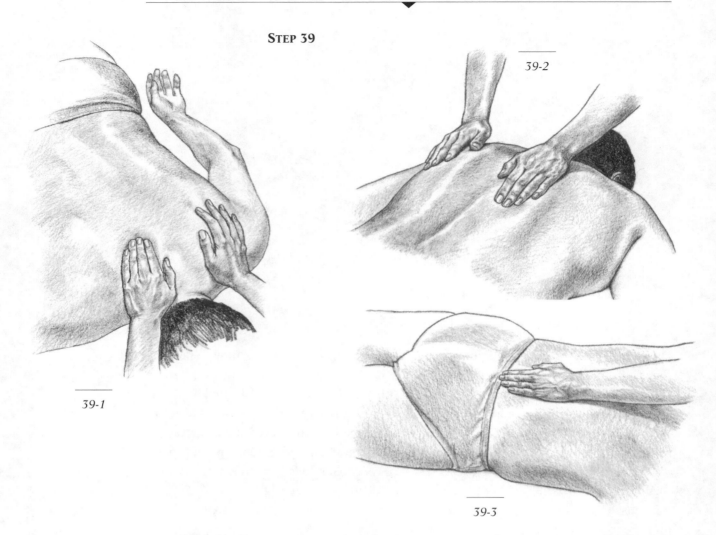

39-1

39-2

39-3

Step 39: Work the muscles of the back from the C7/T1 area down to the posterior superior iliac spine, beginning with circular digital pressure and changing to circular palmar pressure. This manipulation follows the two superficial pathways of the Primary Bladder Channel, each running parallel to the spine. The first pathway lies approximately one inch lateral to the spine and the second pathway lies approximately two inches lateral to the spine, following the medial border of the scapula. The manipulation may be done using alternating hands, beginning with the more medial pathway and followed by the lateral pathway. The manipulation begins with the focus on the palms but increasing emphasis can be placed on the movement of the fingers as the patient's back muscles relax. Repeat the manipulation of each pathway five times.

The major muscles of the back, including the trapezius, the latissimus dorsi, the rhomboids, and the erector spinae group (the spinalis, longissimus, and iliocostalis), are affected by this technique. This manipulation covers a large portion of both the superficial and Tendino-Muscle pathways of the Bladder Channel and portions of the Stomach, Colon, and Small Intestine Tendino-Muscle channels. The treatment of this area is useful for conditions such as back pain, neck pain, headaches, genitourinary dysfunction, and respiratory and cardio-vascular problems.

Step 40: Beginning with circular digital pressure of the right hand and changing to circular palmar pressure, follow the vertebral border of the patient's right scapula, moving from the spine of the scapula around the inferior angle toward the area of Sp21 on the coronal plane. The motion may then be carried down the coronal plane toward the end of the rib cage. The practitioner may switch to the left hand to proceed down the coronal plane. This series of movements is then repeated on the left side, with the left hand working around the patient's left scapula and switching to the right hand, if necessary, for the movement down the coronal plane. Repeat each side five times.

An alternate technique is to complete both movements around the right and left scapula respectively and then move down both coronal planes together. If this is difficult to do from the head of the table, the practitioner may step to one side of the table to complete the movements.

This technique relaxes the trapezius, latissimus dorsi, rhomboids, and serratus anterior muscles. The treatment of these muscles helps to alleviate headaches, neck and shoulder tensions and pain, and upper backache. In addition, the treatment of the Upper Jiao from the posterior position will benefit patients suffering from respiratory and cardiovascular problems. This manipulation covers portions of the Small Intestine, Spleen, Gall Bladder, and Bladder Tendino-Muscle pathways.

STEP 40

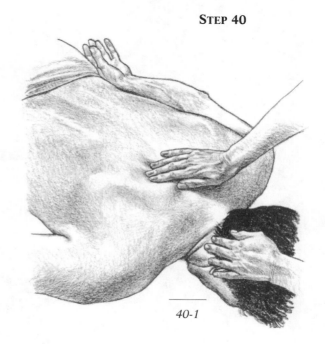

40-1

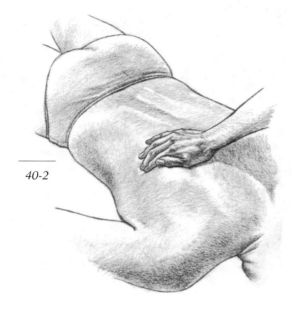

40-2

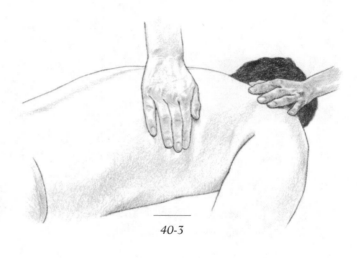

40-3

STEP 41

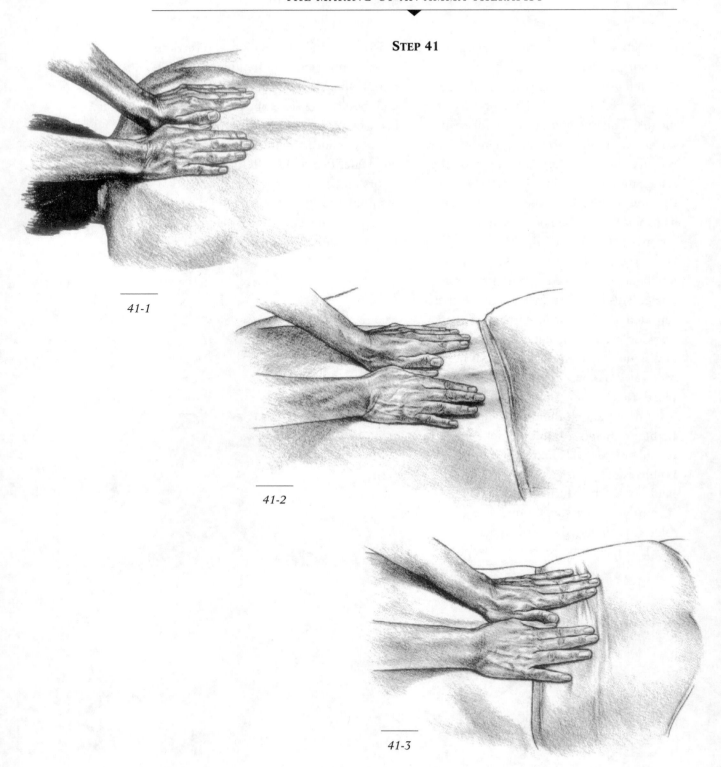

41-1

41-2

41-3

Step 41: Using palmar stroking, simultaneously and with both hands stroke from the level of C7/T1 to the posterior superior iliac spine. When the palms reach the PSIS, both heels rotate over the gluteus medius and the hands move up the coronal plane. The stroke ends as the hands return to the lateral borders of the scapula. Repeat several times, using a continuous flowing motion.

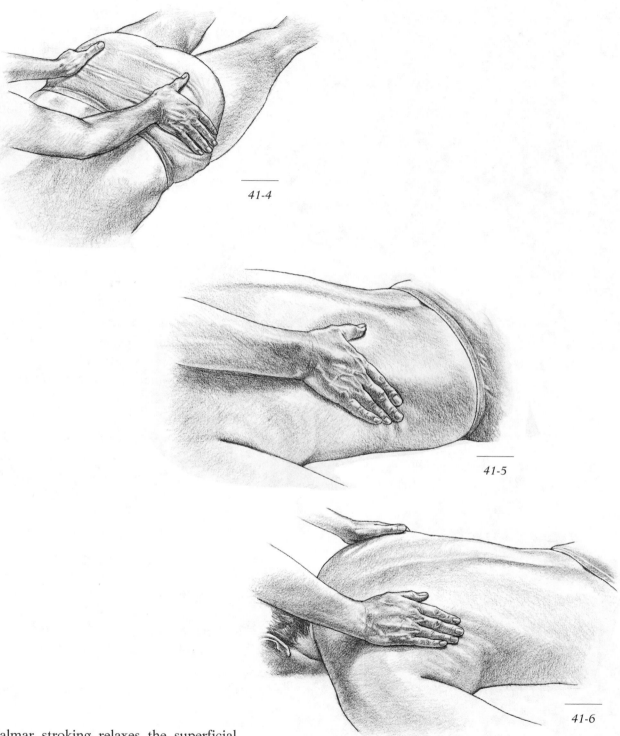

41-4

41-5

41-6

Palmar stroking relaxes the superficial musculature and helps to soothe and calm the patient.

STEP 42

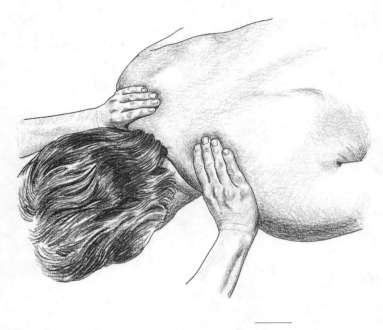

42-1

STEP 43

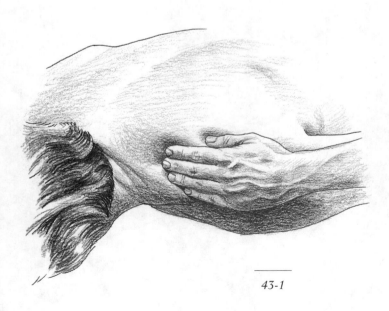

43-1

Step 42: Beginning with palmar embrace and ending with thenar embrace, work along the top of the shoulders, moving the hands from the medial aspect of the shoulder at the base of the neck to the acromioclavicular articulation and the head of the humerus. Both hands may work together or the motion may be done separately on each side. Repeat five times.

This manipulation helps to release tension in the trapezius muscle and is of great benefit to patients suffering from neck and shoulder pain, as well as arthralgia or arthritis in the cervical and shoulder region or bursitis in the shoulders. This manipulation covers portions of the Colon, Stomach, Small Intestine, Bladder, San Jiao, and Gall Bladder Primary channels, as well as portions of the Colon, Small Intestine, Bladder, San Jiao, and Gall Bladder Tendino-Muscle channels.

Step 43: On the last embrace to the shoulders, step to the patient's left side. Switching to circular digital pressure with the left hand, manipulate over the top of the shoulder from the neck to the acromioclavicular articulation. Repeat five times. The right hand rests gently on the patient's back.

As an alternate technique and for a deeper manipulation, switch from circular digital pressure to circular thumb pressure by gently grasping the patient's shoulder, fingers pointing toward the clavicle as the thumb works across the top of the belly of the trapezius muscle.

Step 44: On the last manipulation the motion is continued down the posterior upper arm, moving from the deltoid and the triceps down to the elbow. Continue to manipulate around the elbow with the thumb or all four fingers. Continue the manipulation down the forearm using either your thumb or four fingers. The technique ends with stroking to the patient's metacarpal joints. Repeat five times. This serves to open up the circulation of Qi, Blood, and Fluids to this very important joint area. This technique covers portions of the Small Intestine and San Jiao Primary and Tendino-Muscle channels.

Step 45: Place the hand on the medial aspect of the upper arm, fingers pointing to the axilla. Using circular palmar pressure, manipulate moving distally toward the elbow. If the patient's arm is very tense and is resting palm down, turn your hand perpendicularly so that the palmar aspect of your fingers proceeds down the medial aspect of the upper arm. These techniques affect portions of the Heart and Heart Envelope superficial and Tendino-Muscle channels.

STEP 44

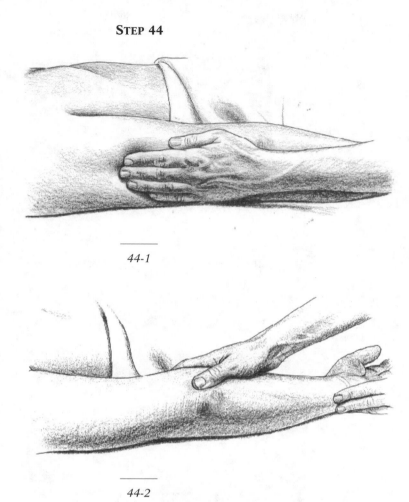

44-1

44-2

STEP 45

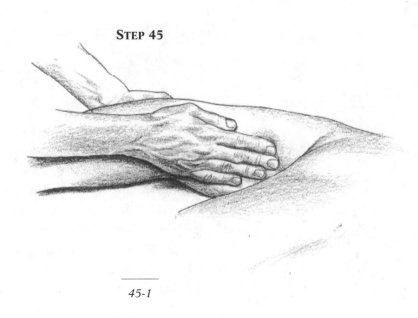

45-1

STEP 46

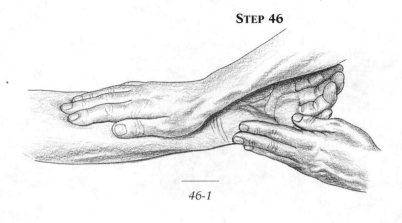

46-1

STEP 47

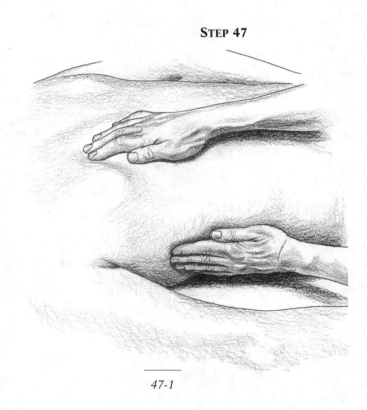

47-1

Step 46: Continue the manipulation down the forearm using either your thumb or your four fingers. The technique ends with stroking to the patient's fingers in the same third-fourth-second-fifth-first sequence. Repeat five times.

This manipulation covers portions of the Lung, Heart, and Heart Envelope Primary and Tendino-Muscle channels.

Manipulation of the fingers helps to keep the movement of the energy free-flowing.

Step 47: Rest your left hand at the Sp21 area and manipulate down the Bladder Channel with your right hand from the neck to the sacrum, using circular digital and circular palmar pressure. Maintain palmar contact throughout the stroke.

This manipulation encourages further stimulation of Qi, Blood, and Fluids of the back and opens up the circulation of the Bladder Primary and Tendino-Muscle channels. It also releases muscular tension of the back. Portions of the Colon, Small Intestine, and Stomach Tendino-Muscle channels are also stimulated.

Step 48: Beginning with the middle finger inferior to the inferior angle of the scapula, manipulate down the intercostals using circular digital pressure with your right hand along the belly of the latissimus dorsi to the floating ribs, raising your palm as you approach the last rib. Continue this movement until you reach the waist. Be careful not to dig your fingers into the rib area. If your hand starts to tire you may use your left hand, supporting the patient with your right hand on the right side of the patient's back. Repeat five times.

This technique provides for continued stimulation of Qi, Blood, and Fluids of the back by opening up the circulation of the Tendino-Muscle Bladder Channel and portions of the Small Intestine and Stomach Tendino-Muscle channels and releasing muscular tension and spasms of the back.

Step 49: Place your two thumbs together on the left side of the spine, beginning one thumb space from the spine at the area of T12. Proceed down to the sacrum using circular thumb pressure. Repeat several times, then return to the T12 area. Move your thumbs laterally an additional space (one thumb width) and repeat the movement, with one thumb slightly above the other. Repeat several times.

An alternate technique is to place your two thumbs together and, depending on the size of the musculature, use either the whole thumb or only the edges of the thumb. Gently stretch the muscle laterally between the two thumbs and continue working down in one-inch increments toward the sacrum. If a spasm is found, stay on that area, concentrating your motion there and encouraging release.

This manipulation emphasizes the lower back area. As the back simultaneously provides support and flexibility, it is easily susceptible to injury through strain, sprain, and trauma. Lower back pain is also a symptom of energy imbalances in the system, which can be alleviated through the techniques applied to this area. The Bladder Primary and Tendino-Muscle channels energize this area, as does a portion of the Stomach Tendino-Muscle Channel.

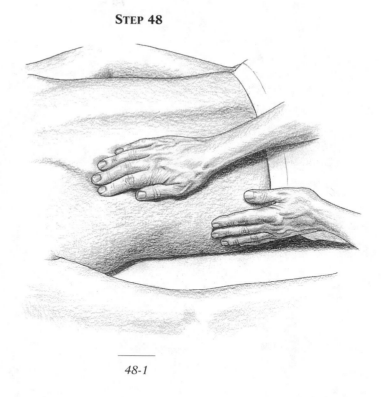

48-1

Step 50: Place both palms directly below the ribs on either side, fingers pointing laterally, and stroke across the lower back. Both sides of the back can be done from this position. Repeat five times.

STEP 49

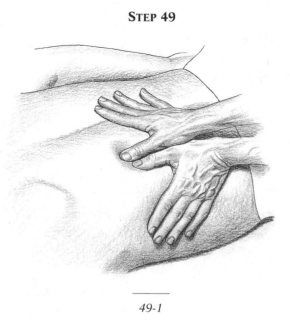

49-1

STEP 50

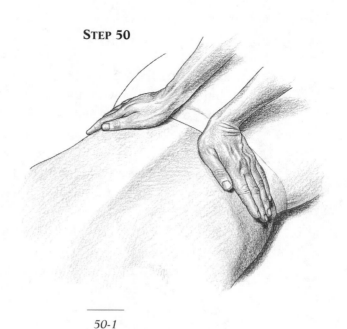

50-1

Step 51

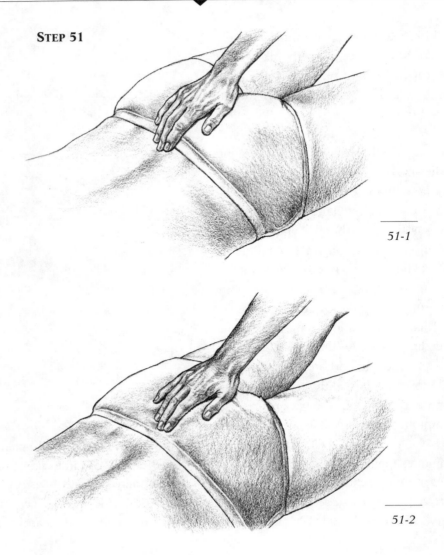

51-1

51-2

Step 51: From the patient's left side, manipulate the sacral area using circular digital pressure with the right hand. Since the spinal cord ends at the level of L2, some pressure can be applied to the midline sacral area. From the superior border of the sacrum work down to the end of the sacrum, raising the palm slightly as you move down. The right hand works the patient's left side. Repeat five times.

There is a concentration of Bladder energy in the sacral area, which contains sixteen Bladder points. Governing Vessel energy is also present, since the Governing Vessel travels the posterior midline of the body from the perineum through the sacral area to the spine. Portions of the Bladder and Gall Bladder Tendino-Muscle channels also energize this area. Manipulation of the sacral region treats back problems, bladder and kidney problems, prostate and menstrual dysfunctions, and constipation.

Step 52: Using circular digital pressure with the left hand, begin at the level of the posterior superior iliac spine and move laterally in an arc across the iliac crest, over the gluteus medius to the hip, around the greater trochanter, and down

STEP 52

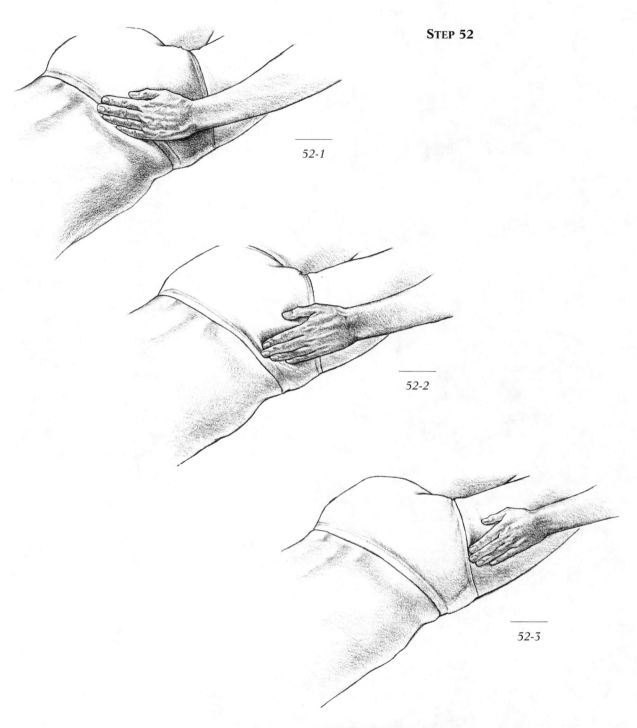

52-1

52-2

52-3

the iliotibial tract to the level of the gluteal crease. The left hand works the patient's left side while the right hand supports, resting on the back of the thigh. Repeat five times.

Manipulation of this area will relax the muscles and facilitate the movement of energy in the Bladder and Gall Bladder Primary and Tendino-Muscle channels. It will also affect a portion of the Stomach Tendino-Muscle Channel. This movement is beneficial for treating hip and lower back problems. It also has a positive affect on genitourinary dysfunctions.

STEP 53

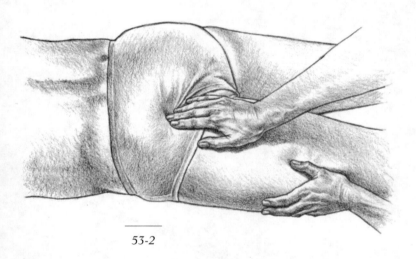

53-1

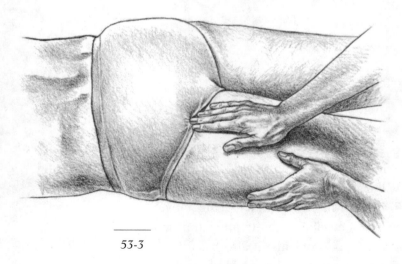

53-2

Step 53: Supporting the thigh with the left hand, use circular digital pressure with the right hand to manipulate the gluteus maximus from the posterior superior iliac spine to the center of the gluteal crease. The right hand works the patient's left side. Repeat five times.

The manipulation of the gluteal area relieves muscle tension in the buttock. It relaxes the lumbar area and treats the upper portion of the hamstrings, allowing for relaxation of the upper thigh. People suffering from genitourinary problems as well as degenerative joint disease of the hip will also benefit.

The energies of the Bladder and Gall Bladder Primary and Tendino-Muscle channels are stimulated with this movement. The treatment of the sacral area and posterior buttock helps to free stagnant energy, which often occurs in the Lower Jiao. It also increases the circulation of Qi, Blood, and Fluids to the lower extremities.

53-3

Step 54: Using circular palmar pressure with the left hand, treat the lateral aspect of the thigh from the greater trochanter of the femur down the iliotibial tract to the knee joint. Support the patient's medial thigh with the right hand as the left hand works down the coronal plane. Repeat five times.

This movement relaxes the tensor fasciae latae, iliotibial tract, and vastus lateralis muscle. It manipulates a portion of the Gall Bladder Primary and Tendino-Muscle channels and a portion of the Bladder and Stomach Tendino-Muscle channels. It will treat hip, thigh, and knee problems, including sciatica, and help to remove obstructions of Qi, Blood, and Fluids in the channels.

STEP 54

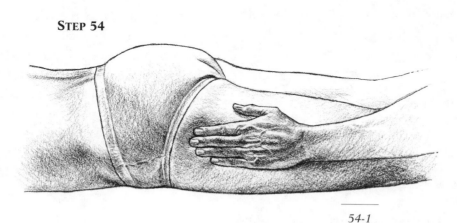

54-1

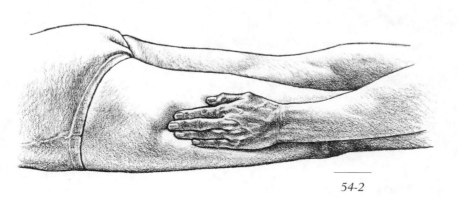

54-2

54-3

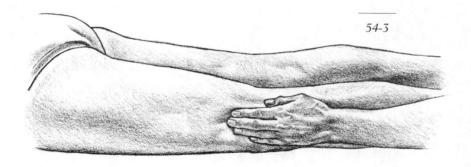

STEP 55

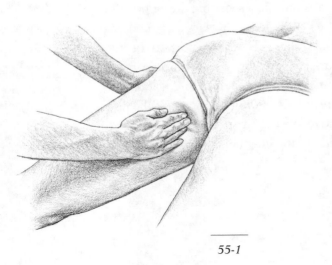

55-1

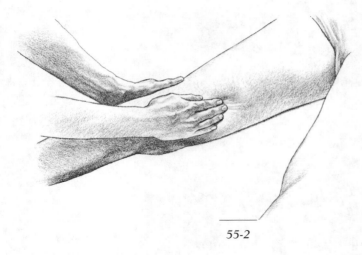

55-2

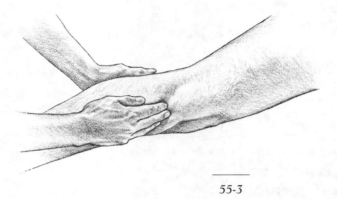

55-3

Step 55: Using circular palmar pressure with the right hand, manipulate the medial aspect of the thigh from the groin to the knee. Repeat five times.

Treatment of this area relaxes the semitendinosus and semimembranosus muscles (two of the three muscles of the hamstring group), as well as portions of the gracilis and the adductor magnus muscles. This manipulation moves energy primarily in the Kidney Primary and Tendino-Muscle channels as well as areas of the Spleen, Liver, and Bladder Tendino-Muscle channels. Treatment of this area benefits patients suffering with genitourinary problems, sciatica, and knee and hip pain or injury.

Step 56: Using circular palmar pressure with the right hand while supporting the lateral leg with the left, manipulate the center of the posterior thigh beginning at the base of the buttock and moving down toward the knee, ending at the popliteal fold. Repeat five times.

An alternate technique is to place the thumbs into a "T" formation with the remainder of the hands gently holding the thigh. Gently and evenly press with both thumbs. Movement is performed in small increments down the posterior thigh while maintaining the "T" formation. These two techniques help to relax the upper thigh, and can be used with patients who are sensitive in this area and cannot tolerate a deeper manipulation.

For patients who require a deeper manipulation, there are two additional techniques. The first is to place the two thumbs together at the base of the buttocks while allowing the hands to gently hold the posterior thigh. Simultaneous circular thumb pressure is used down the posterior thigh to the knee. The second alternate technique is to place one thumb on top of the other while the hands gently hold the thigh. Press into the muscles, moving in increments down the thigh to the knee.

Manipulation of the posterior thigh relaxes the biceps femoris, semitendinosus, and semimembranosus muscles. Energy is stimulated in the Bladder Primary and Tendino-Muscle channels. Treatment of this area is important for patients who suffer with lower back, sciatic, hip, leg, and knee pain as well as genitourinary problems.

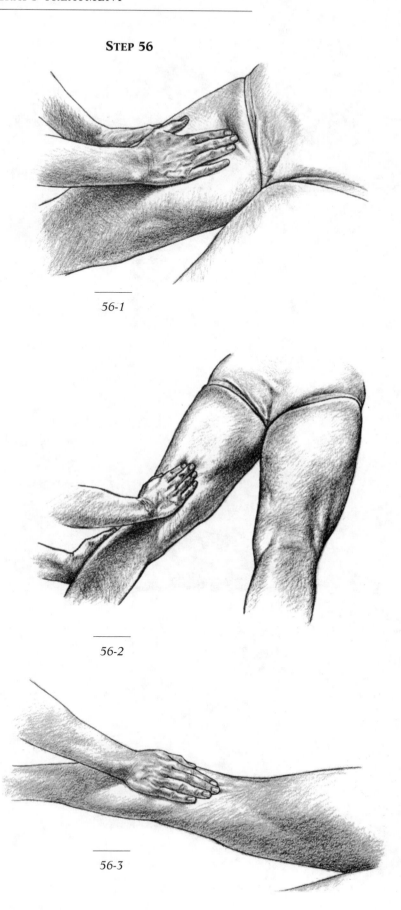

STEP 56

56-1

56-2

56-3

STEP 57

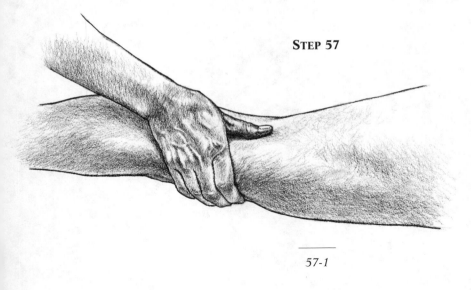

57-1

STEP 58

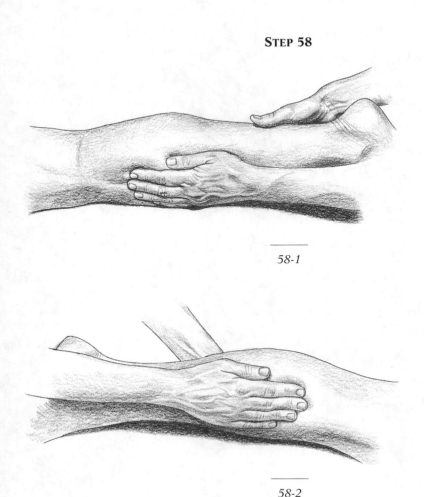

58-1

58-2

Step 57: The popliteal fossa is manip-ulated moving from lateral to medial, using circular thumb pressure with the right thumb arched. Thumbs may be alternated if needed. The medial knee is gently held with the remainder of the right hand while the left hand supports the lateral knee. Repeat five times.

The treatment of the posterior knee helps to relax the hamstring tendons, which insert into this area. This benefits both the thigh and calf muscles. The pos-terior politeal fossa contains two Bladder points and a Kidney point, therefore the manipulation of this area can benefit patients suffering with back pain, hip and knee pain, and genitourinary problems. The Bladder, Kidney, and Gall Bladder Tendino-Muscle channels all move through this area.

Step 58: Using circular palmar pres-sure with the left hand, work down from the lateral popliteal fossa to the external malleolus. Support the leg with the right hand. Repeat this movement with the right hand working from the medial knee to the medial malleolus. Repeat each side five times.

Step 59: Using circular palmar pres-sure with the right hand, move down the middle of the calf, starting inferior to the politeal fossa and ending at the calcaneal insertion of the Achilles tendon. An alter-nate technique is to place the two thumbs together inferior to the popliteal fossa. With the hands gently grasping both sides of the calf, press down the belly of the muscles to the end of the Achilles tendon.

These manipulations help to release and relax the muscles of the calf and remove obstructions from the Bladder, Gall Bladder, Liver, Spleen, and Kidney

Primary and Tendino-Muscle channels. Treatment to this area is useful for knee and lower back problems.

Step 60: Using a palmar embrace, manipulate the musculature of the calf inferior to the popliteal fossa to the base of the Achilles tendon, ending with a thenar embrace to the Achilles tendon. The hands may be alternated. As the practitioner works, the belly of the muscle is drawn into the hand. The flesh of the leg remains in contact with the palm throughout. Repeat five times.

An alternate technique is to grasp the calf with a palmar embrace, and then with a stroking motion bring the thumb to meet the hand. Repeat in intervals down the lower leg.

If the practitioner has small hands and is working on a patient with large calves, both hands can be used simultaneously. The thumbs should stay aligned

STEP 59

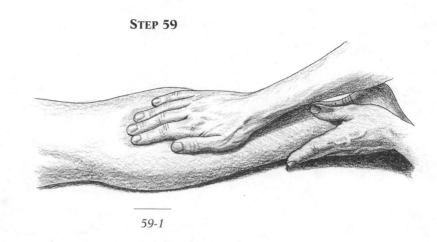

59-1

at the center of the calf while the two bellies of the gastrocnemius muscle are worked together. These manipulations relax the lower leg and also affect the thigh and the musculature of the lower back. They are effective for treating patients with muscular pain as well as sciatica.

STEP 60

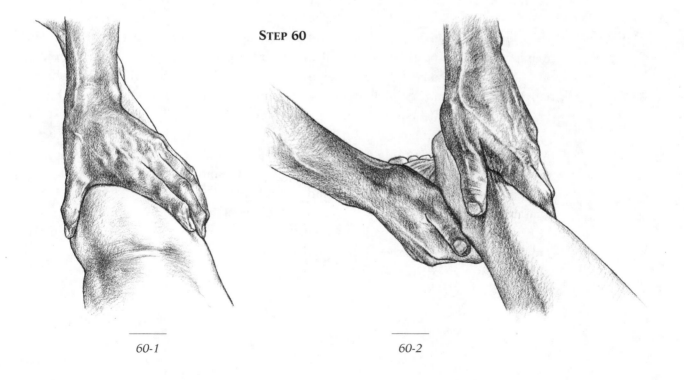

60-1   *60-2*

STEP 61

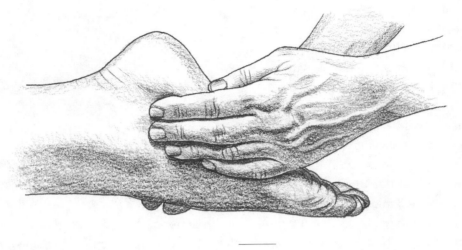

61-1

Step 61: Using the thumb or fingers of the left hand, manipulate around the lateral malleolus several times. Repeat this technique with the right hand, manipulating around the medial malleolus. The area of the heel can be manipulated with the thumb. Stimulation of the lateral malleolus affects the Bladder and Gall Bladder Primary and Tendino-Muscle channels. Stimulation to the medial malleolus affects the Kidney, Spleen, and Liver Primary and Tendino-Muscle channels.

Step 62: Move to the patient's right side and repeat all movements from steps 43 through 61, reversing hands as necessary.

Step 63: Return to a standing position facing the patient's head and repeat steps 39 (circular digital pressure to circular palmar pressure from the C7/T1 area to the PSIS) and 41 (palmar stroking from C7/T1 to the PSIS) in an abbreviated fashion. Repetition of these movements helps to completely relax the trapezius, the rhomboids, the erector spinae, and the latissimus dorsi muscles, while stimulating the flow of energy in the Bladder Primary and Tendino-Muscle channels and portions of the Stomach, Colon, and Small Intestine Tendino-Muscle channels.

STEP 64

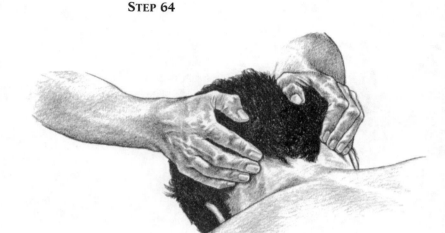

64-1

Step 64: Take a seated position at the patient's head. Place the pads of the fingers of both hands at the base of the occiput and gently but firmly stretch the muscles superiorly. This technique helps to relax both the superficial and deeper neck muscles, such as the sternocleidomastoid, upper trapezius, splenius capitis, longissimus capitis, and spinalis capitis. The relaxation of these muscles helps promote overall relaxation of the neck, shoulders, and back.

Step 65: With the left hand supporting the patient's head and using circular digital pressure with the right, move from the mastoid process to the midline of the occiput. Repeat five times. Repeat this manipulation on the opposite side, using the left hand to work the occiput and the right hand to support the head. This further relaxes the muscles of the neck and upper back and helps to produce emotional calm and physical relaxation.

This area is energized by the Bladder and Gall Bladder Primary and Tendino-Muscle channels and a portion of the Kidney Tendino-Muscle Channel. Manipulation in this area helps patients suffering with tension headaches; migraines; dizziness; and neck, shoulder, and upper back pain.

STEP 65

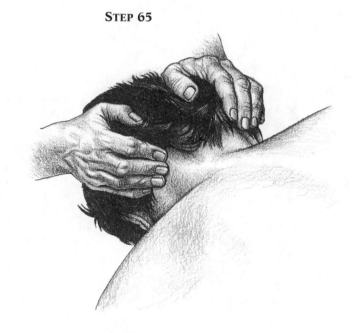

65-1

STEP 66

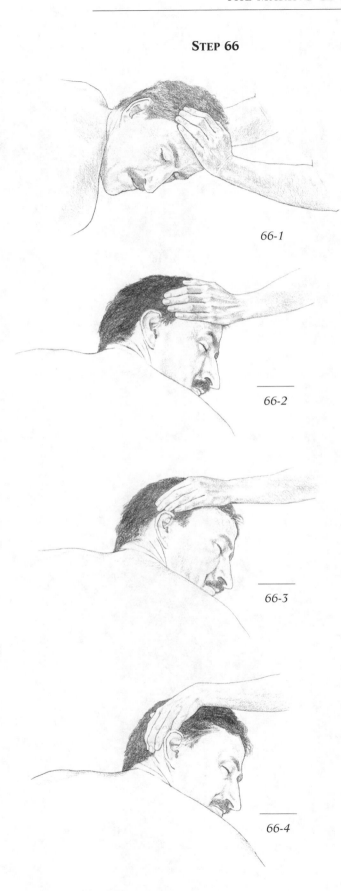

66-1

66-2

66-3

66-4

Step 66: After circular digital pressure to the base of the occiput is completed, treat the area around the ear by one of two methods, depending on the patient's range of motion. If the patient's neck is not in spasm, gently turn the head to the patient's right side. Support the head by cupping the patient's left ear and temple with your right hand. Rest your right arm gently on the table while still supporting the head, and treat the area around the ear using circular digital pressure with the left hand. Repeat five times and then gently turn the head to the left side, cupping the patient's right side of the head with your left hand. Repeat circular digital pressure around the ear with your right hand. When completed, return the patient's head to the central position.

If the patient's neck is in spasm, do not turn the head. Leave the head in the central position and use circular digital pressure with the pads of the fingers, beginning at the temples and following the path of the squamosal suture, moving around the ear and completing the movement at the mastoid process. The third finger guides the movement. Repeat five times on one side of the head and then repeat on the other side. The nonworking hand supports the patient's head.

Both of these techniques follow the superficial pathway and the Tendino-Muscle Channel of the Gall Bladder and San Jiao channels, as well as a deep branch of the Bladder Channel. In addition, the Small Intestine and Colon Tendino-Muscle channels energize this area. The treatment of this area serves to release emotional tension and calm the patient.

Step 67: Repeat palmar stroking to the back as described in step 41.

Step 68: Ask the patient to slowly sit up. Have the patient sit on the edge of the table with her legs dangling over the side. Remind the patient to sit up slowly to prevent dizziness or lightheadedness. Then stand behind the seated patient in order to treat the posterior portion of the patient's neck and shoulders. If the table is too high for this, ask the patient to sit on a chair and then stand behind her.

Using first palmar embrace and then switching to thenar embrace, move across the shoulder from the neck toward the acromioclavicular articulation, completing the movement at the head of the humerus. Repeat five times. Do not squeeze or pinch the muscles but work by molding the hand to the muscles and then drawing the muscle into the hand. Both shoulders may be worked at once. These techniques relax the upper trapezius muscle and treat neck and shoulder discomfort, arthralgia, cervicalgia, arthritis, and bursitis.

STEP 68

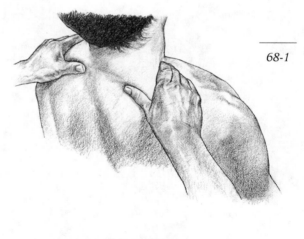

68-1

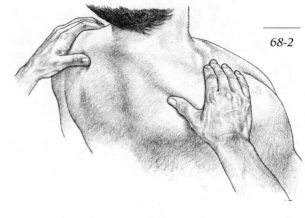

68-2

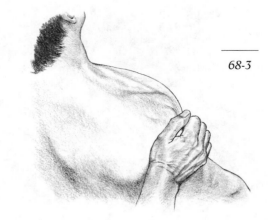

68-3

STEP 69

Step 69: Using circular digital pressure, move across the top of the right shoulder with your right hand while the left hand rests supportingly on the patient's left shoulder. The movement is completed at the acromioclavicular articulation. Repeat five times and then repeat the movement on the left side.

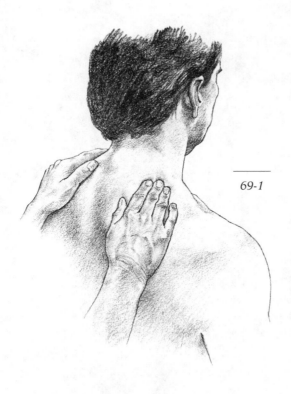

69-1

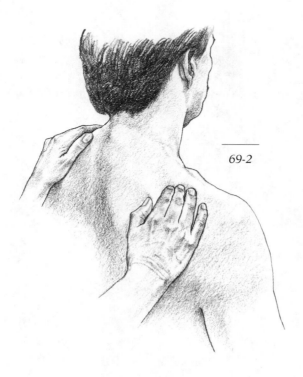

69-2

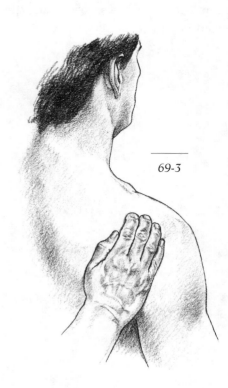

69-3

Step 70: Repeat step 69 beginning at the level of C7/T1, using circular digital pressure and moving across the superior border of the scapula to the acromio-clavicular joint. Repeat five times on the right side and then five times on the left side. As an alternate technique, use circular thumb pressure from the level of C7/T1 across the superior border of the scapula to the acromioclavicular joint.

The manipulations in steps 68, 69, and 70 help to release tension in the upper trapezius and relax the neck and upper back. In addition, step 70 also releases the levator scapulae, rhomboid, and supraspinatus muscles. It is important to note that all of the Yang channels move through the shoulder region to converge at GV14, located between C7 and T1.

STEP 70

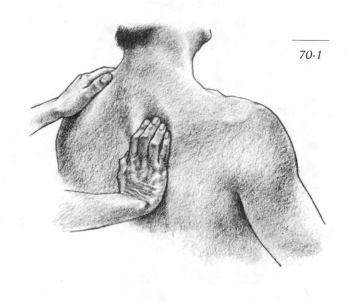

70-1

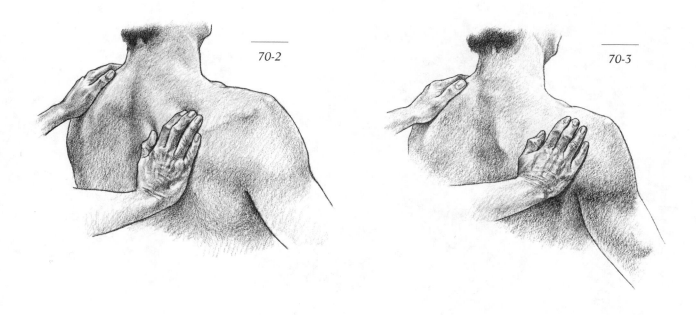

70-2

70-3

Step 71: Move to the patient's left side. Have the patient rest his chin in the palm of your left hand. Instruct the patient to relax his head so that you can feel the weight of his head in your hand.

STEP 71

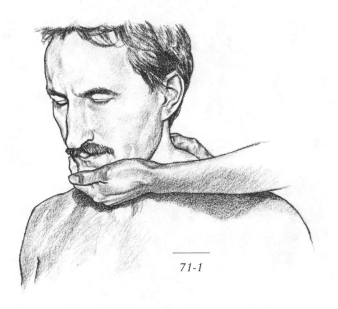

71-1

Cup the chin gently, taking care not to apply pressure to the patient's throat with the blade of your hand. It is important that the patient relax so that the deeper muscles and tendons of the neck can be manipulated. Using circular digital pressure with your right hand, work down the right side of the neck from the base of the occiput to the top of the shoulder. Repeat five times.

Change sides and repeat the manipulation, using your right hand to support the patient's chin and your left hand to manipulate down the left side of the patient's neck. This technique improves the circulation of Qi, Blood, and Fluids to the neck region and benefits patients suffering with cervical pain, arthritis, headaches, and shoulder pain. It also improves and increases the range of motion of the neck.

For patients who can tolerate a deeper manipulation, as as alternate tech-

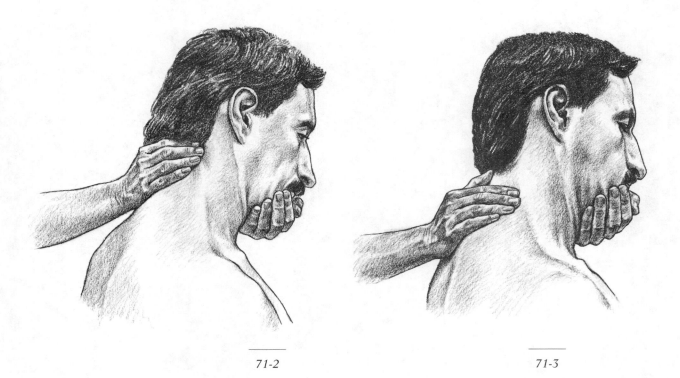

71-2

71-3

nique substitute circular thumb pressure for circular digital pressure. In this case the right thumb works the left side of the neck and the left thumb manipulates the right side of the neck. Each side is repeated five times.

Step 72: Continuing to support the chin, use palmar or thenar embrace to the back of the neck, gently drawing the muscles into the hand. This movement continues to relax the area and to improve the circulation of Qi, Blood, and Fluids.

Step 73: Repeat palmar and thenar embrace to the top of the shoulders to continue to relax this area.

STEP 72

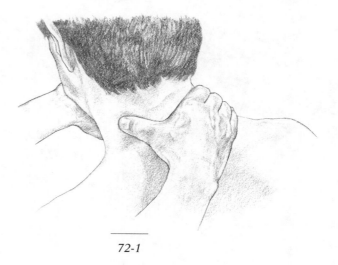

72-1

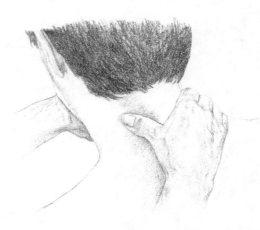

72-2

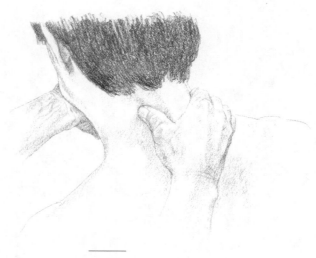

72-3

STEP 74

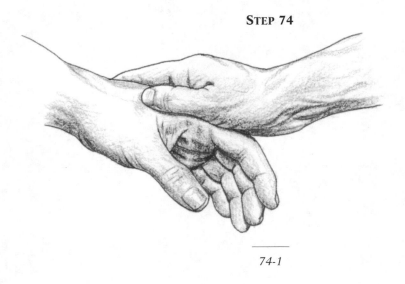

74-1

STEP 75

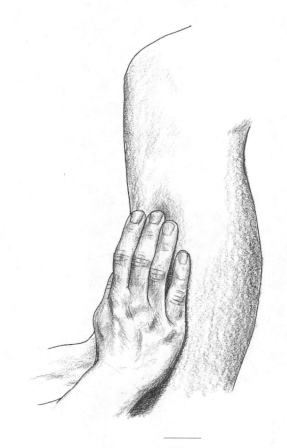

75-1

Step 74: Step to the front of the patient. Lift the patient's left hand and thumb stroke or press the Co4 area. Co4 is located at the high point of the muscle when the index finger and the thumb are drawn together. Then grasp the patient's thumb in the palm of your hand. Gently push up on the palmar aspect of the web that lies between the thumb and the index finger. Using the thumb of the opposite hand, place its lateral side on the radial edge of the second metacarpal bone, then roll the lateral edge of the thumb into the depression on the second metacarpal bone. Pressure is toward the second metacarpal bone. Repeat on the right hand.

Co4 is a major point that has a wide range of functions: it has a strong calming influence, stimulates the Lung's dispersing function, strengthens Wei Qi, and regulates the functions of the Colon. In addition this is a helpful point for influencing the face in invasions of Wind Heat and in treating problems of the face, such as toothaches, headaches, and sinusitis.

Step 75: Using a thumb stroke or circular digital pressure, manipulate St36 on the patient's left leg. St36 is located 3 tsun below St35, which is at the lateral foramen of the patella. Repeat on the patient's right leg. This point has a very strong tonifying effect and has been used since ancient times to build vitality and strength. It regulates and tonifies the Stomach, Spleen, Lung, Kidney, and Colon. It regulates both Wei Qi and Nutrient Qi and therefore strengthens the body's resistance to disease. It can also be used locally for various knee problems.

STEP 76

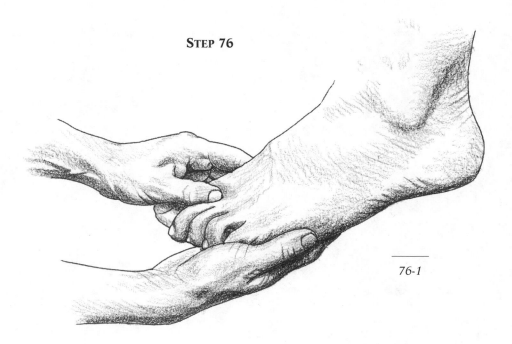

76-1

Step 76: Thumb stroke or gently press Liv2, located 0.5 tsun proximal to the margin of the web between the first and second toes. Grasp the patient's toe with your hand and press into the lateral joint space with your thumb, or thumb stroke the area. This point helps to sedate rising Liver Yang, Liver Fire, and Wind, releases stress, and calms the spirit.

This concludes the basic Amma therapy treatment.

PART FOUR

APPLIED
AMMA THERAPY

AMMA THERAPY ASSESSMENT AND DIAGNOSIS

Amma therapy assessment and diagnosis is a unique synthesis of Western approaches to organ dysfunction and Oriental medical principles. As discussed in part I, Amma therapy shares this basic concept with Oriental diagnosis: that practically every sign and symptom reflects the state of the internal organs and can be utilized in evaluation and assessment, with small areas of the body often seen as a microcosm of the whole. In pulse diagnosis, for example, only a small section of the wrist is palpated and yet fairly detailed information about the channels and their pertaining organs can be obtained. The same is true of observation of the tongue, through which the overall constitutional health of an individual, as well as specific organ problems and dysfunctions, can be ascertained. Tongue diagnosis is an objective data source, whereas pulse diagnosis is more subjective. The skill of the Amma therapist in interpreting the available data depends on the sensitivity and ability that develops from the continual application of knowledge in relationship to palpation. The Amma therapist will also utilize available information from any medical tests that the patient may have taken. Therefore, the results of blood tests, X rays, MRIs, EKGs, and so forth, and even the effects and side effects of medications, are all taken into account. Combined with the wholistic philosophy and principles expressed in this book, Amma therapy assessment and diagnosis integrates all information into a meaningful pattern of disharmony utilizing knowledge and techniques from both East and West.

The approach in Amma therapy is to assess and treat the pattern of disharmony and its symptoms while building the immune function so that the body can defend and heal itself. Given the proper conditions, the body will naturally move toward healing. While uncovering the cause of the problem is important, it is not immediately necessary in order to provide meaningful treatment. Often the patterns observed in the patient will have no direct corresponding Western medical diagnosis. Nonetheless, they are still the cause of pain, discomfort, and deterioration of the physical organism and can be effectively treated through Amma therapy, which addresses the problem from a multidirectional point of view. In some cases, identifying the cause of the pain and dysfunction is helpful in deciding what direction the treatment should take and what recommendations will prevent further injury. In other cases, knowing the cause is but a piece of information that has very little bearing on the course of the actual treatment. For example, a muscle spasm must be treated and released, regardless of its cause. When someone has a cold it matters little how he got it; what must be addressed immediately is the acute condition.

Sometimes the focus of a treatment will be only on the clinical manifestations; other times it will be only on the underlying cause. In Amma therapy the approach is often to treat both the cause and the clinical manifestations. The decision of what, when, and how to treat will depend on the assessment of the therapist and the severity of the signs and symptoms. Generally speaking, if optimum well-being is to be attained, the cause of disease must be addressed. As pointed out in the discussion of the homeodynamic model, a disease often has multi-

ple causes since, over the course of one's lifetime, different conditions of imbalance may have developed at various and/or overlapping times and medications administered along the way, all of which may contribute to the presenting condition. A patient's complete medical history must be taken into consideration when the patient's vitality and resistance to disease is assessed and a treatment plan is formulated.

To properly treat any pain, dysfunction, or illness, the problem must be understood in the context of the patient's whole mindbody condition; the patient's individual pattern of disharmony must be identified and comprehended. In the same way that a good detective gathers his evidence, carefully piecing together the facts to create a picture of a crime, a good therapist gathers as much information as possible about his patient to create a picture of what is wrong and how the mindbody complex is imbalanced. The therapist creates a mindbody portrait of the patient that includes the energetic as well as the structural and emotional imbalances. The Amma therapist skillfully gathers the information from a thorough examination of the patient's medical history, posture, diet and exercise regimen (or lack of one), a tongue and pulse diagnosis, observation of the patient's signs and symptoms, and the patient's complaints. The methods employed by the therapist center around the diagnostic techniques of looking, listening, smelling, asking, and feeling through palpation of the body.

Since the Amma therapist lives in a world of touch, palpating the body to both ascertain and treat disease conditions, the hands and fingers are essential data-gathering devices. When palpating, careful attention must be paid to the location of any areas of sensitivity or pain, as well as to whether the pain is related to any particular position or movement. Attention must also be given to skin temperature, structural deviations, spasms, and any palpable masses or skin changes. The more sensitive the hands and fingers become—first to the material body, and then to the immaterial, energetic body— the more likely it is that the therapist will evolve from an imitator of the master to an emulator, and eventually, into a master himself.

Crucial to the assessment are the expectations or goals that the therapist sets at the beginning of the treatment for both himself and the patient. Holding the proper *li* or notion regarding the outcome of the treatment is essential for realizing that goal. The therapist must always come to a conclusion about what is to be treated first and what can be treated later, about what is of primary importance in treatment and what is of secondary importance. Realistic expectations and objectives in the context of a short-term plan and a long-term plan help set goals that are within the patient's reach. The success of the short-term plan often helps to motivate the patient toward long-term goals. Sometimes an early and easy success becomes an excuse for the patient to deviate from the wholistic path, particularly in the area of diet. However, depending on the illness or dysfunction being treated, it is possible to prevent further pathological changes from taking place with some patients by employing preventive Amma therapy

treatments and proper diet and exercise. In other cases, as with the degeneration of the cervical spine due to aging when a reversal of abnormal changes is not possible, the therapist can at least alleviate the symptoms and pain caused by these changes.

Utimately the degree of success of any treatment depends on several factors, including:

+ the accuracy of the assessment and diagnosis
+ the exactitude with which the treatment is executed by the therapist
+ the severity of the condition
+ the acuteness or chronicity of the condition
+ the span of time between the onset and the treatment sought
+ the patient's medical history, including the residue from past and present medications, illnesses, and injuries
+ the already existing damage to the energy system and the physical body
+ the patient's overall constitutional well-being, a combination of his Pre- and Postnatal Qi.

A patient's constitution reflects in his body's ability to heal itself given the proper conditions. The patient's current diet, level of stress, and—most important—his willingness to comply with the practitioner's recommendations relative to frequency of treatments, diet, supplementation, herbal liniments, stress reduction, and exercise, are all integral factors in the degree of success of any Amma therapy treatment.

INTRODUCTION TO THE AMMA THERAPY TREATMENTS

The following chapters outline treatments that address some of the most common complaints seen by Amma therapists in the clinical setting. Each chapter begins with an Amma therapy etiology incorporating Western and Eastern viewpoints of health and disease and the principles of wholistic health as elucidated throughout this book. Information regarding practical application follows the discussion on etiology. This section on practical application, entitled "Amma Therapy Treatment," is divided into three parts: "Amma Therapy Assessment" describes the basic methods of assessing a patient according to the four traditional methods of Oriental medicine; "Additional Techniques" describes more advanced techniques beyond those taught in the basic Amma therapy treatment, and includes information on moxibustion and the application of herbal liniments; and "Point Location and Action" details specific loci (points) and the general order or pattern in which they should be incorporated into each treatment. The location of each point is presented in conjunction with specific instructions on how to press and manipulate that point and includes the appropriate finger or portion of finger used, angle and amount of pressure, and how to palpate for that point. The actions listed for each point describe the specific functions and indications of that point as they relate to the condition being treated.

Although Amma therapy treatments are not limited to point location and palpation, the use of points is an integral part of each treatment. While successfully locating points ultimately depends on the practitioner's sensitivity to energy, a beginning Amma therapist will necessarily rely on anatomical landmarks and the traditional measurement of a tsun in order to determine point location.

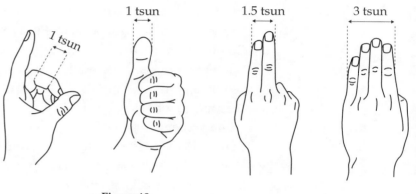

Figure 40

Osteo-inches as measured by units of the finger

As mentioned in chapter 6, a tsun is an acupuncture unit of measurement (AUM) or osteo-inch; it is basically a division of a length of bone. One tsun is approximately equivalent to the width of the thumb or the middle phalangeal bone of the third finger. The width of the index and third fingers together is approximately equivalent to 1.5 tsun, while the width of the second, third, fourth, and fifth fingers together equals approximately 3 tsun (see figure 40). It is important to note that tsun or osteo-inches are measured relative to the *patient's* hand in relation to her body. Since the practitioner's hand and the patient's hand will often not be similar in width, the practitioner must determine and use the width of the patient's osteo-inch and not his own. Of course, using the traditional Chinese method of a specific number of AUMs for a specific extant of a limb or body segment is a more accurate method of point location, especially in tall and thin patients. See the appendix on pages 401–403 for illustrations of the traditional Chinese system of body measurement.

There are three categories of points given for each treatment. These are the points located on the twelve Primary Channels and the Governing and Conception Vessels, the traditional extra points, and Tina Sohn (TS) points. The descriptions of the points located on the Primary Channels and the Governing and Conception Vessels will often have a comment section delineating the category of loci that point belongs to. For the purposes of this text these categories include:

+ Organ (Source or Yuan) points— These points are located at the ankles and wrists and are related to the Yuan Qi that is stored there. Source points directly affect their pertaining organs and are used mostly to tonify the Yin Organs. In addition, Source points may be used in assessment, since changes in the Cutaneous Region over the point may reflect a dysfunction in the pertaining organ. Organ points regulate the energy between the channel and the organ body. They are used in conjunction with the Luo point of their Yin/Yang pair.

+ Luo (Connecting) points—These connect the Luo point of one channel with the Organ point of its Yin/Yang pair. Manipulation of these points balances the energies between the Yin/Yang channels and

Organ pairs. These points can also be used to balance the energies of each of the bilateral Primary Channels. For example, if there is an imbalance between the left and right Lung Channels, the Luo point for the Lung (Lu7) may be used to correct this imbalance. These points may also be used for their individual energetic actions.

+ Mu points—These points are also called Alarm points or Front-collecting points. They are located on the chest and abdomen and are places where the channel Qi collects. Mu points connect directly to their corresponding organs and can be used both for diagnosis and treatment. Mu points are not necessarily located on the channel of the Organ that they affect. Sensitivity or lack of sensation at a Mu point can indicate either an Excess or Deficiency condition in the diseased organ. Their use in treatment is to regulate the affected organ, particularly in acute conditions, although they can also be used with Yu points to treat chronic conditions. Mu points are Yin in nature.

+ Yu points—These are also called Associated points, Shu points, or Back-transporting points. Yu points connect directly to their corresponding Organs; like Mu points, they too can be used for both diagnosis and treatment. The Yu points are all located on the medial pathway of the Bladder Channel, 1.5 tsun lateral to the spine. They are named for the Organ and the Qi of the channel they affect. Used to treat chronic conditions, Yu points can also be used with Mu points to treat acute conditions. The Yu points are Yang in nature, and are used to tonify the Yang energies of the Organs, although they can also tonify the Yin. In addition, they are used to treat the sense organs of their pertaining organs.

◆ Confluent points—These regulate the Extraordinary Vessels, balance the energies between the twelve Primary Channels and the eight Extraordinary Vessels, and can also affect specific regions of the body.

◆ The Five Transporting points (The Sixty Points of Command)—This category consists of five specific kinds of points, all of which are located distal to the elbow and knees on each of the twelve Primary Channels. Each channel contains one point from each category, totaling sixty points. Each of the five subcategories describes the quality of Qi flow using the image of water. Each of the five types of points has specific therapeutic effects.

The Sixty Points of Command also correspond to the Five Elemental Phases. According to this system, the Well points on the Yin channels correspond to Wood and the other points follow accordingly in the Five Element Cycle of Creation, while the Well points on the Yang channels correspond to Metal with the subsequent points following in turn according to the Cycle of Creation. For the acupuncturist, these points can be tonified or sedated according to the Mother-Child law, where the mother tonifies and the child sedates. However, for the Amma therapist

the best clinical application of these points is using them to expel exogenous pathogens, which are always Excess by their nature. This application is more effective with the Yin channels than the Yang channels.

When utilizing these points according to the Five Element theory to treat Excess conditions, Wood corresponds to Wind, Fire corresponds to Fire or Heat, Earth corresponds to Dampness, Water corresponds to Cold, and Metal corresponds to Dryness. Metal points are not used to eliminate Dryness; however, since Internal Dryness is always due to a deficiency of body Fluids and is not an Excess condition. Dryness must therefore be treated by generating fluids.

The five kinds of Transporting points are:

1. Well points—These are located at the ends of the fingers and toes, the area where energy changes from Yin to Yang and Yang to Yin. There is a lot of dynamic activity at these points because it is here that the channel is most superficial; thus, energy can be quickly influenced here. These points are very effective for treatment of acute problems and extreme imbalances of Yin and Yang, such as those found in seizures, loss of consciousness, convulsions, anxiety, and mental illness. Well points are also quite effective in treating problems that are distal to the point.

2. Spring points—These are

located in the metacarpal or metatarsal areas and are always the second point from the Well point along the channel. Like Well points, these points are also more superficial and are analogous to Qi gushing from a spring. They are used to treat febrile disease due to both exogenous and endogenous causes and to clear Heat.

3. Stream points—These are located on or close to the wrists and ankles, the place on the channels where the Qi flows more rapidly and begins to go deeper in the channel. It is here that exogenous pathogens can find their way into the interior, but it is also here that Wei Qi accumulates. Stream points are generally the third point from the Well point on the fingers and toes, except on the Gall Bladder Channel, where they are the fourth point. They are used both locally and distally to treat Painful Obstruction Syndromes, particularly those due to Damp Heat.

4. River points—These are located on the forearms and legs, the place on the channels where the Qi becomes wider and deeper and begins to flow like a river in the channel. These are points where exterior pathogens are turned toward the sinews and joints. River points are used to treat upper respiratory problems, such as asthma, cough, fever, and chills. The River points located on the Yin chan-

nels can also be used to treat Painful Obstruction Syndrome of the joints.

5. Sea points—These are located at the elbows and knees, where the Qi flows more slowly and deeply, like rivers emptying into the sea. Sea points are used to treat Rebellious Qi disorders of the digestive system, which are mostly problems of the Yang channels, such as vomiting, diarrhea, and intestinal disorders. However, the Yin Sea points can also be used to treat the Yang organs. The upper Sea points are also frequently used to expel exogenous pathogens from the skin and muscles and to treat problems of the head, neck, and shoulders.

✦ Influential points—These eight points are named for their influence on the Qi, Blood, Viscera, Bowels, Sinews, Marrow, Bones, and Blood Vessels. These points are used to treat diseases that affect these orbs and substances.

✦ Accumulation points—These points treat acute disorders, in particular when there is pain. They are used to treat Excess patterns of both the channel and its organ. There is one point for each of the Primary Channels and one for four of the Extraordinary Vessels, those being the two Heel Vessels and two Linking Vessels, totaling sixteen points.

✦ Intersecting points—These are points on the body where two or more channels meet. In addition to their other actions, these points can also be used to treat disharmonies between the pertaining intersecting channels.

+ Distal points—These points are located on the hands and feet. Their manipulation reverberates throughout the channel, helping to clear obstructions of Qi and Blood and affecting the areas on the opposite end of the channel.

+ Local points—Since manipulation of a point stimulates the flow of Qi and Blood in that area, local points can treat problems in their immediate vicinity. For example, points located near the eyes treat eye disorders irrespective of the channels they are on. Points located near an organ, the stomach for example, can be used to treat diseases of that organ. Some points are especially powerful and treat an entire area of the body; for example, CV12 can treat the entire Middle Jiao.

The traditional extra points are points generally found off the channels. These points have local and distal effects. Tina Sohn (TS) points are extra points that I have discovered; the table to the right shows the abbreviations and locations for these points. Some of these points are extra points located on the channels; others are located off the channels. They have very specific local and distal effects and treat Organs and channels. These categories of points are by no means all-inclusive. Advanced Amma therapists will also use Ah Shui points, points that become spontaneously sensitive with the arising of an imbalance, and

other point groupings in their treatments.

Since both moxibustion and the use of herbal liniments are discussed in the following chapters, I would like to make some mention of them here. Moxibustion is the application of heat to points and can be done with various types of substances; generally either a moxa stick or heated fresh ginger are used in Amma therapy. A vulnerary is applied to protect the skin. Moxibustion warms the channels, helps to expel Cold, relieves pain, moves Qi, strengthens Yang, activates Blood stagnation, and can help warm the Uterus and stop bleeding in women. No one should attempt this technique without having first been properly instructed by an experienced practitioner.

There are many types of herbal liniments. The major liniment utilized in

TINA SOHN POINT LOCATION

TS-H	Tina Sohn point–head
TS-N	Tina Sohn point–neck
TS-C	Tina Sohn point–chest
TS-Ab	Tina Sohn point–abdomen
TS-B	Tina Sohn point–back
TS-A	Tina Sohn point–arm
TS-E	Tina Sohn point–elbow
TS-FA	Tina Sohn point–forearm
TS-HA	Tina Sohn point–hand
TS-UE-I	Tina Sohn point–upper extremity: thumb
TS-UE-II	Tina Sohn point–upper extremity: index finger
TS-UE-III	Tina Sohn point–upper extemity: third finger
TS-UE-IV	Tina Sohn point–upper extremity: fourth finger
TS-E-V	Tina Sohn point–upper extremity: fifth finger
TS-T	Tina Sohn point–thigh
TS-K	Tina Sohn point–knee
TS-L	Tina Sohn point–leg
TS-F	Tina Sohn point–foot
TS-LE-I	Tina Sohn point–lower extremity: big toe
TS-LE-II	Tina Sohn point–lower extremity: second toe
TS-LE-III	Tina Sohn point–lower extremity: third toe
TS-LE-IV	Tina Sohn point–lower extremity: fourth toe
TS-LE-V	Tina Sohn point–lower extremity: fifth toe

Amma therapy treatments is generically called *teh tah chu*, which translates as "iron palm liquid." Historically, teh tah chu was used as a martial arts liniment to help heal the bruises, strains, sprains, breaks, and fractures induced by martial arts sparring and fighting techniques. The proprietary formula used at the New York College has been handed down for generations in my family and has a wide range of uses for musculoskeletal problems, such as arthritis, bursitis, and muscle sprains and strains. It improves the circulation of Qi, Blood, and Fluids and is widely used in Amma therapy treatments for this reason. In addition, it treats insect bites and can be used preventively as an insect repellent. The liniment is applied sparingly, using the appropriate hand technique with a gauze pad that has been soaked in the liquid. Specific areas may be wrapped using roll gauze and left overnight, to allow the liniment to be absorbed into the affected area. Teh tah chu should not be applied to an open wound as it contains alcohol and will sting the patient.

The following chapter, "General Treatment for Revitalizing and Balancing the Body," incorporates the basic techniques that are the hallmark of Amma therapy with the major points used in an overall tonifying treatment. The basic techniques, in combination with the major energy-balancing points, provide a powerful and profound release of stress and tension, removing energetic blockages due to stagnation of Qi and Blood and thereby moving the body toward balance and health. Once mastered, this protocol can be utilized as the foundation for all other treatments.

Before attempting to learn the treatments that follow, it is important that the reader be practiced in the basic Amma treatment and understand the general responsibilties of an Amma therapy practitioner, all of which are discussed at length in part III.

As discussed on page 252, the success of each treatment depends on several factors. Each treatment can be used effectively as described, or can be further built upon and modified by the therapist based on the immediate needs of the patient. Tailoring the treatment will change the focus from what is outlined here. Nevertheless, the fundamental principles of energy balancing and treatment, and the continuous rhythm and flow of the Amma therapy techniques applied directly to the physical body with specific manipulation of the energies in the Primary and Tendino-Muscle channels and Cutaneous Regions, remain the essence of the Amma therapy treatment and reflect throughout.

CHAPTER
15

GENERAL TREATMENT FOR REVITALIZING AND BALANCING THE BODY

AMMA THERAPY ETIOLOGY

Preventive treatment is a core principle of Amma therapy. Amma therapy seeks to maintain optimum health through the treatment of the physical body, the bioenergy, and the emotions. The techniques of Amma therapy as taught in the basic treatment in chapter 13, in combination with major energy points, comprise this treatment for revitalizing and balancing the body. The purpose of this treatment is to harmonize the body's energy system through manipulation of the energies in the twelve Primary and Tendino-Muscle channels, the two Extraordinary Vessels, the Cutaneous Regions, and specific points. Beginning students often express surprise at the positive results they achieve in the practice of this first general treatment. Despite the fact that they do not yet understand the fundamental principles nor have any real skill, they find that they are able to significantly help people relax and feel revitalized. The patients these students treat in practice clinics regularly express how much more energetic they feel and how their stress appears to have miraculously dissolved.

The reason these changes occur is that, given the proper conditions, the bioenergy has the ability to move toward self-healing. It is important to remember that man is a microcosm of the universe, a universe of Qi, where everything—from the immaterial through increasing levels of density of energy to the material—is all Qi. Qi is energy from the most fine to the most dense. Its manifestations are recognized at the physical level, the emotional level, the mental level, and the spiritual level. There is fundamentally only one Qi, but that energy takes many different forms and manifests in different degrees of activity and coalescing. This is true both in the universe and in man. When Qi fuses or congeals it takes a physical form; this form is able to change depending on location and required function.

Basically, Qi can be divided into the two major categories of Yin and Yang energies—Yin being the vital substances and the substratum of the organs and Yang being the various functional activities that Qi performs. Within these two major categories, Qi takes many forms within the body. Qi is always in motion—without the movement of Qi there is no life. Qi moves in specific directions—ascending and descending, entering and leaving. If any of these functions are obstructed or in stasis, pathological changes will result. Therefore, in this general treatment we seek to activate several different types of Qi, including Vital Energy or Yuan Qi, Defensive/Protective Qi or Wei Qi, Nutrient Qi or Ying Qi, and Blood and Fluids.

The Vital Energy or Yuan Qi is comprised of both Pre-Heaven Qi and Post-Heaven Qi. The former is ruled by the Kidney and the latter by the Spleen and Stomach. It is this energy that motivates or activates the flow of Qi in the channels and acts as the catalyst for all the processes of energy creation and trans-

formation in the body. It motivates the movement of the Blood. When the Vital Energy stagnates, Blood stagnates. When the Vital Energy is free-flowing, the circulation of Blood is facilitated. The basic techniques of Amma therapy in conjunction with special points, such as CV12 and St36, stimulate the functions of the Lung, Spleen, and Stomach, which in turn promote the circulation of the Vital Energy and Blood. This leaves the patient calmer and in a revitalized state.

The extraction and assimilation of the Qi of Air (Da Qi) with the Qi of Grain (Gu Qi) produces Ancestral Qi, which further transforms into True Qi under the influence of Yuan Qi. True Qi is the form that can be used for the various needs of the organism, and further transforms into both Defensive Qi (Wei Qi) and Nutrient Qi (Ying Qi). Wei Qi is the energy that circulates through the most superficial areas of the body, flowing in the Tendino-Muscle Channels and the Cutaneous Regions. This energy is Yang in nature and is responsible for the protection of the body by increasing resistance to attack by exogenous pathogens, which invade the body through the skin and the channels. It is also responsible for opening and closing the pores under the direction of the Lung so that the fluid metabolism and temperature remain in balance. Poor circulation or stagnation of this energy can lead to a weakening of the body's defenses so that a person will be more inclined to feeling cold and becoming ill. Proper circulation is enhanced through the general treatment and this in turn builds the body's defenses and immunity to disease.

The Ying Qi moves through the Organ complex and flows in the blood vessels and channels. Compared to Wei Qi, it is Yin in nature. Through the stimulation of the channels and manipulation of the major points, the practitioner helps to provide nourishment to the entire body and regulate the internal organs. Nutrient Qi in combination with pure Fluids creates Blood. It is Nutrient Qi that is stimulated when we manipulate a point. Poor circulation or stagnation of this energy can lead to a variety of problems stemming from a failure to properly nourish the organs.

Another major substance that is stimulated by Amma therapy is the Blood. The Blood is moved by the Vital Energy, which is the motivating force for its circulation in the blood vessels and channels. Blood and Vital Energy are intimately connected and interdependent. Vital Energy is called the Commander of the Blood and Blood is called the Mother of Qi. Without the Vital Energy, Blood would cease to move. Without the Blood, Qi would not be nourished or rooted to the body.

The main function of Blood, as with the Nutrient Qi, is to nourish the entire body. The ability of the organs to function in their varied capacities and to produce the essential substances of the body is dependent on the adequate supply of nutrients from the Blood. The Blood also has a lubrication activity, being in part responsible for the moistening of muscles, tendons, ligaments, joints, body tissues, eyes, skin, and hair. Blood roots the Mind, nourishing it and preventing the Shen from wandering. Improper circulation of Blood is responsible for many emotional problems, as the Shen or Spirit cannot properly be housed without the sufficient

quality, quantity, and circulation of Blood. Treatment with Amma therapy will improve the circulation of Blood and Vital Energy, thereby helping to prevent disease and calm the emotions.

Various Fluids are also circulated in the Amma therapy treatment. Fluids are closely related to Blood and Qi. Pure Fluids are an important component of Blood and prevent the Blood from becoming too thick and stagnant. In return, Blood helps to nourish the Fluids. Thin Fluids circulate with the Wei Qi in the skin and muscles and moisten these areas, as well as being expelled as sweat and manifesting as tears, saliva, and mucus. Thick Fluids circulate with Nutrient Qi in the Bowels and Viscera and moisten the joints, brain, bones, and spinal cord. The general treatment stimulates the flow of Vital Energy, which moves the Fluids as well as the Blood. Without the stimulation of Qi, Fluids would stagnate and produce disease. Qi also holds the Fluids in the body in the same way that it holds the Blood in the vessels. If the circulation is weak there may be leakage in various forms, such as profuse sweating, incontinence, and bleeding.

The general treatment described here stimulates the circulation of Vital Energy, Wei Qi, Nutrient Qi, Blood, and Fluids, nourishes the Organs, and benefits the muscles, sinews, joints, and bones. Through the application of Amma therapy techniques the patient's energy level is increased, the Shen is calmed, physical strength and well-being are promoted, and the body is strengthened against disease.

AMMA THERAPY TREATMENT

The following protocol is an excellent treatment for the reduction of stress, for building up the body's defensive resources, and for improving the overall well-being and vitality of the organism. The description of the actions of each point pertains to that point's relationship to the treatment for revitalizing and balancing the body. These points have other actions that are not relevant to this particular treatment but will be described in the other Amma therapy treatments that follow.

AMMA THERAPY ASSESSMENT

Before treating any patient the practitioner must first try to assess the patient's condition. Even the novice practitioner should practice the art of assessment, utilizing and analyzing the information gleaned from the patient's complaints, medical history, diet, medication, and lifestyle. Even at the most rudimentary level, all students should be practicing pulse and tongue diagnosis once they have been taught the basics of these diagnostic techniques.

ADDITIONAL TECHNIQUES

This treatment is a bridge between the basic treatment as taught in chapter 13 and the more advanced treatments that follow. No additional or advanced techniques are provided here so that the student can continue to focus on and perfect the basic manipulations, the practice of point location, and the development of palpatory skills.

POINT LOCATION AND ACTION

1. Bl2

Location: In the depression proximal to the medial end of the eyebrow, directly above the inner canthus.

Pressure is activated with the pad of the index finger or middle finger in the sulcus of the bone, pressing toward the posterior skull. Pressure is held for approximately 15–30 seconds. Support the opposite side of the head while executing this technique.

Action: Due to its location, this point is used for a variety of eye, sinus, and nasal problems. It is important to note that Bl2 is located at the beginning of the Bladder Channel, the largest channel in the body and the one that covers the entire back. The proper flow of energy through this channel is imperative not only to the health of the eyes, but also for the musculature of the back and the overall health of the Bladder and Kidney Organs.

2. CV17

Location: Midway between the nipples at the center of the sternum.

Pressure is activated with the pad of the middle finger gently pressing directly toward the table.

Action: This is a very important point for releasing stagnant emotional energy trapped in the chest and for tonifying the energy of the Upper Burner, energy that relates to the Heart and the Lung. This point helps the function of breathing by opening up and expanding the chest. It is also useful in Lung problems when there is a chronic cough.

Comment: This is the Mu point for the Upper Burner and the Heart Envelope. It is also an Influential point for tonifying Qi, especially of the Heart and Lung. It is an Intersecting point with the Spleen, Small Intestine, Kidney, Triple Burner, and Heart Envelope channels.

3. CV12

Location: Midway between the end of the sternum and the umbilicus, or 4 tsun above the umbilicus on the anterior midline of the body. The point is activated with the thumb or third finger.

Gently place one hand above CV12, palm down, to help stabilize the point pressure of the thumb or third finger of the opposite hand. Ask the patient to inhale and exhale slowly. As the patient exhales, pressure is applied directly toward the table until a slight pulsation is felt. The point is held for 15–30 seconds and then slowly released. As you release pressure, begin circling your finger.

Action: This is a major point for any digestive problem since it tonifies both Stomach and Spleen Qi. It is particularly helpful for calming Rebellious or Deranged Stomach Qi (Stomach energy that is ascending instead of descending) and for resolving Damp Spleen. It is also helpful for bringing the emotional energy down from the chest toward the feet and opening up the chest, since the Lung Channel begins deep to CV12.

Comment: This is the Mu point for the Stomach as well as for the Middle Burner. It is also an Intersecting point of the Small Intestine, San Jiao, and Stomach chan-

nels, and as such is an important point for the Yang Organs that deal with digestion. In addition, CV12 is an Influential point used to tonify the Yang Organs.

4. Lu5

Location: With the elbow slightly bent, this point can be found lateral to the biceps tendon at the cubital crease.

Grasp the patient's arm with your hand, place your thumb alongside the lateral side of the biceps tendon in alignment with the Lung Channel (the top of your thumb is level with the cubital crease), and press gently with the pad of the thumb directly toward the table. Hold the point for 15–30 seconds and then gently release, circling as your pressure lightens.

Action: A local point for elbow pain, Lu5 is a major point for regulating and tonifying the Lung. Healthy Lung function is essential for overall health and vitality, since the Lung is responsible for the extraction of the Qi of Air, which is then utilized to make Nutrient Qi. This point also stimulates the descending function of the Lung, helping to expand and relax the chest and thereby also releasing stress and tension commonly held in that area. This is a useful point for both acute and chronic Lung conditions.

Comment: Lu5 is both the Sea and Water point for the Lung Channel.

5. Ht3

Location: With the elbow bent, this point can be found between the medial end of the transverse cubital crease and the medial epicondyle of the humerus.

Grasp the elbow with your hand that is closest to the patient's body. Using the pad of your thumb, press laterally directly toward the joint space of the medial epicondyle of the humerus. Hold the point for 15 seconds or longer, depending on the emotionality of the patient.

Action: This is a major point for calming the Shen and therefore the emotions. It helps clear Heat or Fire from the Heart and regulates the flow of Blood and Qi. It can also be used locally for elbow pain.

Comment: Ht3 is both the Sea and Water point for the Heart Channel.

6. Co4

Location: In the center of the flesh between the first and second metacarpal bones, closer to the second metacarpal bone.

Grasp the patient's thumb so that the second and third fingers fall on the palmar aspect of the patient's hand. Gently push up on the palmar aspect of the web that lies between the thumb and index finger. Using the thumb of the opposite hand, place its lateral side on the radial edge of the second metacarpal bone. Then roll the lateral edge of the thumb into the depression on the second metacarpal bone. Pressure is toward the second metacarpal bone.

Action: This major point has a wide range of functions. In the general treatment its use is primarily as a soothing influence on the mind and emotions, particularly when combined with Liv2. It has a strong influence on the Lung's dispersing function, helps to balance ascending and descending energies, and strengthens Wei Qi, thereby increasing the body's resistance to attack by exogenous pathogens.

Comment: This is the Organ point for the Colon.

7. Sp21

Location: On the midaxillary line, 6 tsun below the axilla and midway between the axilla and the free end of the eleventh rib.

This point can be manipulated bilaterally with the patient in either the supine or prone position. The point is activated with the pads of the third fingers pressing directly into the intercostal space.

Action: This is one of the major points of Oriental medicine. It is the Great Luo (Connecting) point of the Spleen. This point helps to regulate Qi and Blood via its connection to the minute Blood Luo channels throughout the body and is used as a general tonification point in this treatment.

8. St36

Location: 3 tsun below St35, 1 tsun lateral to the anterior crest of the tibia. (St35 is at the lateral foramen of the patella).

Stand alongside the patient facing the patient's knee. Place the pad of the thumb of the hand closest to the patient's head on the point. Gently hold the foot with the other hand and tilt the leg toward your body as you press toward the tibia. This will give more pressure into the point. Hold the point for 15–30 seconds. Circle as you release your pressure.

Action: This point has a very strong tonifying effect and has been used since ancient times to build vitality and strength. It regulates and tonifies the Stomach, Spleen, Lung, Kidney, and Colon. It regulates both Wei Qi and Nutrient Qi and therefore strengthens the resistance of the body against disease. It can be used locally for various knee problems.

Comment: St36 is both the Lower Sea and the Earth point of the Stomach Channel.

9. Sp6

Location: 3 tsun proximal to the vertex of the medial malleolus, just posterior to the tibial border.

Stand at the foot of the table. Grasp the patient's leg with your hand and place the pad of the thumb on the point. Gently press toward the tibia until you feel a sulcus in the bone. Hold the point for 15–30 seconds and then slowly release, circling as you lighten your pressure. This point can be pressed bilaterally.

Action: This is an important point with a wide range of functions. Three major Yin channels meet at this spot—the Spleen, Liver, and Kidney channels. This point serves to strengthen the Spleen, which extracts the Qi of Grain necessary for the creation of Nutrient Qi. It also tonifies the Kidney, regulates genitourinary functions, and promotes the smooth flow of Liver Qi. In this last regard it has an important effect on calming the emotions and relieving irritability.

10. Liv2

Location: 0.5 tsun proximal to the margin of the web between the first and second toes.

Grasp the patient's toe with your hand and press into the lateral joint space with your thumb. Angle your thumb to fit into the joint space. This point may be more tender than others and should be pressed gently at first, then with increasing pressure. Hold for 15–30 seconds and then slowly release, circling as you lighten your pressure.

Action: Liv2 helps to sedate rising Liver Fire and Wind. It releases stress and calms the Spirit, particularly when used in combination with Co4.

Comment: This is both the Spring and Fire point of the Liver Channel.

CHAPTER 16

TREATMENT FOR STIFF NECK WITH SHOULDER PAIN

AMMA THERAPY ETIOLOGY

Pain and dysfunction of the neck and shoulders are among the most common conditions seen in the clinical setting. Of all the musculoskeletal and neuromuscular conditions that can cause pain and disability, neck and shoulder pain is a frequent complaint, exceeded only by lower back pain. Since the causes of neck and shoulder pain are many and varied, the degree of success of the following treatment will depend on the many factors discussed in chapter 14. Neck and shoulder pain reflect both internal and external imbalances. Amma therapy etiology encompasses both Western and Eastern considerations of cause.

As the therapist enters the treatment room, she can gain some preliminary sense of the patient's posture and emotional states simply through a first visual impression. A major component of a patient's posture is his genetic inheritance through which congenital postural problems are passed on from generation to generation, as happens with some types of scoliosis. Certain conditions, such as Parkinson's disease or osteoporosis, also cause structural abnormalities. However, perhaps the most destructive influences upon posture are emotions and habits. Posture is often a reflection of our emotional state, since we stand, sit, and move in accordance to how we feel internally. Our posture often unconsciously depicts our inner attitudes about ourselves. The person who is trying to hide from others may stand with a rounded upper back, leading to thoracic hyperkyphosis and scapular protraction. In compensation the neck is excessively arched, like a giraffe's neck, producing a cervical hyperlordosis and causing strain and fatigue of the muscles and ligaments as well as pain. A tall child who hovers over his peers and is self-conscious about his height or a young girl who is self-conscious about her developing breasts will hold these thoracic and cervical distortions, and such abnormal posture will lead to and indeed accelerate degenerative changes over time. Unless there is a conscious effort to change such configurations through body therapy and proper exercise, abnormal postures developed in childhood may become fixed and lead to further structural distortions and pain in adult life.

In cases where there has been no obvious trauma, neck and shoulder pain may be due to muscular strain from holding an awkward position for prolonged periods of time. This can occur during sleep, or when propping oneself up to watch television or read in bed, or when looking up while working overhead. Muscular strain and spasm can also occur when normal activities are performed under emotional stress. Neck problems can be catalyzed or aggravated by occupations that require keeping the head fixed in the same position for long periods of time, such as the computer operator or assembly-line worker does. Often it is only upon questioning the patient that information related to these types of postures is elicited.

Emotional tension usually affects the neck more than any other aspect of the musculoskeletal body. The muscular tone of the neck and upper back reflect the emotional stress and tension of the

patient. Palpation of the muscles of the neck and shoulders often details the depth of a patient's stress. The tense person who fails to relax his muscles sustains contractions that produce a viselike tightness of the neck and shoulders. Myalgia of the neck due to emotional tension is particularly painful and disabling.

The development of neck pain from sustained muscle contractions is multifactorial. Sustained traction at the periosteal site of muscular attachment produces local pain and tenderness. Sustained contractions also increase intramuscular pressure, which can result in muscle fiber tears and changes in microcirculation, themselves leading to inflammation and ischemia. The combination of tissue ischemia and accumulated metabolic wastes from the sustained contractions leads to a cycle of pain and disability that affects the muscle and its contiguous tissues. Muscular contractions can also irritate the cervical nerve roots in the intervertebral foramen, producing pain that radiates to the shoulder, arm, hand, or head. The soft tissues of the cervical spine, the thoracic outlet region, and the upper extremities—the nerves, muscles, tendons, ligaments—as well as the joint capsules, synovial fluid, and cartilage of the joints are all subject to numerous stresses and strains. Pain in and from the neck can be caused by pressures on these areas and their nerve endings, ischemia of the tissue, and subsequent impairment of movement, together leading to a loss of function or disability.

Disc degeneration caused by repetitive mechanical stress and subsequent inadequate nutrition to the disc is a common cause of neck pain. The weight-bearing forces of the neck are almost equally distributed between the triple joint complex of the cervical spine—the intervertebral disc joint and the two articular facet joints. Degeneration of the anterior disc joint puts increased stress on the vertebral bodies, resulting in osteophyte formation and hypertrophic changes in the posterior facet joints and associated ligaments. These structural aberrations are referred to as degenerative arthritis or osteoarthritis. Due to their close proximity, such changes in the vertebral bodies can result in compression and ischemia of the nerve roots, a condition that produces radiating pain. Barring traumatic impact, nerve compression from disc herniation is not likely to occur in the cervical spine, due to certain bony elevations of the vertebral bodies and the protective barrier between the nerve roots and the disc formed by the thick, double-layered posterior longitudinal ligament. All discs ultimately undergo some degenerative changes, depending on the aging process, the stresses of daily life, injuries, work habits, posture, and emotional tensions. All of these factors will affect the supply of Blood and Qi to the disc. This degeneration can ultimately result in the tearing of the annulus fibrosus of the disc and a protrusion of the nucleus pulposus through the annulus. Because the annulus is pain sensitive, the tearing and irritation of its fibers will cause acute neck pain.

Subluxations of the cervical spine are another source of neck pain. Vertebral misalignments and their compensatory biomechanics will accelerate the degenerative process and may directly irritate the nerve roots, causing neck and shoulder pain. The cervical spine, having the greatest range of motion, is the most eas-ily injured region of the spine during neck strain/sprain and hyperflexion or hyperextension traumas, such as whiplash. The extent of the injury to the neck depends upon the force of impact, the exact position of the head at the moment of impact, and the preexisting health of the tissues of the neck. Trauma to this area can have long-ranging effects depending on the extent of the damage, the patient's overall constitutional health, and preexisting propensities. Injury sustained by a cervical spine that has resilient muscles, ligaments, and discs will be less traumatic than that sustained by a compromised degenerative spine, which will find much less resiliency and a smaller margin of safety in the same situation. Preexistent degeneration may be present and show no symptoms until a seemingly minor trauma impinges on its tenuous margin of safety, and pain results.

Another potential cause of neck pain is thoracic outlet syndrome. This syndrome is a compression of the neurovascular bundle consisting of the brachial plexus and the subclavian artery as they pass from the cervical region to the axilla. These structures are susceptible to compression as they exit the neck between the anterior and middle scalene muscles, pass between the clavicle and first rib, and pass under the pectoralis minor insertion on the coracoid process of the scapula. The nerve irritation and ischemia that result from the compression of these structures at any of these sites can produce neck and shoulder pain, and numbness, tingling, and pain in the upper extremity. The presence of a cervical rib (an extra rib attached to the seventh cervical vertebra) can also produce thoracic outlet syndrome.

When we look at the source of neck and shoulder problems from the homeodynamic perspective we see that one of the common causes is invasion by exogenous influences (climatic forces), particularly Wind, Cold, Heat, and Dampness, which often enter through the back of the neck and cause occipital pain and stiffness. Wind is the most pernicious of these influences, often being the vehicle through which the other pathogens enter. Wind is a major cause of Painful Obstruction Syndrome, or Bi Syndrome. If the pathogenic factors are stronger than the body's Defensive Qi at any particular time, they can lodge in the channels and move into the joint spaces, causing Painful Obstruction Syndrome. Pain results from the obstruction of the circulation of Qi and Blood in the channels by the exogenous pathogens.

The joints are important areas where pathogens can enter and obstruct the flow of Qi and Blood; they are also the areas where Qi and Blood meet and interact. If a joint is already weakened through overuse due to sports, occupation, or improper Qi and/or Blood nourishment, the joint will be predisposed to invasion by exogenous forces.

Since all of the Yang channels converge at GV14, located in the C7/T1 area, an invasion of an exogenous influence will generally take place in the Yang channels that move through the neck and shoulder areas. These are the more superficial channels and the easiest to penetrate. Because these pathways all pass through the neck area, it is easy for an exogenous influence to cause obstructions in these channels, thereby affecting the digestive channels and subsequently the processes of assimilation, digestion, and elimina-

tion. Conversely, problems in the Yang Organs can produce blockages in the channels that can manifest as pain in any of the areas that the channel traverses, in this case most notably the neck and upper shoulder areas. It is important to remember that the Organs and their pertaining channels together constitute an indivisible energetic unit. A problem in an organ can affect its channel or a blockage in a channel can make its way into the interior of the body and be transmitted to its pertaining organ. In addition, after invading the superficial channels first, exogenous pathogens, such as Cold, Wind, Heat, or Damp, can then settle in the joints, causing Qi and Blood to stagnate. Painful Obstruction Syndrome is frequently not visible on the results of tests prescribed by Western doctors. Standard Western diagnostics, such as X rays, MRIs, and so forth, often show no positive indications of the same etiological information found by an Oriental medical practitioner, since these tests are unable to uncover energetic disturbances and are limited to discovering structural imbalances only.

Accidents can also be a cause of Painful Obstruction Syndrome, even if the patient states that the accident happened years ago and he had a full recovery. Often the areas impacted by an accident sustain some Blood Stagnation that predisposes the area to invasion by exogenous pathogens years later. It should also be noted that Phlegm can lodge in the channels and joints and contribute to Painful Obstruction Syndrome.

In chronic cases of Painful Obstruction Syndrome, such as in the elderly, we must look more toward Qi and Blood deficiencies as important factors in the condition. From the traditional Chinese medical viewpoint, the sources of chronic muscle and bone problems are generally to be found in disharmonies of the Spleen, Liver, and Kidney, since these Organs rule the muscles, sinews, and bones respectively. The Spleen is responsible for extracting the Qi of Grain from the food, which is the foundation for Qi and Blood. The Qi of Grain mixes with the Qi of Air to form first Ancestral Qi, and, through further transformations, Nutrient Qi. It is the Nutrient Qi that is transported throughout the body by the Spleen and is sent to nourish the muscles and limbs. If the Spleen Qi is deficient, this Qi cannot be transported to the muscles and the person will feel fatigued. In severe cases there will be atrophy of the muscles.

More important are the kind of nutrients the person is ingesting, from which the extraction of the Qi of Grain takes place. If an individual eats food laden with chemicals, such as artificial flavors, chemical substitutes for sugar, artificial colorings, preservatives, pesticides and the like, then there will be poor quantity and poor quality Qi of Grain available for extraction. Sweets, cold foods, and mucus-forming foods also negatively affect the Spleen. All will affect the quality and quantity of the Ancestral and later Nutrient Qi created for the organism—what is then being transported is failing to nourish and sustain the body. In time the transformation and transportation functions of the Spleen will become impaired and even less Nutrient Qi will reach the limbs and organs, resulting in a depletion of the overall immune system.

Since we are what we eat, the importance of proper nutrition in the maintenance of the body's health cannot be overemphasized, no matter what the condition being treated. The conditions under which we eat are also important. Eating irregularly, eating on the run, eating under stress, eating while worrying, arguing at mealtimes, or sparse or excessive eating all put a strain on the Spleen and can lead to Spleen Qi Deficiency or Spleen Yang Deficiency, resulting in fatigue and weak limbs.

Another important factor to be considered about the Spleen is its relationship to Blood, since the Spleen transports both the Qi of Grain and pure Fluids, the basic components of Blood. It is not only the transportation of Qi that is vital to the muscles and the flesh, but also the transformation and transportation of the Blood. Any weakness or dysfunction of the Spleen, usually termed a Spleen Blood Deficiency, will therefore have a profound effect on other Organs and on the muscular system, resulting in numbness or tingling sensations.

The Liver works closely with the Spleen and controls the state of the sinews (the tendons, ligaments, and to some extent the joints, since the extension and flexion of the sinews allows the joints to move). The sinews, which alternately contract and relax, affect the ability of our muscles to move with ease or difficulty. They are dependent on the smooth flow of Blood and Qi to keep them moistened and supple.

The Liver feeds the sinews in two ways. One way is through the smooth flow of Qi and Blood throughout the entire body, including the organs. Since the nature of Liver energy is ascending and spreading, it can affect all parts of the organism. The Liver is easily made dysfunctional by negative emotions, which constrain and stagnate Qi. This interferes with the flowing and spreading function of the Liver and results in tight and inflexible sinews. When people become upset their negativity is often directly translated into a tightening of the sinews and, in turn, the muscles. The Gall Bladder, which is paired with the Liver, is also easily affected by negative emotions. The Gall Bladder Channel moves through the neck and shoulders—common areas of muscular spasm. The more the Liver energy is impeded the more emotional negativity will be experienced, resulting in more Liver and Gall Bladder dysfunction.

The Liver also controls the volume of Blood circulating through the system. It therefore works with and relies upon its relationship with both the Spleen's transformation and its transportation of Blood to maintain the proper flow of Blood throughout the body. When the Liver Blood is deficient, the sinews lack the nourishment and lubrication they need. This lack of nourishment and moistening can lead to muscle spasms and cramps; tightness of the sinews, which affects their ability to extend and flex; numbness; tremors; and joint degeneration. Liver Blood Deficiency is more common in women, while Liver Qi Stagnation or Liver Yang Rising is more common in men. In the elderly we generally see Liver Wind or Liver Fire as the predominant cause of these symptoms.

The last of this trio, the Kidney, is perhaps the most important for a variety of reasons, one of which is the Kidney's rule of the bones through their production of Marrow, which in TCM is a substance that forms the bones, bone marrow, brain, and spinal cord. The Essence of the Kidney produces the Marrow, which is the basis for bone marrow. If the Kidney Essence is strong, the bones will also be strong; if the Kidney Essence is weak, the bones will be brittle. Declining Kidney Essence is the cause of increased bone degeneration in the elderly. In addition, according to the Five Element theory, the Kidney is the Mother of the Liver; therefore, Kidney Essence feeds the Liver. Kidney Essence Deficiency could in turn lead to a Liver Blood Deficiency, which would affect the health of the Spleen and Kidney as well as the whole organism. The connection between the production of Marrow and the production of Blood cannot be underestimated, for it defines one of the essential relationships between the Kidney, Spleen, and Liver. Clearly the creation of Blood, its transportation, and its importance to the health of the musculoskeletal body is dependent on the success of the relationship of this important triumverate.

Acute neck pain is usually due to an exogenous invasion, usually Wind, or to trauma or spasm and strain of the neck. In these cases there is a sudden onset and restricted range of motion of the neck. If the patient has a propensity toward a Liver disharmony, he will be more susceptible to this problem. Chronic neck pain evolves over a long period of time and is due to frequent acute attacks that do not receive proper treatment. It can also be due to a predisposition to Liver, Spleen, and Kidney disharmonies. Patients who suffer from chronic neck pain will find their problems exacerbated during periods of windy weather or unseasonal weather where wind predominates.

Shoulder pain is often due to invasion of the shoulder by exogenous Cold, which can cause the muscles and sinews to contract and thereby cause pain. Cold and damp weather will often aggravate this problem. If this problem is not treated in a timely fashion, such invasions can evolve into chronic problems. Shoulder pain can also be caused by excessive repetition of movements involving the shoulder, such as those of a carpenter or bricklayer. And of course accidents will cause stagnation of Qi and Blood to the local area. We must also consider the channels that flow through the affected areas. Sometimes organ dysfunctions can express themselves as pain along the pertaining channel. For example, shoulder pain along the Colon Channel can be a reflection of a problem with the colon.

With all of the above in mind, a patient's "simple" complaint of pain in the neck and shoulder region must be closely examined within the assessment strategies outlined below. In some patients the site of pain may also be the source of pain; it may also merely be the area to which the pain is referred. A thorough investigation of the problem is always warranted.

The following basic neck and shoulder treatment will always assist in conditions of Qi and Blood obstruction and help to relieve the immediate symptoms regardless of the cause. However, in chronic conditions where there is more present than the obstruction of Qi—where there are Spleen, Liver, and/or Kidney energetic imbalances more deeply affecting the Yin and Yang energies of the body—more advanced techniques and point locations are necessary.

AMMA THERAPY TREATMENT

The patient is assessed through the application of the Four Traditional Methods.

The therapist begins assessing from the moment he sees the patient—observing how the patient walks, sits, and lies down on the table looking for signs of misalignment, such as one shoulder being higher than the other, the neck tilting to one side or rotated to one side, the shoulders bowling forward, or the visibility of a winged scapula. The therapist then palpates for areas of thickness of the muscles, sinews, and bones; tightness; spasms; muscle weakness; atrophy; misalignment of the vertebrae or the shoulders; any existing arthritic conditions (thickening of the vertebrae); or fusion of the vertebrae.

Once the problem has been identified, the next step is to determine the course of treatment and the proper nutritional, herbal, and exercise recommendations. The following treatment is one that can be incorporated into or integrated with other treatments where stiff neck and pain occur. Recommendations will vary, of course, and will be modified depending on the pattern that is identified. For example, if a patient is suffering from a stiff neck as a result of an invasion by an exogenous influence, such as Wind Cold, treatment must include emphasis on the Lung Channel and related points, as well as treatment of the stiff neck.

AMMA THERAPY ASSESSMENT

The treatment of the neck and shoulder includes manipulation of the Tendino-Muscle Channels found in those areas, as well as palpation of specific points on the superficial pathways of the Primary Channels.

1. Check for tightness under the occiput. The therapist should be able to feel some space between the occiput and the insertion of the muscles. Some patients' muscles are so tight and in spasm that this space has been lost and this area needs to be relaxed. Deep manipulation may be required. One side of the trapezius muscle is generally tighter than the other. Pay more attention to the tighter side.

2. Check for temporomandibular joint (TMJ) problems, which can move the neck out of alignment. Ask the patient if they have any dental fixtures, as these often cause misalignment of the TMJ. Place the palms bilaterally on the TMJ, with the fingers resting on the neck and throat. Ask the patient to slowly open his mouth while monitoring the movement of the mandible with the palms of the hands. Listen for clicking noises, check for tenderness and swelling, and see if he can open his mouth without it deviating to one side. Manipulation in the joint spaces of the TMJ helps to relieve spasms and pain.

3. Advanced Amma therapists should palpate for swollen thyroid (goiter). Sometimes simply looking at the neck will reveal thyroid swelling, which can cause neck pain. Palpation is done with palms placed on the TMJ and the pads of the second, third, and fourth fingers resting gently on both sides of the throat. Ask the patient to swallow. As the patient swallows, gently alternate the second, third, and fourth fingers as you palpate for swellings.

Students should practice palpation on their own throats so that they can distinguish between a normal and a swollen thyroid. Practice is also essential for developing sensitivity and for learning how to apply the appropriate amounts of pressure. Care must be taken not to jab the patient's neck and throat with the fingers. Should a swollen thyroid be present, apply teh tah chu. If the condition was previously unknown to the patient, suggest that he see his physician. Thyroid problems are also treatable through advanced Amma therapy, which includes specific dietary recommendations, herbs, and supplementation. This option should also be suggested to the patient.

4. Check for spasms in the sternocleidomastoid (SCM) muscle. One side will often be tighter than the other. The tighter side will feel thin and hard, like a taut rubber band; the side that is not in spasm will feel wider and softer. Spasms in the SCM are often the cause of a great deal of neck and shoulder pain.

5. Palpate the shoulder for tightness, stiffness, heat, calcification, or swelling of the joint spaces.

6. Look at the shoulders and see if they bowl forward, or if one is higher while the patient is lying in the supine position.

7. Perform passive range of motion of the shoulder. This should be done gently and slowly, and no sudden movements should be made. When the arm is abducted to the shoulder level be very cautious about raising it any higher, especially in elderly patients. Then have the patient

perform active range of motion. Both of these techniques are performed to observe and assess restrictions of movement.

8. Palpate the posterior aspect of the shoulder joints for calcification. If calcification is found, manipulate with teh tah chu.

ADDITIONAL TECHNIQUES

1. If the patient's shoulders bowl forward, an extra point located on the anterior aspect of the shoulder may be used. The point is located halfway between the acromioclavicular articulation and the anterior axillary fold, and should be used only if the muscle feels tight upon palpation. This point is useful for pain, inflammation, restricted movement of the shoulders, and frozen shoulder. If your finger seems to fall into a hollow space it indicates muscle atrophy. In such cases do not use this point but instead concentrate your technique on manipulation of the upper shoulder.

2. If the patient's shoulders are bowling forward, gently push the shoulders toward the table, with the palms of both hands resting on the pectoralis muscles. Keep the elbows straight and push down toward the table, gradually increasing your pressure. Use a rocking motion as you alternate from side to side to prevent the patient from further tightening and resisting.

3. For very tight necks and for "crane's neck," traction the neck with both hands, the index fingers pressing up into GB12 and the fourth fingers pressing up into GB20. The patient's chin should be gently tucked when performing this technique. If your hands tire, you may traction one side at a time, however you should work toward being able to traction the neck using both hands at the same time to provide a deeper release and more balanced stretch.

4. For a very tight SCM muscle, walk approximately one-third of the way down the SCM, with the third finger leading while using the second and fourth fingers as guides. Then stretch the muscle in one-space increments, walking back up to the occiput.

5. If the neck muscles are extremely thick and tight and the range of motion is limited, turn the head slightly to one side and, while tractioning with the hand that is supporting the head, use the other hand to manipulate the muscles next to the cervical spine. All fingers are in contact but the third finger leads, moving down the muscle.

6. If there are spasms in the SCM, place your thumb at the clavicle where the clavicular head of the SCM originates and move laterally across the clavicle to the shoulder manipulating above the clavicle as you move across.

7. Stroke down the SCM with the thumb to release it. Be careful not to jab your thumb into the supraclavicular fossa.

8. Using the third fingers, simultaneously stretch both SCMs up toward the occiput.

9. Abduct the shoulder and with your

thumb manipulate the anterior, medial, and posterior portions of the deltoid muscle. The tightness will change as the arm is moved and rotated. As the areas of tightness change, manipulate those areas.

10. Apply circular thumb or circular digital pressure to the triceps. This is useful when the patient's forearm is too tense to relax down to the table.

11. If the patient suffers with radiating pain from the neck into the shoulder and the range of motion is limited, advanced Amma therapists may tilt the head slightly and, with the other hand, apply direct thumb pressure into the muscles along the cervical spine, which insert under the occiput. Starting from the occiput, move down the musculature in 1-tsun increments.

12. Palpate the GB21 area and check for swelling. If you feel a spasm, press directly into it using thumb pressure. The direction of force is inferior and slightly medial.

13. Standing at the head of the table, observe the chest muscles from the shoulders to the nipples. Look for differences between the left and right sides. Spasmed muscles will appear shorter and thicker. If one side appears shorter and thicker, advanced Amma therapists may use the heel of the palm to press and rotate in order to release the spasm. With female patients, always take care not to press directly on breast tissue.

14. With the patient in the prone position manipulate around the scapula, with particular attention on the glenohumeral joint. Manipulate this area

using circular thumb pressure, then rotate the patient's arm while continuing to manipulate.

15. For patients with upper back spasms, manipulate alongside the medial scapula with one palm on top of the other. This is a more forceful technique and should only be used by advanced Amma therapists on patients who can tolerate deeper manipulation.

POINT LOCATION AND ACTION

The actions listed for each of the following points pertain to each point's relationship to the treatment of neck pain and stiffness. These points have other actions that are not relevant to this particular treatment but that will be explored in other advanced Amma therapy treatments. These points are by no means exclusive, as there are other points that may be useful for this treatment and that can be incorporated, depending on the etiology and the skill of the therapist.

1. GB12

Location: In the depression posterior and inferior to the mastoid process.

Whether the patient is in the supine or prone position, this point can be accessed bilaterally with the third finger pressing up toward the occiput. If the third finger is not strong enough by itself, it may be combined with the second finger, with the two fingers together hooking up under the occiput.

Action: GB12 relaxes muscle spasms, helps expel exogenous Wind, and calms the emotions. It is useful for headaches due to rising Qi in the Liver/Gall Bladder complex, and for pain behind the ear.

Comment: GB12 is the Intersecting point for the Gall Bladder and Bladder channels.

2. GB20

Location: In a depression between the SCM and the upper portion of the trapezius.

Whether the patient is in the supine or prone position, this point can also be accessed bilaterally with the third finger pressing up toward the occiput. If the third finger is not strong enough by itself, it may be combined with the second finger. Use the pads of the two fingers together to hook up under the occiput.

Action: GB20 eliminates exogenous Wind Cold or Wind Heat, which cause headache and stiff neck; eliminates Interior Wind; and is used to treat dizziness, vertigo, eye problems, and hearing problems resultant from rising Liver Yang or Fire.

Comment: GB20 is the Intersecting point of the Gall Bladder and San Jiao channels.

3. GB21

Location: Midway between GV14 and the acromion, on the highest point of the shoulder.

This point is pressed bilaterally from either the supine or prone position, using the thumbs. The force is slightly medial and down toward the feet.

Action: GB21 relaxes the sinews, treats Painful Obstruction Syndrome of the neck and shoulders, and expels Wind and Cold.

Comment: GB21 is the Intersecting point of the Gall Bladder and San Jiao channels.

4. Co11

Location: In the depression at the lateral end of the transverse cubital crease, midway between Lu5 and the lateral epicondyle of the humerus when the elbow is half-flexed.

Bend the patient's elbow and place your thumb on the point. Gently open the arm and press. The force is straight into the joint.

Action: Co11 expels exogenous Wind and Wind Heat. It benefits the sinews and joints and can therefore be used in treating Painful Obstruction Syndrome of the neck and shoulders. Co11 is also useful for elbow and arm pain, and for treating motor difficulties due to stroke.

Comment: Co11 is the Earth and the Sea point of the Colon Channel.

5. TS-FA1

Location: 1 tsun below Co11 when the forearm is pronated.

Using the thumb, slightly hook your finger into the point with pressure straight into the arm.

Action: This point benefits the neck and shoulders and benefits Painful Obstruction Syndrome.

6. Co15

Location: At the anterior and inferior border of the acromioclavicular joint, inferior to the acromion, when the arm is abducted. The point is in the depression of the acromion when the arm is in full abduction.

While the patient is lying in the supine position, use your thumb and press into the depression.

Action: Co15 helps the sinews; it also treats Painful Obstruction Syndrome of the shoulders and shoulder bursitis, pain, stiffness, and inflammation; stimulates the circulation of Qi in the channel; helps expel Wind; and treats muscular spasms.

Comment: If the patient is suffering from bursitis, this point will be extremely painful upon pressing. In this case, release your pressure immediately and instead use teh tah chu to generally manipulate the area.

7. Co16

Location: In the depression between the acromial extremity of the clavicle and the spine of the scapula.

With the patient lying in the supine position, use your thumb to hook into the depression.

Action: Co16 benefits the joints and shoulders, treats upper extremity pain, helps remove obstructions from the channel, and stimulates the local circulation of blood.

Comment: This point is also useful for stimulating the descending of Lung Qi and can assist in the treatment of asthma and coughs that are due to a failure of the Lung Qi to descend.

8. St38

Location: 8 tsun below St35, 2 tsun below St37.

The therapist may use his thumb or knuckle; the force is toward the tibia.

Action: St38 reduces pain and stiffness of the shoulder, relaxes the tendons and ligaments, and helps to dispel Wind and Cold.

Comment: The patient should gently rotate his shoulder while the therapist is manipulating this point. If the patient's movement is severely restricted, an addi-

tional person may help the patient to gently rotate the shoulder. Distal points are useful for helping to remove obstructions from the involved channel.

9. Sp5

Location: In the depression distal and anterior to the medial malleolus, halfway between the tuberosity of the navicular bone and the vertex of the medial malleolus, between Liv4 and Ki6.

Use the pad of the third finger to manipulate directly into the depression.

Action: This is a very useful point for relieving Painful Obstruction Syndrome due to Dampness, and while it is often used locally for pain in the ankle and foot, it can be used as an overall River point for any channel that is suffering from Painful Obstruction Syndrome due to Dampness.

Comment: Sp5 is a River and Metal point of the Spleen Channel. The patient should gently rotate his shoulder while the therapist is manipulating this point.

10. TS-LE-I1

Location: Lateral side of the proximal phalange of the great toe at the midpoint of the shaft.

Grasp the toe and use your thumb to manipulate. After manipulation, gently thumb stroke the shaft a few times.

Action: This point treats the neck. The Liver Channel starts on the lateral side of the great toe and proceeds up the dorsum of the foot. Manipulation of the beginning of the channel helps to promote the free flow of Qi, one of the Liver's major functions and that which is necessary for the proper nourishment of the sinews.

11. TS-LE-I2

Location: On the medial side of the proximal phalange of the great toe at the midpoint of the shaft.

Grasp the toe and use your thumb to manipulate. After manipulation, gently thumb stroke the shaft a few times.

Action: The Spleen Channel begins on the medial side of the great toe. Manipulation of the beginning of the channel helps to promote the free flow of Spleen Qi necessary for proper nourishment of the muscles and flesh. This point treats the shoulder.

12. TS-LE-I3

Location: On the lateral side of the great toe, between Liv2 and TS-LE-I1.

Grasp the toe and use direct thumb pressure.

Action: This point treats the area where the neck and shoulder meet. It is excellent for stiffness and pain in the neck and shoulders.

13. TS-LE-I4

Location: On the medial side of the great toe, between Sp2 and TS-LE-I2.

Grasp the toe and use direct thumb pressure.

Action: This point treats neck and shoulder problems.

14. TS-LE-IV1

Location: Plantar surface of the fourth toe, on the proximal interphalangeal joint.

Grasp the toe with your thumb and palpate for the ball of the bone. Manipulate that area (the proximal interphalangeal joint) using circular thumb pressure. This point is pressed when the patient is lying prone.

Action: This point treats pain in the back of the neck that radiates over the top of the head.

15. Sp21

Location: On the midaxillary line, 6 tsun below the axilla and midway between the axilla and the free end of the eleventh rib.

This point can be manipulated bilaterally, with the patient in either the supine or prone position. The point is activated with the pads of the third fingers pressing directly into the intercostal space.

Action: Sp21 treats general muscular aches and pains due to stagnation of Blood.

Comment: This is the Great Luo (Connecting) point of the Spleen.

TREATMENT FOR LOWER BACK PAIN

AMMA THERAPY ETIOLOGY

According to the principles of Amma therapy, back pain is generally not an isolated symptom but part of a set of symptoms that define a particular pattern of imbalance, which is often the result of combinations of internal and external causes of disease. Therefore the therapist must, as always, conduct a thorough diagnostic assessment in order to establish whether the pain is stemming from simple muscular strain or if it is part of a larger, more complex pattern of disease. Back pain is a frequent problem seen in the clinical setting. It is estimated that 88 percent of the population will experience neck or back pain at some point in their lives. Seventy million Americans have experienced severe backache more than once in their lifetime and twelve million patients receive medical treatment of some kind for it every day. There are two million new cases of back pain added to these statistics each year.

Lower back pain is generally defined as any pain located from the level of the twelfth thoracic vertebra to the area of the gluteal crease. If we look at lower back pain from a musculoskeletal point of view, we see that the back is a complex structure that serves weight-bearing and locomotor functions. Since the lumbar area is fairly mobile and supports the weight of the trunk, injury occurs here quite frequently. The discs, ligaments, and muscles in this area of the spine have to both support the weight of the upper body and control movements in the lower back.

Fluid movement of the spine requires good neuromuscular coordination, sufficient elasticity of tissues (muscles and ligaments), and capability of the participating joints. The limits of the range of motion of the spine depend on the flexibility of the ligaments, joints, and muscles and the fluidity of the discs. It is important to remember that the flexibility, elasticity, and fluidity of these tissues are also determined by the amount of movement and activity in which they are engaged. Proper movement of the joints helps to keep them lubricated and also helps to keep the ligaments supple and properly nourished. Since both the discs and ligaments have little or no blood supply, they rely on the motion of the joints to pump tissue fluids to them in order to provide necessary nutrients. Adhesions in the joints and ligaments and malnutrition of the tissues result when there is improper movement, which in turn accelerates their degeneration. This produces stiff and painful joints with limited range of motion. Regular exercise in which the joints are properly put through their full ranges of motion is essential for the health of the back as well as the neck.

Because the back must provide both support and flexibility, it is easily susceptible to injury through strain, sprain, and trauma. From a Western viewpoint, there are two basic categories of back injuries: peak overload trauma and cumulative trauma. Peak overload trauma is a single severe stress to the spine, such as a fall or blow, an automobile accident, lifting a heavy weight, and so forth. The more common cumulative trauma is repetitive small traumas to the spine (microtraumas), such as stress and tension; poor standing, sitting, sleeping, or bending postures; improper lifting technique; poor nutrition; obesity; and so forth. Many of the sources of these microtraumas to the neck and back originate from personal lifestyle habits at home and at work. Occupational or daily hazards can include poor posture or sleeping positions and physical overwork of the back, such as excessive standing, sitting, reaching, bending, crouching, twisting, and lifting. Improper bending and lifting and excessive twisting are the most common causes of injury in the lower back.

An example of an occupational hazard is the excessive lifting done by a delivery man or the excessive standing of a salesperson or waitress. These activities tend to weaken, strain, and imbalance the muscles of the lower back, which are the primary stabilizers of the spine. The muscles of the back extend from the base of the skull to the buttocks and are arranged in a series of layers in which the larger muscles are superficial and the smaller, shorter muscles are deep. No individual muscle extends from the head to the buttock; instead, smaller muscles are arranged in an overlapping, stair-step fashion from the pelvic bones up to the skull. Weakness of the back muscles produces an unstable back and predisposes an individual to injury. Since the back is always working, proper muscle tone and flexibility are essential to prevent injury.

The intervertebral foramina allow for the exit of nerves traveling to and from the spinal cord to all the structures of the body. In addition, connective tissue, fat, and blood and lymph vessels are located inside these spaces. Any encroachment or narrowing (stenosis) of the intervertebral foramina will compress the structures within the foramina and produce ischemia of the nerve roots, causing pain in the lower back; hip; perineal, gluteal, or inguinal regions; and the lower extremities.

The intervertebral discs that lie between the vertebral bodies comprise 20 to 25 percent of the total length of the vertebral column. Vascularity of the discs decreases beginning at age eight, the discs becoming more avascular in adulthood. Degenerative changes in the discs begin after the second decade of life. With the decrease in the amount of fluid contained within each disc, the disc becomes thinner, more immobile, and prone to trauma because of its increased brittleness.

Disc herniation (bulging or protrusion) can occur from peak overload trauma or, more commonly, from cumulative trauma in which repetitive strain continually weakens the annular fibers of the disc leading to herniation of the nucleus pulposus. A herniated disc in which the annular fibers are still intact is called a contained disc. A noncontained or prolapsed disc occurs when the annular fibers tear and are no longer able to restrain the nucleus pulposus. This allows the nuclear material to sequester or free-fragment into the vertebral canal.

Disc herniation is a frequent cause of intervertebral foramina stenosis. The most common areas of disc herniation are the L4/L5 and L5/S1 discs because of their great weight-bearing load and the high degree of motion occurring at these levels of the lumbar spine. Acute onset of radiating pain down either leg is the main sign of a disc herniation. The pain may continue for months or years and become chronic, and could cause progressive neurological deficits, such as numbness or muscular atrophy.

As the discs degenerate their shock-absorbing abilities diminish and more stress is placed on the bodies of the vertebrae and the articular facets, which undergo changes (lipping and spur formation) as a result of this increased load. These hypertrophic changes of the articular facets and thickening of the surrounding ligaments can lead to encroachment on the nerve roots and/or spinal cord and contribute to radicular pain either with or in the absence of disc herniation. Misalignment of the vertebrae, increasing or reversal of the spinal curves, and degenerative arthritis of the spine can all lead to changes in the intervertebral joint complex, resulting in the narrowing of the intervertebral foramina or spinal canal and producing nerve compression.

Many people have been diagnosed as having "arthritis" of the spine—this is a catch-all diagnosis for degenerative changes. These changes can generally be avoided with proper posture and good body mechanics, which place less stress on the vertebrae and discs by evenly distributing and minimizing the wear and tear on these structures. Proper diet is also important to provide nutritional support to these tissues. Amma therapy, chiropractic manipulation, acupuncture, and appropriate exercises like hatha yoga or t'ai chi chuan can help to relieve discomfort and assist the patient in correcting degenerative conditions.

Another source of lower back pain is sciatica. The sciatic nerve is formed by the nerve roots of the lower lumbar and upper sacral nerves. The sciatic nerve is the largest nerve in the body, supplying the posterior thigh muscles and all the muscles of the leg and foot. The condition known as sciatica is an irritation or inflammation of the sciatic nerve, characterized by pain radiating from the back into the buttock, and possibly down the back of the leg and into the foot, depending upon the degree of irritation to the nerve. Prolonged irritation of the sciatic nerve can produce muscle atrophy and skin changes in the leg and foot.

The most common cause of sciatica is lumbar disc herniation. One sign of disc involvement with sciatica is pain on sneezing, coughing, and straining during defecation. Pain in all three of these actions is a good indicator of herniation of a contained disc. (Sneezing, coughing, and straining upon defecation will not exacerbate the pain of a noncontained disc.) Irritation to the sciatic nerve can also come from problems with the piriformis muscle, a deep muscle of the buttock that extends from the sacrum to the greater trochanter of the femur. Anatomical variations show that the sciatic nerve passes under, over, or through this muscle. Due to its close proximity to the sciatic nerve, any spasm or flaccidity of this muscle may irritate the nerve, producing a sciatica-like pain that can mimic the pain of a disc herniation. This is called piriformis syndrome.

Another type of lower back syndrome is called facet syndrome. The facets are the small joints on the neural arch of the vertebrae that help guide vertebral movement and provide minimal weight-bearing support. When these joints are irritated or inflamed they swell and can compress the contents of the intervertebral foramina, producing sciatica-like pain that radiates down the leg to the knee. Any condition that increases the lumbar curve will place more weight on these small joints, joints that are not

built for such support. Men with protruding abdomens and pregnant women or women who wear high-heeled shoes exhibit increased lumbar curves and are prone to developing a facet syndrome. One distinguishing characteristic of this syndrome is increased pain on extension of the lumbar spine.

Other problems manifest in a condition known as spondylolisthesis which translates as "spinal slipping" or "spinal falling," a condition in which the neural arch is not completely formed or undergoes degeneration, thus allowing the body of one vertebra to slip forward onto the segment below. This condition occurs most frequently with the fifth lumbar vertebra moving forward over the sacrum. In most instances this condition is asymptomatic until the second or third decade of life, when the person may experience low back trauma. Pain then develops in the lower back in the area of the sacroiliac joints, and sometimes radiates into the thighs. This condition is easily seen on an X ray. Some authorities feel that placing an infant in an upright posture before the spine has matured appropriately may predispose the child to the development of a spondylolisthesis. However, this condition rarely progresses, and in fact most backaches that patients experience are due to other causes unrelated to the level of the slippage. Appropriate stretches and conservative care consisting of Amma therapy, and chiropractic manipulation when necessary, will manage this condition.

Scoliosis is a lateral curvature of the spine. This condition may be symptomatic or asymptomatic. Most are of idiopathic cause and are treatable through conservative measures. However, the more serious progressive types of scoliosis can lead to impairment of lung and heart function and require more aggressive treatment. Scoliosis, which first develops between the ages of seven and eleven, is more common in young girls, and there can be a congenital tendency to developing scoliosis. The success of the treatment of this condition depends on how early it is detected and how severe the degree of curvature is. Amma therapy, in conjunction with appropriate chiropractic manipulation and exercise, is extremely beneficial and can produce significant improvement in many cases of scoliosis. This will depend on the patient's level of compliance, the severity of the scoliosis, and how early therapy is instituted.

From a homeodynamic perspective, lower back pain, which may be acute or chronic, results from energetic imbalances within the system. For thousands of years, lower back pain has been diagnosed and treated successfully without the use of X rays and MRIs. (The latest research shows that these imaging studies have little or no influence on the clinical decisions relative to the treatment of lower back pain.) The channels that most directly influence the lower back are the Bladder and Kidney channels and the Governing Vessel. The Bladder Channel, the largest channel within the body, flows in four pathways—two on either side of the spine, both sides having a medial and lateral branch. At Bl23, located 1.5 tsun from the lower border of L2, the Bladder Channel goes deep to connect with the Kidney Channel before reemerging at the same point to continue the superficial pathway flow. Other channels also energize the back area. The Bladder Tendino-Muscle Channel energizes the muscles of the back

and the Bladder Divergent Channel also flows on both sides of the spine. The Kidney Channel has a deep pathway that flows up the spine to connect with the bladder and the kidneys. The Kidney Tendino-Muscle Channel connects to the anterior aspect of the spine and the Kidney Divergent Channel flows with and connects to the Bladder Channel. The Governing Vessel, considered by many ancient texts to be a branch of the Kidney Channel, flows up the spine.

We have already established that one of the common causes of lower back pain is occupational. Occupations that require repetitive movements of one particular part of the body will generally tend to cause a stagnation of Qi and Blood to that area. This is also true for the back. In chronic situations, Qi to this area can also stagnate through excessive use, such as excessive lifting, standing, reaching, or bending. When the muscles of the lower back are strained, the Kidney Qi will become deficient.

When one part of the body's structure is worked in excess of the rest of the body, three major Yin Organs—the Spleen, the Liver, and the Kidney—will generally be affected. Each Organ has a special relationship with a particular tissue of the body. This relationship between certain tissues and Organs is an active and functional relationship. Therefore the state of the Organ is reflected in the health of the tissue and, conversely, problems with the tissues can affect the Organs. In cases of lower back pain, the relationships are that of the Spleen Qi ruling the muscles and the flesh, Liver Qi ruling the sinews (tendons, ligaments, and to some extent the joints), and the Kidney Qi ruling the bones. The Spleen Qi transports vital nutrients and Fluids as well as Blood to the muscles and flesh. Obstructions of Spleen Qi that result from repetitive movements can block the transport of these vital substances, causing muscle weakness and, in severe cases, muscle atrophy in the area. Conversely, a weak Spleen, common in our culture due to poor diet and lack of exercise, can fail to transport vital substances to the muscles, resulting not only in muscle atrophy but in general fatigue.

The health of the Spleen is a major influence on how much energy is available. The Liver in turn influences the sinews by insuring that there is a smooth flow and circulation of Qi, Blood, and vital substances to the ligaments, tendons, and joints where these tissues originate and insert. Obstruction of Liver energy can cause spasms, numbness, and difficulty in bending and stretching, or simply bring on weakness in a particular area. The Kidney produces the Marrow, which creates the spinal cord and the brain and is the foundation for the formation of bones. Weak Kidney Qi can be responsible for congenital problems of the spine and joints. Stiffness of the spine is often related to deficiency of Kidney Qi. Activities that obstruct or deplete the Qi and Blood to the lower back area can progress to dysfunctions of the channels and then to the Organs themselves. For example, what begins as lower back pain due to strain and sprain of the area may over time progress to dysfunctions of the Kidney and Bladder Organs and their orbs of influence.

The wrong kind of exercise can be another cause of obstruction and stagnation of Qi and Blood, causing pain or muscle strain to the lower back, which in turn influences and weakens the Kidney Qi. While exercise is necessary and beneficial to a person's well-being as it pumps the Blood and vital substances throughout the vessels and channels, the proper form of exercise is essential. Certain types of exercise that concentrate and strain a particular area of the body can be as detrimental to that area as occupational stress. In the case of the lower back, weight lifting can have a negative effect in the same way that tennis can instigate problems with the elbows, weight lifting causing stagnation of Qi and Blood in the lower back, as well as muscle strain. High impact aerobic exercise with excessive repeated impact trauma from jumping can damage the joints and muscles. Exercise that is excessive during the time of puberty can cause menstrual dysfunction for young girls later in life, and lower back pain often appears as a major symptom.

Lack of exercise can also be a cause of disease, since consistent exercise is necessary for the proper circulation of Qi and Blood. The "couch-potato syndrome" can lead to stagnation of essential energetic substances, as can obesity, which puts additional strain on the spine. Lack of exercise can result in weakening of the spine and its supporting ligaments and muscles. This is why Oriental forms of exercise, such as qi kung, t'ai chi chuan, and hatha yoga, are so beneficial, for they greatly improve the circulation of Qi and Blood and speed the transport of vital essences through the system to nourish the organs, bones, muscles, and flesh.

Excessive sexual activity can also weaken the lower back, since it depletes Kidney Qi. When Kidney Qi is deficient, both the bones and muscles of the lower back will be affected, resulting in chronic lower back pain.

Lower back pain takes on an added dimension in relationship to menstruation, pregnancy, and menopause. Lower back pain, a frequent complaint of PMS, can often result from deficiencies of the Liver and Kidney. In these cases pain begins after the onset of menstruation. Pain can also result from Excess conditions, such as stagnation of Liver Qi, in which case the pain begins before the onset of the period. Lower back pain can result during pregnancy in women with weak constitutions, women who have too many pregnancies or too many pregnancies close together, women who do not rest sufficiently during or after childbirth, or women who have a deficiency of Blood. Due to the increased weight gain and excessive lordosis of the spine, pregnancy will naturally put stress on the spine and tax the Kidney energies, which must support both the mother and the fetus. However, if a woman takes good care of herself with appropriate rest and diet, she can actually strengthen herself during pregancy.

During menopause, the Kidney Essence is in decline and therefore the bones do not get the same nourishment they did previously. This too can lead to lower back pain. Combined with continuous stress, physical and mental overwork, insufficient relaxation, lack of proper exercise, and poor nutritional habits, the Yin energies of the body become depleted and force the Kidney to compensate, thereby depleting the precious energies of the Kidney even further and weakening the lower back area.

In the homeodynamic model of health we see the negative influence of exogenous pathogens (the climatic factors of Cold, Damp, Wind and Heat), which can invade the body and cause obstructions and stagnations of Qi, Blood, and Fluids in the joint spaces and can catalyze Painful Obstruction Syndrome. Since the joints are areas where Qi and Blood aggregate, they are also places where Qi can migrate from the exterior to the interior and from the interior to the exterior. These are areas where exogenous influences can easily enter and collect, upsetting the circulation of Qi, Blood, and Fluids and causing them to stagnate, resulting in pain. Patients often complain that their pain is aggravated at night or when they lie in bed for long periods of time; in this case the lack of movement contributes to the stagnation and subsequent pain.

Cold and Damp are two of the most common sources of lower back pain. The Gate of Vitality, which lies between the two kidneys, should be kept warm and protected from injury. When the back is exposed to pathogenic Cold and Damp, this area can be easily invaded, resulting in either acute or chronic lower back pain. For example, lower back pain that has plagued a person for several years may have begun when the patient lived in a cold, damp, basement apartment, demonstrating an invasion of Damp Cold into his lower back area that subsequently lodged there. People who are exposed to damp weather, such as swimmers or joggers who run in all types of weather, make themselves susceptible to invasion by Damp and Cold. If these pathogens are not appropriately expelled, they can lead to chronic weakness of the Kidney.

In a Damp Cold condition, the pain

is more acute in the morning and improves with a little exercise. This is due to the fact that the flow of Blood and Qi has slowed when the person is lying down, creating more of a stagnation problem. In these cases, proper exercise will help diminish the pain as the flow of Qi and Blood increases and helps to remedy stagnation. Applying wet heat, such as from a hydroculator or a hot-water bottle, is helpful. This condition will feel worse when the weather is cold and damp. If there is more Cold than Damp, there will be more stiffness and pain, since the muscles will contract from the Cold. If the Dampness is greater than the Cold, there will be swelling, a sense of heaviness, and perhaps some numbness.

If the lower back pain is due to Qi and Blood Stagnation, the patient will complain of a sharp, stabbing pain that is worse when sitting, standing, or lying down but improves with some exercise (although too much exercise will exacerbate the pain). Such a condition is not influenced by the weather, does not respond to the application of heat, and is sensitive to palpation. The patient's lower back muscles are often stiff, tense, and inflexible, with limited range of motion due to the obstruction of energies. Acute stagnation of Qi and Blood is brought on by trauma, such as a sprain or strain to the area. Improperly treated exacerbations of this condition can result in a chronic problem, with repeated attacks of lower back pain. If the patient already has a propensity for a Kidney Deficiency, this problem will certainly become chronic and easily exacerbated.

From an Amma therapy perspective, Deficient Kidney Qi is a major cause of chronic lower back pain when the pain is dull and reoccurs in repeated "attacks." Such back pain improves with rest and worsens with too much work, stress, or sexual activity. If the lower back is Cold due to a Kidney Yang Deficiency, some heat applied to the lower back area may temporarily bring relief, but this will not be permanent. Kidney Qi Deficiency weakens the lower back so that exogenous pathogens find an easier entrance into this area; then, with increasing weakness of the musculature, the area becomes more prone to injury. Improper diet, lack of exercise, and heredity are major factors in the onset and progression of this illness. As a person ages, there is a concurrent decline in Kidney Qi, which forms and influences the bones. This is why arthritic tendencies show up more often in the elderly. There may also be inherited tendencies toward unnatural kyphosis, scoliosis, and lordosis, curvatures of the spine that can be exacerbated by poor posture, diet, and exercise.

Genitourinary problems can also result in lower back pain. Pathological conditions of the kidneys, such as infections, stones, and so forth, will usually manifest as lower back pain due to the location of the kidneys in this area, as well as the disruption of energy in the Bladder Channel, which traverses the entire back of the body. These conditions fall under the category of Painful Urinary Syndromes. They can often be attributed either to the accumulation of Damp Heat in the Lower Burner, which negatively affects Bladder functions, fluid circulation, and urination; to Liver Qi Stagnation in the Lower Burner; or to the deficiency of Kidney and Spleen Qi, which must work together in the transportation of Fluids. In such cases the collection of symptoms and signs will give the necessary information to determine whether there is an organ problem. For example, if the patient was suffering from an acute kidney condition, such as kidney stones, this would be obvious from the intense pain and its radiation into the groin; in cases of nephritis, the patient would be complaining of fatigue, edema, and urination problems, all of which would be tested with urinanalysis and cultures.

Finally, we must not overlook the effects of long-standing emotional disturbances that disrupt the mindbody complex and deplete the energies of the Kidney, Liver, and Spleen, the Organs that are responsible for the proper nourishment and maintenance of the musculoskeletal structures. Long-standing emotional worries, fears, anger, and resentments can all deplete the energies of their respective Organs, which in turn affect the tissues that these Organs nourish. Depending on preexisting propensities, history of trauma and exacerbations, age, and occupation, specific areas such as the lower back may become targeted for problems.

Following is a treatment for lower back pain due to strain, sprain, muscle spasms, and general obstruction of Qi and Blood. The additional techniques presented in this treatment are to be utilized in the context of the basic Amma treatment, in conjunction with the techniques previously taught.

AMMA THERAPY TREATMENT

Prior to treatment the therapist will have examined the patient's written medical history. As the physical assessment begins, the therapist continues questioning the patient as to the onset of his condition, how long the condition has persisted, and whether he has had a recent exacerbation. Other information that must be elicited includes the circumstances around which the problem first began, the location and nature of the pain, the associated symptoms, and the time of day the symptoms are better or worse.

After eliciting this information from the patient, the therapist proceeds to observe the musculoskeletal structure and Cutaneous Regions, and to palpate.

AMMA THERAPY ASSESSMENT

1. Ask the patient whether this is an acute or chronic problem, or an exacerbation of a chronic problem. A chronic problem will require a longer amount of time and more treatments to heal.
2. Ask the patient about the quality of her pain; certain types of pain characteristically originate from certain types of injuries.
   + Sharp, stabbing, well-localized pain suggests a superficial lesion of the muscles or fascia due to Qi and Blood Stagnation.
   + Bone pain tends to be deep and boring.
   + Muscle pain is often dull and aching and aggravated by active (but not passive) movements. A Kidney Qi Deficiency will also produce dull, aching pain.
   + Ligament pain is sharp and

localized and aggravated by active and passive movements.

* Vascular pain tends to be throbbing, diffuse, aching, and poorly localized.
* Nerve pain tends to be sharp, burning, and radiating.
* Excruciating, unrelenting, intolerable, deep, boring pain that does not shift with rest, activity, or postural changes suggests serious pathology.

3. Can the patient exercise, or is the patient completely restricted regarding exercise?

* If the pain improves with movement, it indicates a stagnation problem related to a musculoskeletal condition.
* If the pain improves with rest, it points to a Kidney Qi Deficiency or a condition of vascular insufficiency.

4. Is the pain worse in the morning upon arising?

* Lower back pain that is worse in the morning but improves as the day progresses is due to an exogenous Cold or Damp Cold invasion. Arthritic conditions show the same pattern.
* If the pain is better upon awakening and worsens as the day goes on, it is due to a Kidney Deficiency. Osteoarthritis in weight-bearing joints will cause fatigue and produce this pattern of pain.

5. Does the pain change in relation to the weather?

* If the pain worsens with Cold and Damp weather changes, an exogenous invasion is the cause; arthritic conditions are often aggravated by weather changes.
* If the pain has no relationship to the weather, it is due to either trauma or some type of Kidney Deficiency.

6. Does the patient feel better with the application of heat? If so, this indicates an invasion of Cold or Damp Cold or a Kidney Yang Deficiency.

7. With the patient in the prone position, examine the spine for structural abnormalities: scoliosis, hyper- or hypokyphosis, hyper- or hypolordosis, or prominence of the rib cage unilaterally. Be aware that some postural distortions will only be evident when the patient is standing in a weight-bearing posture.

8. Check to see if one side of the back is raised more than the other, indicating spasms of the erector spinae group, imbalances in muscular development, or scoliosis. Hard and stiff muscles indicate Blood and Qi Stasis.

9. Check for dowager's hump. This curvature causes stagnation of Qi and Blood and interferes with the flow of energy in the Yang channels, which all converge at GV14.

10. See if one shoulder is higher than the other or if a winged scapula is present. A winged scapula indicates a weak serratus anterior muscle.

11. Check for any swelling in the lumbosacral area. Check for spider veins in this region, which indicate either an injury or a weakness resulting in Blood Stasis.

12. Look to see if the pelvis is misaligned, as one ilium may be raised or

one posterior superior iliac spine may be more posterior in relation to the other. Check for leg length discrepancies by comparing the relationship of the medial malleoli to each other. A short leg occurs on the side of posterior misalignment of the pelvis, while a long leg occurs on the side of anterior pelvic misalignment.

13. Check to see if one hip is rotated abnormally. This indicates a spasm in the hip region or some degree of misalignment of the hip, both of which can affect the lower back. Ankle pronation and other leg and foot abnormalities may also cause rotation of the hip and lower back pain.

14. Palpate for skin temperature and see if there are any differences in temperature between the different areas of the lower back. For example, is the left side colder than the right side? Is the temperature uneven under your hands? Changes in skin temperature can indicate circulation problems, that is, obstruction of Qi and Blood in the channels of the back; a cold lower back can be a sign of a Kidney Yang Deficiency or an invasion by exogenous Cold and Damp.

15. Palpate for areas of tightness and atrophy of the muscles. If the upper back muscles are very tight and the lower back muscles are weak and lack tone, this can be an indication of a constitutionally weak back, a prior injury to the area leading to weakness, an obstruction of Qi and Blood to the lower back area due to the tension in the upper back, generally poor muscular development, or chronic constipation. If the lower back is weak, the upper back may seek to compensate by trying to take some of the strain off the lower back, resulting in spasms and upper back strain.

16. Palpate for any spasms in muscles that are obviously tight and in muscles that appear weak. Weak muscles can often be deceiving in their appearance. Superficially they feel soft but upon deeper palpation, strands of muscle can often be felt in spasm. These must also be attended to.

17. Palpate the vertebrae for misalignment. This is done by feeling the spinous processes to make sure they are properly aligned. When palpating the vertebrae, pay attention to their thickness and any other changes that may indicate an arthritic condition.

18. Check for skin discoloration in the lumbar area.
    + A local area of darker coloration may indicate stagnation due to long-standing muscle tension.
    + An area of pale skin may indicate local ischemia or Cold.

19. Check for scars and adhesions from prior surgeries, which can block the flow of Qi and Blood.

20. Palpate the hip and gluteal regions for areas of tightness or tenderness. Hypertonicity of the gluteal muscles and iliotibial tract may indicate increased weight-bearing strain of these areas due to a weak lower back.

21. Check the Kidney pulse on the left wrist in the proximal position. In cases of severe pain, this pulse will feel wiry and floating, particularly if the condition is acute or is an exacerbation of a chronic problem.

+ If the pulse feels tight, it can indicate an exogenous invasion of Damp Cold in the Bladder Channel.
+ If the pulse is weak, floating, thin, and slightly wiry, it can be a sign of chronic lower back pain due to Dampness in the channels.
+ If the pulse is both rapid and wiry, it can indicate Damp Heat in the Bladder Channel.

These pulses can also indicate Organ dysfunctions, however these conditions would be accompanied by corresponding symptoms.

ADDITIONAL TECHNIQUES

1. If the patient has a slight scoliosis with one side of the back higher than the other, manipulate the high side from the upper scapula to the sacrum by using deep circular digital pressure while feeling for the presence of any spasms. If the therapist finds hard fibers in the belly of the muscle, place the two thumbs together and use even circular thumb pressure to manipulate down the spasm.

2. If the patient has a slight scoliosis or hyperkyphosis, locate the areas of tightness. If the tightness is directly next to the spine, use deep circular thumb pressure, placing the top of the pads of the thumbs on either side of the spine, in between the transverse processes. The thumb pressure should be focused and directed down toward the table and obliquely toward the spine. Then walk the thumbs slowly down the spine, in between the transverse processes.

3. In cases of severe scoliosis the tight, high side of the back and the weaker, lower side must both be palpated and manipulated. Spasms on either side of the back should be located and treated. Circular digital pressure can be used.

4. In cases of severe scoliosis, after treating the back an advanced Amma therapist may place her thumb pads on the convex side of the curve at its apex, and apply gentle pressure to "straighten" the spine.

5. If one hip is higher than the other, the gluteal muscles and erector spinae group on that side will be in spasm. In this case, manipulate the gluteus medius and the tensor fascia lata (both areas are energized by the Bladder and Gall Bladder Tendino-Muscle channels), beginning with a combination of circular palmar pressure and following with circular thumb pressure, from the iliac crest, through the hip region, and along the iliotibial tract to the lateral knee. Rest the supporting hand on the back of the thigh. If the hamstring muscles tighten, release them by using circular palmar pressure while continuing with the other technique. The therapist may switch to circular thumb pressure as needed in the iliotibial tract, ending at GB34. The therapist may also manipulate with circular thumb pressure in between the Bladder and the Gall Bladder Primary channels, between the posterior thigh and the coronal plane.

6. If the patient suffers from a winged scapula or uneven scapulae, manipu-

late along the medial border of the scapula with either circular digital or thumb pressure. Advanced therapists can then place the entire palm on the scapula and manipulate with the palm in an effort to bring the scapula back into alignment. If one scapula is very high, two thumbs can be used on the superior border of the scapula, with circular thumb pressure directing the force diagonally toward the inferior angle of the scapula to relax it downward.

7. A dowager's hump should be treated as taught in the basic treatment.

8. If there is a swelling in the sacral area, it is important to use teh tah chu and manipulate in the middle of the sacrum with the palmar aspect of the fingers in an effort to disperse the swelling. In these cases the upper back is often very tight, and it is therefore important to release the upper back as well.

9. In areas that are particularly tight, areas that show discoloration due to prior, long-standing stagnation, and areas that are calcified or where there are arthritic changes, use the technique of placing the thumbs on either side of the spine, in between the transverse processes, and directing the force down and inward.

10. Advanced Amma therapists may do a deep manipulation of the psoas muscle, which originates at the transverse processes, bodies, and discs of the lumbar vertebrae and inserts into the lesser trochanter of the femur. The psoas muscle is responsible for flexing the thigh and adducting and rotating the thigh medially. It is innervated by lumbar nerves L2–L3. This muscle

is often strained when there is a lower back problem. In female patients, start the manipulation with deep circular thumb pressure lateral to the pubic bone in the inguinal crease and manipulate inferiorly along the Liver Channel to the medial side of the knee. In male patients the manipulation begins at CV2 and moves laterally to the inguinal region and inferiorly along the Liver Channel.

11. Place the thumbs into a "T" formation on the midline of the posterior thigh, with the remainder of the hand gently holding the thigh. Gently and evenly press with both thumbs. Movement is performed in small increments down the posterior thigh and leg while maintaining the "T" stroke to release the muscles and stimulate the energy in the Bladder Channel.

12. Thumb stroke across the popliteal fossa to clear blockages from the Bladder Channel, relax the sinews, and strengthen the lower back.

13. Beginning at Bl64, use circular thumb pressure to manipulate along the lateral edge of the cuboid bone toward the calcaneus, following the arch formed by the tarsal bones. The manipulation ends in the depression inferior to the external malleolus. Manipulation of this area will help to relax the muscles of the back.

POINT LOCATION AND ACTION

1. TS-C1

Location: At the junction where the body of the sternum meets the xiphoid, and the rib cage separates.

Gently rest your left hand above the rib cage separation to stabilize the right hand as it locates and presses the point. Locate the point with the middle finger of the right hand and press lightly in and down and slightly superiorly toward the body of the sternum while maintaining pressure. Be careful not to move the surface skin or you will be off the point. If your third finger is too weak to maintain the pressure, place your second finger on top of your third finger for added strength and support.

Action: This point relaxes the rib cage anteriorly and posteriorly, and releases the thoracic and abdominal muscles. This point can also be used for emotional release.

2. TS-F1

Location: In the depression posterior and superior to the base of the fifth metatarsal, 1 tsun superior to Bl64.

With the patient in the supine position, grasp the foot with the opposite hand and manipulate the point with the thumb. This point should also be manipulated when the patient is in the prone position.

Action: This point strengthens the lower back, relaxes the muscles of the lower back, and relieves swelling and Qi and Blood obstructions of the lower back.

3. TS-T1

Location: Level with Liv11, 5 tsun below the iliac crest between the Stomach and Gall Bladder channels, in the interstice between the lateral edge of the quadriceps muscle and the tensor fascia latae.

Using direct thumb pressure, direct the force to the opposite side and hold for 20 seconds, then rotate the thumb toward the opposite hip and press. Hold for another 20 seconds and release, then generally massage the area.

Action: This point releases lower back muscles.

4. TS-T2

Location: 3 tsun above the medial epicondyle of the femur, between the vastus medialis and the sartorius muscles, and 1 tsun inferior to Liv9.

Using the pad of your thumb, press directly into the muscle.

Action: This point releases lower back muscles.

5. Ki3

Location: Midway between the tip of the medial malleolus and the calcaneal tendon.

Using the thumb, apply pressure directly in toward the bone with a slight medial hook.

Action: Ki3 is the Organ point for the Kidney. Since the Kidney rules the lower back and the bones, this point can be used to alleviate lumbar pain.

Comment: This is the Organ, Stream, and Earth point of the Kidney Channel.

6. Sp6

Location: 3 tsun proximal to the vertex of the medial malleolus, just posterior to the tibial border.

Stand at the foot of the table. Grasp the patient's leg with your hand and place the pad of the thumb on the point. Gently press toward the tibia until you feel a sulcus in the bone. Hold the point for 15–30 seconds, then slowly release, circling as you lighten your pressure. This point can be pressed bilaterally.

Action: Sp6 helps to promote the smooth

flow of Liver Qi and therefore helps to calm the patient. It also promotes the proper flow of Blood and Qi to the muscles and sinews.

Comment: This is an Intersecting point of the Spleen, Liver, and Kidney channels.

7. Liv5

Location: 5 tsun proximal to the vertex of the medial malleolus, in a depression on the medial aspect of the tibia.

Pressure is applied with the pad of the thumb directly into the depression.

Action: Liv5 regulates the smooth flow of Liver Qi and treats lower back pain.

Comment: This is the Luo point of the Liver Channel.

8. Bl60

Location: Level with the vertex of the lateral malleolus, in the depression between the lateral malleolus and the tendocalcaneus.

Press with the third finger directly into the depression, or manipulate the area with your thumb.

Action: Bl60 strengthens the lower back, relaxes the sinews, and treats chronic low back pain. It also treats the upper part of the back.

Comment: Bl60 is the River and Fire point of the Bladder Channel.

9. Bl61

Location: 1.5 tsun inferior to the external malleolus, directly below Bl60.

Press with the thumb directly into the calcaneus with a slight downward hook while the patient is in the prone position.

Action: Bl61 strengthens the lower back, relaxes the muscles, and removes obstructions.

10. Bl23

Location: 1.5 tsun lateral to the Governing Vessel at the level of the lower border of the spinous process of the second lumbar vertebra.

This point may be manipulated bilaterally with the thumbs. Press directly toward the table and, while maintaining the pressure downward, pull the muscle slightly upward.

Action: Bl23 tonifies the Kidney, strengthens the lower back and sacral area, and benefits the bones.

Comment: This is the Yu point for the Kidney.

11. Bl24

Location: 1.5 tsun lateral to the Governing Vessel, at the lower border of the spinous process of the third lumbar vertebra.

This point may be manipulated bilaterally with the thumbs. Pressure is straight down toward the table.

Action: Bl24 treats lower back pain and stiffness and helps to regulate Qi and Blood in the Lower Burner.

Comment: This point is the back's Sea of Qi and relates to CV6 in terms of its regulation of Qi and Blood within the Lower Burner.

12. Bl25

Location: 1.5 tsun lateral to the lower border of the spinous process of the fourth lumbar vertebra, approximately at the level of the upper border of the iliac crest.

Pressure is applied bilaterally with the thumbs, straight down toward the table.

Action: Bl25 activates the excreting function of the Colon. It is very good for treating chronic constipation and lower back pain resulting from constipation.

Comment: This is the Yu point for the Colon.

13. GB30

Location: At the point one-third of the distance between the highest point of the greater trochanter of the femur and the hiatus of the sacrum.

Pressure is toward the ASIS of the opposite hip, applied with the third finger or the thumb.

Action: GB30 strengthens the lower back, particularly in the treatment of sciatica. It is also beneficial in treating Painful Obstruction Syndrome of the hip. GB30 benefits the circulation of Qi and Blood to the leg and strengthens the sinews.

Comment: GB30 is the Intersecting point of the Gall Bladder and Bladder channels. This point may be used in combination with Bl36 for the treatment of sciatica.

14. Bl36

Location: Located at the center of the gluteal transverse crease.

Use the third finger or the thumb to press upward into the ischial tuberosity.

Action: Bl36 strengthens the lower back, is beneficial in the treatment of sciatica, and helps the circulation of Qi in the Lower Burner.

Comment: This point may be used in combination with GB30 for the treatment of sciatica.

15. Bl39

Location: At the lateral edge of the popliteal crease, on the medial side of the tendon of the biceps femoris.

Pressure is with the third finger or the thumb. Support the medial knee with the opposite hand.

Action: Bl39 treats lower back pain secondary to bladder dysfunction, and benefits the Bladder.

Comment: Bl39 is the local point for knee pain and stiffness. It is also the deep ending of the Triple Burner Channel, affecting the elimination function of the Lower Jiao.

16. Bl57

Location: Inferior to the belly of the gastrocnemius muscle on the line connecting Bl40 and the calcaneal tendon, approximately 8 tsun below Bl40.

Pressure is straight down with the thumb or third finger. This point can be extremely sensitive, so carefully palpate the calf muscles first. If they are very tight, gently manipulate the area with circular digital pressure rather than applying direct pressure to the point.

Action: Bl57 treats lower back pain and sciatica and strengthens the lower back.

17. Bl58

Location: 7 tsun directly above Bl60 on the posterior border of the fibula, approximately 1 tsun inferior and lateral to Bl57.

Pressure is straight down with the thumb or third finger.

Action: Bl58 treats lower back pain and sciatica.

Comment: This is the Luo point of the Bladder Channel.

TREATMENT FOR THE COMMON COLD

AMMA THERAPY ETIOLOGY

Everyone is familiar with the symptoms of the common cold—acute inflammation of any or all parts of the mucous membranes of the respiratory tract, which includes the sinuses, throat, larynx, trachea, and bronchi. Symptoms of the common cold include congestion of the nasal mucosa, which may cause partial or complete obstruction of the nasal passages, a mucus discharge from the nose that may be clear and watery or yellow or green, sniffling and frequent blowing of the nose, sneezing, tearing of the eyes, sore throat (pharyngitis), chills, and lethargy. Sometimes earaches accompany these symptoms, and fever may also be present.

Western medicine has no conclusive evidence on the etiology of the common cold. Today approximately one hundred distinct common cold viruses (called rhinoviruses, *rhin* being the Greek word for nose) have been isolated as the potential source of the common cold and upper respiratory tract infections. Rhinoviruses have often been cited as the major cause of the common cold, in spite of the fact that rhinoviruses were isolated in only 15 to 40 percent of adults with these illnesses and only found in 5 percent of common colds in children. In addition, these viruses can also be found in healthy, asymptomatic people. The fact is that, from a Western perspective, much remains unknown about the common cold. We do know that a strong immune system is the best defense against acute rhinitis. Factors such as stress, fatigue, depression, and overwork can all contribute to a weakening of the body's defenses and cause an individual to be more susceptible to becoming sick. The common cold has the potential to become a more serious illness in children and the elderly, in whom it can lead to complications such as ear infections, sinusitis, bronchitis, and pneumonia.

Acute rhinitis usually has a sudden onset, with an inflammation of the nasal mucosa, a congested runny nose, sneezing, and general discomfort, and perhaps a sore throat and a low or moderate fever. Colds are generally highly contagious during the first twelve to seventy-two hours after onset and do not result in any kind of immunity from future colds. Despite the fact that the common cold does not cause permanent physical illness, the economic toll taken by the common cold has been well-documented in studies done of absenteeism in schools and industry. Treatment from the Western standpoint consists of an attempt to relieve symptoms through the use of nose sprays (which can become addictive), analgesics, antihistamines (which may produce side-effects), and cough suppressants or expectorants. Physicians concur that antibiotics have no value in the treatment of the common cold, and the efficacy of antihistamines in the treatment of acute rhinitis is still being debated.

From a TCM perspective the common cold is caused by an invasion of exogenous Wind. Wind is the most active pathogen among the Six Pernicious Influences and is frequently accompanied by either Cold or Heat. (In this way the TCM perspective corroborates the Western medical viewpoint that viruses are not the causative agents of colds, since virus-type infections in traditional Chinese medicine are considered to be Fire and not Wind.) Invasions by exogenous pathogens take place when there are sudden changes in the climate or abnormal deviations in the weather and the body's defensive energy cannot adapt quickly enough. Often these invasions take place during the transition from one season to the next, when the weather can be unpredictable, or if a person is exposed to manmade, artificial temperature extremes, such as exposure to air conditioning in the summer. Basically an exogenous invasion can take place at any time if a person's Wei Qi is low due to stress, overwork, and poor diet, or if an individual suffers from a weak constitution. If a person suffers from weak Lung Qi, his Lung will not disperse enough Wei Qi to the exterior of the body, resulting in an insufficient defense or immune system.

The Lung is called the delicate Organ because it is the most easily injured by invasion of exogenous pathogenic influences, usually Wind Cold or Wind Heat, although Damp and Dry can also affect the Lung. The major function of the Lung is the descending and dispersing of Qi, Blood, and Fluids in the body. In particular, it is the dispersing function that sends Wei Qi, the protective energy, to move through the skin, muscles, and flesh. This energy keeps the body temperature stable and also protects the body against invasion by exogenous pathogens. Pathogens that break through this protective barrier disturb the flow of the Wei Qi, causing obstructions. Wind often combines with Heat or Cold, penetrating through the skin, nose, and mouth and thus blocking the circulation of Wei Qi. Wind also interferes with the dispersing function of the Lung and blocks its movement, which is exactly how we feel when we have a cold and our heads and noses feel "stuffed up." Because the Lung's functions of descending and dispersing are impeded, the person suffers with a runny nose as well as other symptoms depending upon whether Wind is combined with Cold or Heat. A combination of Wind and Cold will obstruct the movement of Wei Qi and produce severe occipital pain and stiffness, a runny nose with clear or white mucus, an aversion to cold, an absence of sweating, no fever or a slight fever, marked body aches, clear urine, no thirst, a floating and tight pulse, and a tongue that looks basically normal with a thin white coating in the early stages. A combination of Wind and Heat will prevent the descending of Lung Qi, producing a marked fever, slight body aches, aversion to cold, and occipital pain and stiffness, and give rise to sweating, thirst, dark urine, a floating and rapid pulse, and the tongue showing redder at the tip and sides (although in the early stages there may be no noticeable change). These exogenous pathogens frequently enter through the skin, nose, and mouth, and at the back of the neck, since the Yang channels all congregate at the area of GV14 and, as the most superficial channels, they are the most easily accessed by external pathogens. There are specific points on the sides and back of the neck where the chill often enters. We instinctively hunch and raise our shoulders in cold weather to discourage Cold from entering those points.

A deficiency of Lung Qi can be due to propensities inherited from the parents, particularly if one parent had a chronic lung problem. A deficiency of

Lung Qi can also be created from postural problems, when the shoulders bowl forward either from tension or occupation. Furthermore, a deficiency of Lung Qi can be produced by an attack of Wind Cold or Wind Heat that has not been completely removed from the body, where some of the pathogen remains lodged within the system and festers to create a chronic weakness. This condition is frequently stimulated by the widespread use of antibiotics for a cold or flu. Antibiotics are often responsible for locking the pathogens deeper into the system and creating a chronic lung problem, inhibiting the descending and dispersing functions of the Lung. Long-term Deficiency of Lung Qi may progress to a Yin Deficiency of the Lung—a deficiency of the fluids of the Lung—resulting in a dry cough, thirst, and dry throat.

Recurrent colds and upper respiratory infections can also cause chronic rhinitis or chronic sinusitis. Chronic rhinitis is continuous inflammation of the mucous membranes of the nose. Chronic sinusitis is continuous inflammation of the sinuses. Both conditions can be caused by failure to expel the pathogen from the system. Pathogenic factors can move from the upper respiratory tract into the sinuses, impairing sinus drainage and possibly allowing for infection by a rhinovirus. When improperly treated, usually with antibiotics, which serve to lock the pathogen deeper into the system and weaken the immune system, the condition can turn into a chronic one. Examination of the tongue shows the aftereffects of lung disease treated incorrectly with antibiotics. The tongue coating will be partially peeled, red, dry, and shiny after antibiotic use, as antibiotics are injurious to the Stomach Yin. The coating can also lose its root from antibiotic use. In children the tongue will become partially peeled as a result of antibiotic use, again indicating injury to the Stomach Yin. After prolonged use of antibiotics there can be retention of Dampness in the Lung, which manifests as a yellow hue just behind the tip of the tongue.

Overuse and addiction to decongestants and nasal sprays or exposure to harmful chemicals and pollutants will aggravate this condition, as will smoking and exposure to passive smoking. Changes in altitude can also have a negative effect on the sinuses and the eustachian tube. Consequently, people should avoid flying whenever possible when they are suffering from a cold.

In any discussion of the common cold it is imperative to mention the role of diet in the onset and progression of this annoying and potentially debilitating illness. Ingestion of dairy products, in particular milk (beyond what might be appropriate in a cup or two of coffee each day) and cheese, produces excess mucus that obstructs the nasal passages and produces phlegm, which obstructs the lungs. Excessive consumption of cold and raw foods and sweets will weaken the Spleen and produce internal Dampness. Since the Spleen and Lung work together in the production of Nutrient Qi—the Spleen being responsible for the transformation and transportation of Fluids while the Lung helps to descend and disperse them—any weakness of the Spleen will affect the Lung. Thus a Damp Spleen can give rise to phlegm in the lungs.

Nasal cleansing is very helpful for nasal obstruction that arises as a result of the common cold. Nasal cleansing and irrigation are best accomplished with either a touch of sea salt or baking soda in warm water. The water is gently and slowly poured into one nostril while the head is tilted over the sink. The use of a special ceramic pot, called a neti pot, is very helpful, but a paper cup can be substituted. The patient blows his nose periodically to remove the dislodged, purulent materials and open up the air passages. After the technique is repeated a few times, the water will come out the opposite nostril, indicating that the passageway is clear.

Nasal cleansing, a yogic cleansing technique, is very beneficial to sufferers of chronic and acute sinusitis and rhinitis. Gargling with warm water and juice from one-half of a fresh lemon will soothe a sore throat. Herbal liniments that use natural oils, such as menthol, peppermint, and eucalyptus, can be rubbed into the chest, dotted under the nose, or sprinkled on the sheets at night—the fumes help to open up the nasal passages. When they are prescribed by a qualified health practitioner, herbs may be taken internally for sinus congestion and cough.

The following treatment is excellent for working with patients who have common cold symptoms.

AMMA THERAPY TREATMENT

Before treating the patient, the therapist will first have thoroughly reviewed the patient's medical history to see if there are any prior conditions that would contribute to the current problem, such as a history of frequent colds or recurrent bouts with bronchitis, pneumonia, asthma, allergies, and so forth. The therapist is also interested in any medications that the patient may have taken in the past or may currently be taking that could have weakened the immune system and lessened resistance to disease. Of special concern in this regard is the long-term use of antibiotics; other such medications can include steroids, immunosuppressants, anti-inflammatory medications, and chemotherapeutic drugs. This information is important in determining the types of recommendations that will be made. While the aim of the treatment is to alleviate the immediate symptoms and discomfort of the cold, for individuals with a prior history of weakened immune system, subsequent treatments would then focus on strengthening and tonifying the energy system to prevent further exacerbations.

AMMA THERAPY ASSESSMENT

1. Look at the color of the patient's complexion, check whether his eyes are watery, and check the color of nasal discharge if his nose is runny.
   + If the patient's complexion is pale and his nasal discharge is clear or white, it indicates a Cold condition.
   + If the patient's complexion is flushed and his nasal discharge is yellow, green, or blood-streaked, it indicates a Heat condition.
2. Take the pulses to ascertain if the cold is due to a Wind Cold attack or an attack of Wind Heat.
   + In a Wind Cold attack the pulse will be floating, slow, and tight, particularly at the Lung position.
   + In a Wind Heat attack the pulse will be floating and rapid, particularly at the Lung position.
3. Look at the tongue coating for any confirmation of the pulses. If the patient has come for a treatment in the very early stages of a cold, the tongue will not show any changes. However, if he has had a cold for several days and/or if the pathogen was very strong, the tongue will show the progress of the pathogen, how far it has penetrated into the interior, and whether, if it began as Wind Cold, it has transformed into Heat.

   A normal tongue coating is thin, white, and slightly moist, and remains so in the early stage of an exogenous attack. In the acute stages of a Wind Cold attack, the coating may be thicker on the front portion of the tongue or along the rim of the tongue. Both of these areas reflect the exterior of the body. As the pathogen moves deeper into the body, the thickness of the coating will migrate to the center, indicating the movement of the pathogen into the interior. Its strength is made manifest in the coating thickness. If the pathogen is Wind Cold and is not treated properly and expelled, it can move deeper into the system and manifest as a thick, white tongue coating that is more wet than normal. If the Wind Cold transforms into Heat, which is common, the coating will change to yellow.
4. Does the patient have a fever and, if

so, has it been high or only slightly elevated?

- A high fever indicates a Wind Heat condition.
- A slight fever or absence of fever indicates a Wind Cold condition.

5. Ascertain if the patient's aversion to Cold is severe or slight.
- A strong aversion to Cold indicates a Wind Cold condition.
- A slight aversion to Cold indicates a Wind Heat condition.

6. Ask the patient about body aches and pains and establish the degree of intensity.
- Severe body aches and pains indicate a Wind Cold condition.
- Slight body aches and pains indicate Wind Heat.

7. Does the patient have a headache? If so, how severe is it and where is it located?
- Severe occipital pain indicates a Wind Cold invasion.
- Slight occipital pain indicates Wind Heat.

8. Ask if there is any perspiring and to what degree.
- There is an absence of sweating in a Wind Cold attack.
- There is sweating in a Wind Heat attack.

9. Ask if the patient has been noticeably thirsty.
- There is an absence of thirst in a Wind Cold attack.
- The patient will feel thirsty in a Wind Heat attack.

10. Question the patient about the color of his urine.
- Clear urine reflects a Wind Cold condition.
- Dark urine reflects a Wind Heat condition.

11. Does the patient have a productive cough?
- Thin, whitish sputum suggests the presence of Cold and is called Cold sputum.
- Thick yellow or green, usually purulent sputum indicates Heat and is called Heat sputum.
- Scanty, sticky sputum implies the presence of dryness and is called Dry sputum.

12. Ask the patient if his throat is sore and painful and if he has difficulty in swallowing. Examine the pharynx by asking the patient to extend his tongue and say "ahh" while shining a light at the back of the throat. In some cases it is necessary to use a tongue blade to depress the tongue so that the back of the throat is visible.
- A very red throat indicates a Wind Heat invasion.
- If the arch of the pharynx is red with white spots, it may indicate strep throat.

13. Ask the patient if he has an earache or stuffiness in his ear, or if his hearing seems muffled or obstructed.

14. Ask the patient if his bowel movements are normal. Frequently patients will experience constipation when they have a cold. This is resultant from the disruption in the Lung's descending of Qi, Blood, and Fluids to the Colon.

15. Palpate the tonsillar, submandibular, and cervical lymph nodes for any swelling or tenderness.

16. As you start treating the patient and begin palpating, you may find that his neck is stiff, which could be an indi-

cation of blocked Qi in the channels due to exogenous invasion. Treatment will then incorporate techniques used for the neck as discussed in the treatment for neck and shoulder problems.

17. If the patient complains of an earache, use an otoscope to examine the ear for excess wax accumulation and/or inflammation of the tympanic membrane. It is important to validate one's suspicions with the otoscope, as toothaches and temporomandibular joint dysfunction can also cause a quality of pain in the ear that is very similar to otitis media. A normal eardrum will be a pearly white color. If otitis media is present, the eardrum will be inflamed and red. Bacterial infections, such as strep, staph, pneumococcus, or Haemophilus influenza, are usually the cause of otitis media, as the bacteria migrate from the nasopharynx through the eustachian tube into the middle ear. In recent years new strains of these bacteria have mutated, becoming resistant to conventional medications.

Young children from infancy to six years of age are the most prone to otitis media because the eustachian tubes, which connect the middle ear with the nasopharynx, are almost horizontal, allowing for the easy passage of bacteria from the nasopharynx to the middle ear. In adults the eustachian tubes are more vertical, enhancing the natural drainage of fluid from the middle ear and also making the passage of bacteria into the middle ear more difficult. Adults can still become infected if the nose is blown harshly and with force, which will push bacteria up the eustachian tubes.

It is interesting to note that studies have shown that antibiotics do not hasten the healing process, nor do they prevent hearing loss. Children who do not take antibiotics do not suffer from hearing loss and heal at basically the same rate as children who do. In fact, antibiotics weaken the immune system and increase the chances of repeated infections, resulting in chronic otitis media.

ADDITIONAL TECHNIQUES

1. If there is swelling in the forehead due to sinus inflammation, use extra thumb stroking and extra circular digital pressure to the forehead to disperse the blockage of Qi and Fluids.

2. If there is tenderness and swelling in the maxillary sinuses, use thumb stroking above and below the zygomatic bone.

3. If there are swollen glands along the sternocleidomastoid muscle, use teh tah chu and, with circular digital pressure, manipulate directly on the glands in a clockwise motion with the right hand and a counterclockwise motion with the left hand, moving from the mastoid process to the clavicle in an effort to drain the glands.

4. If there are swollen submandibular glands, tilt the head backward so that the chin is elevated and, using teh tah chu, manipulate the glands with circular digital pressure, moving from posterior to anterior.

5. If the throat is swollen and painful, using teh tah chu, manipulate on both sides of the throat with circular digital pressure, moving from the jaw line to the clavicle. This movement should be repeated three times, each time asking the patient to swallow as the manipulation is being done.

6. If there is tightness in the chest and the patient complains of stuffiness or fullness in the chest, use extra circular digital pressure down the sternum and in the intercostal spaces.

7. If the patient is constipated, extra attention should be paid to the manipulation of the colon.

8. To relieve pain and tightness in the occiput and upper back due to obstruction of Qi from the exogenous invasion, utilize techniques discussed in the neck and back treatment.

9. Using the pad of your third finger, stroke from Bl1 to Bl2, coming slightly out to the medial eyebrow, following the ridge of the bone, and then holding at Bl2.

10. Using the thumb stroking technique, stroke laterally over the nose and cheekbones toward the temples. Begin with the pad of each thumb in contact with the nasal bones, with the thumbs molding to the contours of the superior aspect of the maxilla and zygomatic arch while the rest of the hand gently grasps the chin. End the stroke at the temple, using the hairline as a guide. Repeat the stroke again, this time following the inferior aspect of the maxilla and the zygomatic arch. This manipulation helps to drain the maxillary sinuses and reduce swelling. It is beneficial to those suffering with chronic or acute sinusitis and rhinitis and treats sinus headaches. In addition, manipulation of this area relaxes the facial muscles as well as promotes general relaxation.

POINT LOCATION AND ACTION

1. Bl1

Location: In the slight bony depression, 0.1 tsun medial and superior to the inner canthus at the orbital border.

Using the tip of the little finger, press into the depression. Hold the patient's head steady with the opposite hand.

Action: While treating all eye disorders, this point is also used for tearing, itching, and swelling of the eyes, as well as headaches due to colds, sinusitis, and nasal obstructions. This point expels exterior Wind and clears Heat from the eyes.

Comment: Bl1 is the Intersecting point of the Bladder, Stomach, Small Intestine, and Triple Burner channels and the Governing Vessel.

2. Bl2

Location: In the depression proximal to the medial end of the eyebrow, directly above the inner canthus.

Pressure is activated with the pad of the index finger or middle finger in the sulcus of the bone, pressing toward the posterior skull. Pressure is held for approximately 15–30 seconds. Support the opposite side of the head while executing this technique.

Action: Like Bl1, Bl2 brightens the eyes

and can dispel exterior Wind from the face.

3. Extra point (yu yao)

Location: In the middle of the eyebrow, on the supraorbital ridge.

Rest the palm on the patient's forehead so that the pad of the index or third finger extends slightly over the midpoint of the eyebrow. Curve the pad of the finger under the ridge and hook up into the depression.

Action: This local point treats frontal and sinus headaches and all eye disorders; it opens and brightens the eyes.

4. GB14

Location: 1 tsun above the midpoint of the eyebrow, directly above the pupil.

Using the pad of the index or third finger, press directly into the point.

Action: This is a local point for frontal and sinus headaches and all eye disorders. It opens and brightens the eyes.

Comment: This point is an Intersecting point between the Stomach and Gall Bladder channels.

5. St1

Location: Directly inferior to the center of the pupil, on the midpoint of the infraorbital ridge.

Ask the patient to close his eyes. While sitting at the head of the table take the thumb of one hand and gently pull the skin down away from the infraorbital ridge. Then, using the thumb of the other hand, lean the lateral edge onto the top of the infraorbital ridge and roll the thumb into the depression.

Action: This point treats all eye disorders and helps with tearing, eye pain, and

swelling due to colds, sinus, and nasal congestion. It expels Wind Cold and Wind Heat from the eyes.

Comment: St1 is the Intersecting point of the Conception Vessel and the Stomach Channel.

6. St2

Location: Directly below St1, on the inferior ridge of the orbital cavity.

Using either the pad of the index finger or the third finger, press into the depression on the ridge of the orbit.

Action: St2 is used to brighten the eyes and expel exterior Wind. It also opens the nasal passages.

7. Extra point (bi tong)

Location: In the depression below the nasal bone at the superior end of the nasolabial sulcus.

Support the patient's head with one hand. Using the edge of the third finger of the other hand, rotate your finger toward the nose in the depression between the nasal bone and the cheekbone.

Action: This point clears the nasal passages. It is useful for all nasal and sinus problems, including rhinitis, sinusitis, allergies, and nasal polyps.

8. Co20

Location: At the midpoint of the ala of the nose, in the nasolabial groove.

Move the nostril to the side and press directly into the sulcus with the little finger.

Action: Co20 is a local point used to clear the nose from colds, rhinitis, sinusitis, loss of sense of smell, nasal polyps, and epistaxis. It is also helpful for runny nose or sneezing. This point expels exterior Wind Cold or Wind Heat.

Comment: This is the Intersecting point of the Stomach and Colon channels.

9. TS-H1

Location: At the ala of the nose in the corner of the nasolabial groove.

With the pinky or index finger, press into the corner of the nasolabial groove, moving the nostril to the side. The force is directed toward the opposite corner of the mouth.

Action: This is a local point to clear the nose from colds, rhinitis, sinusitis, loss of sense of smell, nasal polyps, and epistaxis. It is also helpful for runny nose or sneezing, and for expelling exterior Wind Cold or Wind Heat.

10. St3

Location: Directly below St2, level with the lower end of the nasal ala, lateral to the nasolabial groove.

Using the index finger or the pad of the third finger, hook up under the cheekbone.

Action: St3 treats nasal congestion and obstruction and expels Wind from the eyes.

11. SI19

Location: With the mouth slightly open, in the depression between the tragus and the temporomandibular joint.

Using the index finger or the pad of the third finger, press directly into the point.

Action: SI19 benefits the ears with any type of ear problem, such as otitis externa, otitis media and interna, ear pain, tinnitus, vertigo, deafness, TMJ problems, or arthritis.

Comment: The Gall Bladder, Small Intestine, and San Jiao channels intersect here.

12. SJ21

Location: With the mouth slightly open, in the depression in front of the anterior notch of the auricle and slightly superior to the condyloid process of the mandible.

Using the index finger or the pad of the third finger, press directly into the point.

Action: SJ21 benefits the ears with any type of ear problem, such as otitis externa, otitis media and interna, ear pain, tinnitus, vertigo, deafness, TMJ problems, and arthritis.

13. GB2

Location: With the mouth slightly open, located in the depression anterior to the intertragic notch directly below SI19.

Using the index finger or the pad of the third finger, press directly into the point.

Action: GB2 benefits the ears with any type of ear problem, such as otitis externa, otitis media and interna, ear pain, tinnitus, vertigo, deafness, TMJ problems, and arthritis. It also expels Wind Heat.

14. Lu1

Location: On the lateral aspect of the chest, in the interspace between the first and second ribs, 6 tsun lateral to the midline of the chest.

Using the pad of the index finger, third finger, or thumb, press down and direct the pressure toward the center of the chest.

Action: Lu1 regulates the Lung, catalyzes the descending function of the Lung, opens up the chest, and helps to expel exogenous Wind Heat. This point is used when the exterior pathogen has moved to the interior and there is fullness in the chest. It is not used when the pathogen is still in the exterior regions of the body. Lu1 is useful for treating coughs and retention of phlegm in the lungs.

Comment: This point is the Mu point for the Lung and is used to treat acute conditions. It is also the Intersecting point of the Lung and Spleen channels.

15. Lu5

Location: With the elbow slightly bent, this point can be found lateral to the biceps tendon at the cubital crease.

Wrap the patient's elbow with your hand, place the top of your thumb at the cubital crease next to the lateral side of the biceps tendon, in alignment with the Lung Channel, and press gently with the pad of the thumb straight down toward the table. Hold the point for 15–30 seconds and then gently release, circling as your pressure lightens.

Action: Lu5 catalyzes the descending of Lung Qi and opens and relaxes the chest. It expels Wind Heat from the Lung, the symptoms of which include yellow or green sputum, cough and fever; it also expels Cold Phlegm, the symptoms of which include profuse white sputum and chills.

Comment: Lu5 is the Sea and Water point of the Lung Channel.

16. Lu7

Location: In a slight depression at the origin of the styloid process of the radius, 1.5 tsun above the transverse crease of the wrist.

Grasp the patient's hand and, using your thumb, press into the depression between the tendon and the bone.

Action: This point catalyzes the descending and dispersing of Lung Qi; expels exogenous influences such as Wind Cold and Wind Heat; stimulates opening of the pores and sweating; helps circulate Wei Qi; opens up the nasal passages; and aids sneezing, nasal congestion, loss of sense of smell, runny nose, and headaches from colds. Lu7 is helpful in the early stages of the common cold or flu.

Comment: This is the Luo point for the Lung Channel and a Confluent point for the Conception Vessel.

17. Lu10

Location: On the radial border at the midpoint of the first metacarpal bone.

Grasp the patient's thumb with your hand, leaving your thumb free. Pull the patient's thumb toward you and press directly into the metacarpal bone using your thumb.

Action: Lu10 clears Heat from the Lung, especially in acute conditions. It also treats sore throat.

Comment: This is the Spring and Fire point of the Lung Channel.

18. Co4

Location: In the center of the flesh between the first and second metacarpal bones, closer to the second metacarpal bone.

Grasp the patient's thumb so that the second and third fingers fall on the palmar aspect of the patient's hand. Gently push up on the palmar aspect of the web that lies between the thumb and index finger. Using the thumb of the opposite hand, place its lateral side on the radial edge of the second metacarpal bone, then roll the lateral edge of the thumb into the depression on the second metacarpal bone. Pressure is toward the second metacarpal bone.

Action: Co4 expels Wind Heat from the Lung. It treats the face and head, and is helpful for nasal congestion, runny nose, tearing eyes, and sneezing, since it stimulates the dispersing function of the Lung. Co4 also treats cough and stiff neck. Because it strengthens Wei Qi, Co4 is very helpful in treating the beginning stages of the common cold or flu.

Comment: This is the Organ point for the Colon.

19. St36

Location: 3 tsun below St35, 1 tsun lateral to the anterior crest of the tibia (St35 is at the lateral foramen of the patella).

Stand alongside the patient, facing the patient's knee. Locate the point and place the pad of the thumb of the hand that is closest to the patient's head on the point. Gently hold the foot with the other hand and tilt the leg toward your body as you press toward the tibia. This will direct more pressure into the point. This point may be held for 15–30 seconds. Circle as you release your pressure.

Action: This point has a very strong tonifying effect and has been used since ancient times to build vitality and strength. It regulates and tonifies the Stomach, Spleen, Lung, Kidney, and Colon. It regulates both Wei Qi and Nutrient Qi and therefore strengthens the resistance of the body against disease. It is useful in attacks of exterior Wind Cold.

Comment: This is the Sea and Earth point of the Stomach Channel.

20. Sp6

Location: 3 tsun proximal to the vertex of the medial malleolus, just posterior to the tibial border.

Grasp the patient's leg with your hand and place the pad of the thumb on the point. Gently press toward the tibia until you feel a sulcus in the bone. Hold the point for 15–30 seconds and then slowly release, circling as you lighten your pressure. This point can be pressed bilaterally.

Action: This important tonifying point has a wide range of functions, since three major Yin channels (the Spleen, Liver, and Kidney channels) meet at this spot. This point serves to strengthen the Spleen, which in turn enhances the Spleen's interactions with the Lung. It also tonifies the Kidney, which assists the Lung with the grasping of Qi. In addition this point promotes the smooth flow of Qi by strengthening the Liver. The Lung depends on the Liver for the free flow of Blood and Qi.

Comment: Sp6 is the Intersecting point of the Liver and Kidney channels with the Spleen Channel.

21. Bl12

Location: 1.5 tsun lateral to the lower border of the spinous process of the second thoracic vertebra.

Standing at the head of the table, use the pads of the thumbs to apply pressure straight down into the point.

Action: Bl12 is useful in treating the early stages of exterior Wind Cold or Wind Heat. It helps relieve clogged nose and sneezing and catalyzes the dispersing function of the Lung.

Comment: Bl12 is the Intersecting point

of the Governing Vessel with the Bladder Channel.

22. Bl13

Location: 1.5 tsun lateral to the lower border of the spinous process of the third thoracic vertebra.

Standing at the head of the table, use the pads of the thumbs to apply pressure straight down into the point.

Action: Bl13 regulates and tonifies the Lung Qi. It activates the descending and dispersing functions of the Lung, thus helping to release exogenous pathogens to the exterior. It expels both Wind Cold and Wind Heat and helps to govern Wei Qi and Nutrient Qi. It also clears Hot sputum from the Lung and is helpful in both acute and chronic Lung conditions.

Comment: This is the Yu point (Associated point) for the Lung.

19

TREATMENT FOR INDIGESTION

AMMA THERAPY ETIOLOGY

Digestive disorders are among the most frequent patient complaints. Virtually everyone has experienced indigestion or dyspepsia, and the widespread promotion of antacids and alkalizers in the media demonstrates how commonplace this problem is. Expressions such as "I feel sick to my stomach" or "my stomach is killing me" are often used to describe this condition. Indigestion consists of a group of symptoms that are associated with poor nutrition, bad eating habits, and emotional stress. These symptoms include heartburn, nausea, excessive flatulence, mild abdominal distress, and fatigue. These symptoms are frequently simple responses to digestive abuses that can be easily corrected through treatment and dietary change.

The stress of a contemporary, fast-paced lifestyle often dramatically affects our eating habits and digestive functioning. Quarreling, worrying, or working while eating; improper eating habits, such as eating quickly at a fast-food counter (and generally eating too fast); overeating; smoking before, during or after meals; and eating shortly before bedtime all help contribute to indigestion. We must also consider the effects of poor nutrition, which include eating foods with little or no nutritional value; foods laden with chemicals, such as pesticides, artificial flavorings and colorings, artificial preservatives, and so forth; contaminated and improperly prepared foods; and foods that have been prepared by microwaving, which alters the energy levels of the food.

Proper digestion is necessary for the absorption of Qi and nutrients by cells, so that old cells and tissues can be replaced and precious energies can be generated by the human machine. Although an individual may in fact follow a nutritious and healthful diet, if digestion, assimilation, and elimination are not properly accomplished, malnutrition and indigestion will result.

The most common symptom of indigestion is heartburn, a burning, painful sensation usually centered in the middle of the chest near the sternum and at the lower portion of the breastbone, caused by the reflux of acidic stomach fluids that enter the lower end of the esophagus, causing irritation, inflammation (esophagitis), a bad taste in the mouth and, in severe cases, ulceration. Heartburn is the most common manifestation of gastroesophageal reflux disease. The onset of heartburn may be accompanied by sudden pain on the left side of the chest, inability to take a deep breath, and palpitations that simulate cardiac distress. The pain can come on rapidly and, while initially lasting only for a minute or two, can reoccur sometimes hours later. Oftentimes an acid or sour stomach may build slowly after the completion of the meal, or it may occur suddenly and continue for an hour or two.

There are two dysfunctions of the esophageal sphincter that may also be associated with the reflux of gastric acids. One is a sphincter with very low muscle tone and the other is inappropriate relaxation of the sphincter. Substances such as nicotine, caffeine, and alcohol, ingested with or independent of food, can overstimulate the production and secretion of gastric juices, which then reflux into the esophagus. Chronic heartburn can therefore result from the use of these substances and can lead to the development of more serious digestive conditions, such as ulcers.

At one time the presence of a hiatal hernia was considered to be a major factor in the reflux of gastric juices into the esophagus, resulting in heartburn. It is now thought to be much less of a factor, since radiologists report finding hiatal hernias in a large percentage of patients who are asymptomatic for reflux and under treatment for unrelated problems. They conclude that the important factor to investigate and focus on is reflux, not hiatal hernia.

Swallowed air expands once it enters the body due to the body's warm temperature. This can produce belching with sufficient force to reflux stomach acid into the esophagus, causing inflammation of the esophageal mucosa. Excessive swallowing of air (aerophagia) is a common problem in people who eat quickly and under stress, and can contribute to heartburn. Gases in carbonated beverages such as beer and soda can contribute to heartburn; patients should be advised to avoid drinking such fluids during meals.

Nausea, the second symptom of indigestion, is that unpleasant, queasy sensation that often precedes a desire to vomit. Ginger, a stomachic herb, has traditionally proven to be very helpful for the treatment of nausea, even when it is catalyzed by motion sickness. (At one time ginger ale was made with real ginger and was the drink of choice for nausea). Green clay mixed with water is also beneficial for settling the stomach and relieving this annoying symptom.

Flatulence, the third symptom of indigestion, occurs due to an excess amount of gas or air in the stomach or intestines which is alleviated by belching or by the passage of flatus through the intestines. Like heartburn, flatulence can be caused by aerophagia or by drinking carbonated drinks. Certain foods, such as cabbages, beans, and milk products, can cause flatulence due to the production of intestinal gases. Methane is created by decaying and rotting bacteria that are living in the undigested food of a sluggish stomach. A temporary increased production of gases is also sometimes experienced as a side-effect of a high fiber diet. Fermented foods, such as yogurt, can assist in the assimilation of high fiber and increase the amount of beneficent bacteria in the colon, thereby decreasing the production of gas. Mild abdominal distress is often the result of these excess gases, which can cause abdominal distention and pain.

Fatigue often accompanies or is the result of the other symptoms of indigestion. When the body's metabolism has been unduly influenced by stress, poor diet, and improper eating habits, lassitude naturally results. Without the proper quantity and quality of nutrients and energy entering the body, the necessary substances cannot be produced to supply the organs, muscles, sinews, and bones. In addition, nutrients and essential substances and energies cannot be transported easily. Hence the person feels weak and exhausted from little or no activity.

It is important for the therapist to understand that indigestion can also be a sign of, or the forerunner of, more serious digestive problems, in which case it will be accompanied by different sets of signs and symptoms. The two more serious problems commonly seen in the clinical setting are acute or chronic gastritis and ulcers. If the patient is suffering from gastritis, which is an inflammation of the mucous lining of the stomach, he will be prone to acute attacks that can be triggered by stress, medications, spicy foods, or too much alcohol. In addition to indigestion, the patient will complain of a severe, burning pain or pressure in his stomach, loss of appetite, lassitude, headache, nausea, and perhaps vomiting. Chronic gastritis may follow from repeated acute attacks.

Ulcers are defects in the gastrointestinal wall that penetrate the muscularis mucosa. Patient complaints will include indigestion characterized by a gnawing, burning pain that concentrates between the breastbone and the navel, and feelings of hunger, often absent in the morning but present at night and sometimes strong enough to wake the person up. The pain has an episodic pattern—it can last for minutes or hours, and will be interspersed with long symptom-free periods. Oversecretion of hydrochloric acid, which peaks about an hour to two hours after eating, is also a symptom. In particular, the esophagus and the duodenum are not geared for operating in the presence of gastric juices. As stated earlier, gastric juices that reflux into the lower part of the esophagus or into the upper part of the duodenum can cause inflammation and ultimately ulceration. Aggravation of pain one to two hours after a meal is characteristic of a duodenal ulcer; the alleviation of pain after eating is more indicative of a gastric ulcer.

The same factors that can catalyze indigestion—anxiety, anger, stress, poor diet and bad eating habits, smoking, caffeine, and alcohol—all play a major role in the creation and exacerbation of both gastritis and ulcers. Medications such as steroids and antibiotics can erode the walls of the stomach and induce these conditions. Recent studies have shown that certain strains of bacteria can also cause ulcers. The therapist must therefore conduct a differential diagnosis to make sure that he is treating only indigestion and not a more serious problem.

From the TCM viewpoint, indigestion due to emotional upset, poor diet, or improper eating habits is a reflection of dysfunctions of the Stomach and Spleen. The Stomach and the Spleen together constitute the root of Postnatal Qi, meaning that their combined functions provide the vital nutrient energies after birth. The downward function of the Stomach is to rot and ripen the food, while the upward function of the Spleen is to transform and transport Food Qi up to the Lung, where it combines with the Qi of Air to produce first Ancestral Qi and then True Qi (Wei Qi and Nutrient Qi). Any disruptions in the natural flow of energies of these two Organs will produce problems of the Middle Burner, often resulting in the energies flowing in the wrong direction. This condition is known as Rebellious or Deranged Qi.

Many of the problems of the Stomach from an Oriental perspective have to do with diet. This includes how much food is ingested, the quality of that food, and the conditions under which food is being eaten. In our modern-day society we often see two opposing or contradictory situations regarding food—either people are overeating or they are dieting. Overeating leads to food stagnation in the Middle Burner—the Stomach Qi cannot descend, resulting in indigestion, acid regurgitation, and abdominal distention. Dieting can produce varying degrees of

malnutrition due to insufficient intake of nutrients.

Inadequate nutritional intake can run the gamut from simply not eating enough food to eating foods laden with chemicals, preservatives, and pesticides that have no nutritional value. Stomach Qi is also weakened by illnesses such as anorexia or bulimia where there is a failure to take in and absorb food essences. Stomach Qi Deficiency can result from any chronic illness where the overall Qi of the body has been depleted. If a Stomach Qi Deficiency progresses, it will transform into a Stomach Yin Deficiency. This means that the Fluids, which are the Yin of the Stomach and necessary for digestion of food, will become scarce, causing constipation, pain in the epigastrium, dry mouth, dry throat, and loss of appetite. These symptoms are not due to Excess Heat but rather to the depletion of Fluids.

According to traditional Chinese dietary principles, people who adhere to vegetarian diets may also be unknowingly depriving themselves of vital nutrients and energies. Vegetarians often have a lot of dairy in their diets. Dairy produces mucus and phlegm, which injures the Spleen. They also often eat too many salads and raw foods, which promote Dampness, also injurious to the Spleen. The Spleen likes warm and dry foods and needs a certain amount of animal protein to produce enough Blood for the organism. In particular, women who are vegetarians often suffer from Blood Deficiency, which interferes with their menses and leads to conditions such as amenorrhea or dysmenorrhea. Senior citizens who live alone often will not cook only for themselves and frequently suffer from some level of malnutrition. When the body does not get enough nutrients, fatigue, lack of tonicity in the muscles, and mild epigastric pain will ensue. The quantity of food eaten should reflect how much activity a person engages in daily and what type of occupation he has. People who engage in heavy physical labor will obviously require more food intake than those who do sedentary work.

The quality of the food eaten is also of great importance, and patients must be educated on avoiding not only chemicals in their foods but antibiotics and hormones that are frequently added to meats and milk. Shopping for organic foods and natural meats should be encouraged. Foods that are harmful to the Stomach and Spleen should naturally be avoided. These include raw and cold foods, which tend to produce internal Cold conditions; hot or spicy foods, red meat, and alcohol (for persons who suffer from Stomach Heat); greasy fried foods; dairy products, which lead to the creation of Dampness and Phlegm; and heavy consumption of sweets, which can weaken the Spleen and Pancreas and contribute to Heat and Dampness in the Stomach.

In Amma therapy we also stress that the conditions under which food is eaten have a profound effect on the functioning of the digestive system. Meals should be eaten at regular intervals to maintain proper blood sugar levels throughout the day and to assist the Stomach and Spleen with digestion. Breakfast in particular is important, since the hours when the Stomach is most active are between 7 A.M. and 9 A.M. Eating breakfast helps to provide enough energy for our daily activities; not eating breakfast will cause

a Stomach Qi Deficiency.

Eating too fast, eating on the run, or eating under stressful conditions causes Stomach Qi to stagnate, resulting in food retention. Eating late at night can cause a Stomach Yin Deficiency, since the evening is the time when Yin energies have the most influence and a person who eats late at night is using up Stomach Yin energies instead of Stomach Qi energies. Constant eating throughout the day does not give the Stomach a chance to empty itself and can also lead to stagnation of Stomach Qi. Eating irregular amounts of food from one day to the next can also interrupt the normal functioning of the Stomach and lead to a Stomach Qi Deficiency. When people travel to different places or different countries, the change in eating habits and climate can also induce Stomach disorders. Periodic detoxifying in the summer, when the body requires less food intake, is often beneficial for cleansing the body of unwanted toxins and helping the Stomach and Spleen restore their natural balance.

Aside from the effects of diet on digestion, the emotions also play a major role in Stomach problems. Negative emotional states often catalyze or accompany indigestion. The reverse is also true, for an Organ dysfunction can have a major effect on the emotions associated with that Organ. In the case of indigestion, anger and its associated emotions of frustration, irritability, and resentment will cause either Liver Yang or Liver Fire Rising if the negativity is manifested, or stagnation of Liver Qi if the emotions are repressed. The smooth and free flow of Liver Qi is essential for assisting and supporting the Spleen in transforming and transporting the Qi of Grain, Blood, and Fluids and in assisting the Stomach in the rotting and ripening of food; anger and its affiliated emotions upset the smooth flow of Liver Qi, which either invades or stagnates in the Middle Burner, disrupting the descending flow of Stomach Qi and the ascending flow of Spleen Qi. Rising excessive Liver Qi will affect the Stomach and result in Rebellious Stomach Qi, manifesting as belching, acid reflux, a sour or bad taste in the mouth, nausea, abdominal distention, and epigastric pain which may radiate on either side of the hypochondriac region.

When the Liver Qi stagnates in the Middle Burner it affects the Spleen more, resulting in loose stools and fatigue. When there is a Spleen Qi Deficiency in conjunction with obstructed Liver Qi and the Spleen Qi Deficiency is greater, diarrhea will result. If the Liver Qi obstruction is greater, there can be constipation with small and difficult-to-pass feces. When the Liver energy negatively influences the Middle Burner, the condition is known as the Liver overcontrolling the Middle Burner. This is one of the most common patterns seen in the clinical setting.

Through its relationship with the Gall Bladder the Liver also promotes the even secretion of bile, a Yin substance considered a pure Fluid essential for the metabolism of fats during digestion. If Liver Qi is obstructed or stagnant and the bile cannot move smoothly, the functions of both the Stomach and the Spleen will be adversely affected and indigestion can result.

Patients will manifest different combinations of the above-named symptoms, and will rarely experience all of them at the same time. Liver Yang or Liver Fire Rising and Liver Qi Stagnation can originate from a Liver Blood Deficiency. This again demonstrates the importance of diet. A diet heavily laden with fried foods, alcohol, nicotine, and hot and spicy foods can create the syndrome of Liver Fire, while a diet that is deficient in meat can contribute to a Liver Blood Deficiency.

The Stomach is also adversely affected by the emotions of worry and anxiety. These emotions knot Qi and induce Qi Stagnation. Subsequent symptoms are indigestion, burning, regurgitation, and nausea. Excessive worrying and ruminating as well as excessive mental work, such as over-studying or intense work at a computer, knot the Qi and block its movement. When accompanied by poor and irregular eating habits, this can manifest as Spleen Qi Deficiency and ultimately Stomach Yin Deficiency.

Another factor that may influence a person's proclivity to indigestion is an inherited constitutional weakness of the Stomach and/or Spleen. Often children who demonstrate digestive problems carry such problems into later life. Other factors involved are stress and overwork (particularly physical overwork, which can deplete Stomach Qi), and iatrogenic-induced indigestion from the side effects of many Western medications, such as antibiotics, steroids, and anti-inflammatory drugs. There are many other medications from which digestive upset is a side-effect. The therapist should always check a patient's medication in the Physician's Desk Reference to discover the possible influence of the drug on the patient's condition.

Many patients who suffer from

indigestion use over-the-counter antacids and alkalizers, which are heavily promoted in the media. These medications are only a temporary solution to the problem and may even be harmful and habit-forming. Antacids place an extra burden on the stomach to secrete more acid in order to counteract the neutralizing effects of the drug. The result is a rebound effect—the stomach is left with excess acid, causing the very symptoms that the patient was initially trying to alleviate. Promoting proper digestion is better served through a change in lifestyle and good dietary habits, encouraging the patient to eat leisurely in a calm atmosphere and where possible to take a walk after a meal. Proper treatment, natural digestive enzyme supplementation at mealtimes, and the intelligent use of appropriate natural herbal supplements, such as green clay, that may be used as natural digestive aids will all serve to improve the patient's condition. Energy-balancing exercises such as t'ai chi chuan will help harmonize the digestive system.

The following treatment will relieve indigestion due to emotional upset, poor nutrition, or bad eating habits. It is important to remember that each person's dietary needs must be evaluated individually, for each person has his own constitutional differences, and age and medical history must be taken into account.

AMMA THERAPY TREATMENT

Prior to treatment the therapist will have examined the patient's written medical history. As the physical assessment begins, the therapist continues questioning the patient regarding the onset of his condition, how long the condition has persisted, and whether it has recently been exacerbated. In treating digestive problems the therapist must question the patient's diet, the nature of the patient's pain, and when and how the discomfort is alleviated or aggravated. Detailed information about the patient's diet, what he eats, when he eats, the conditions under which he eats, and his bowel movements is essential both for proper treatment and for making recommendations that will avoid future recurrences. The therapist is also interested in any medications that the patient may have taken or may be taking. While the aim of the treatment is to alleviate the immediate symptoms and discomfort of indigestion—the heartburn, nausea, fatigue, and abdominal pain and distention—subsequent treatments would then focus on strengthening and tonifying the Stomach and Spleen.

AMMA THERAPY ASSESSMENT

1. Question the patient about eating habits and diet.
2. Question the patient as to the nature of the pain:
   + A severe epigastric pain will indicate an Excess condition.
   + A dull pain indicates a Deficiency condition.
   + A stabbing pain indicates Blood Stasis.
   + A burning pain indicates Heat.
   + A swollen feeling of fullness in the abdomen is an indication of Dampness. If the pain is dis-

tending pain it indicates stagnation of Qi.

3. Ask the patient if there is a particular time of day that the condition worsens:
   + Deficiency conditions will usually feel worse in the mornings.
   + Conditions due to stagnation of Qi will feel worse in the afternoons.
   + Conditions due to Blood Stasis will feel worse in the evenings.

4. Does the patient feel generally better after eating?
   + If so, this points to a Deficiency condition which may be related to a gastric ulcer.
   + If the patient feels worse after he eats, this points to an Excess condition which may be indicative of a duodenal ulcer.

5. Does the patient feel better with the application of heat or when drinking hot liquids? If so, it indicates a Cold condition.

6. Does the patient feel better after resting? This indicates a Deficiency condition.

7. Does the patient feel better after moving around? If so, this indicates stagnation of Qi or Blood.

8. Is it a Heat condition?
   + Excess Heat conditions are characterized by intense burning pain that is worse after eating, and a dry red tongue with a yellow coating.
   + Deficiency Heat conditions are characterized by dull pain, a slight burning feeling, a dry mouth and a desire to slowly sip fluids, and a peeled, red tongue.

9. Is it a Cold condition?

   + Excess Cold conditions are characterized by acute pain; no thirst; vomiting; a thick, white tongue coating; and a full, tight pulse.
   + Deficiency Cold conditions present with a dull pain, a desire for warm drinks, no thirst, and the vomiting of clear, thin fluids. The pulse feels empty.

10. Does the patient feel thirsty but is averted to drinking fluids? This indicates Damp Heat.

11. Question the patient as to the taste in his mouth.
    + A bitter taste indicates Heat, usually of the Liver if the bitter taste is somewhat constant.
    + A sweet taste indicates either a Spleen Deficiency or Damp Heat.
    + A sour taste is an indication of food retention in the Stomach or Liver Qi invading the Stomach.
    + An absence of taste indicates Spleen Deficiency.
    + A sticky taste indicates Dampness.
    + A salty taste can indicate a Kidney Yin Deficiency.

12. Listen for the patient's belching sounds, or question him about his belching patterns.
    + If the patient feels better after he has belched, this indicates stagnation of Qi.
    + If the patient has loud belching, this indicates an Excess condition.
    + Low-key belching indicates a Deficiency condition.

13. Does the patient experience sour

regurgitation? This reflects food retention in the Stomach or Liver Qi invading the Middle Burner and stagnating there.

14. Does the patient feel nauseous? If the patient feels nauseous, it indicates a Deficiency condition or food retention.

15. Does the patient vomit?
    + Vomiting soon after eating, vomiting food, or vomiting loudly are all indications of Excess.
    + Vomiting a while after eating or vomiting thin fluids both indicate a Deficiency condition.
    + A sour taste when vomiting indicates that the Stomach has been invaded by Stagnant Liver Qi.
    + Blood in the vomit indicates Heat.
    + A bitter taste when vomiting means there is Heat in the Liver and Gall Bladder.

16. Does the patient feel better after vomiting?
    + If so, this indicates an Excess condition. The pulse is rapid and overflowing.
    + If the patient feels worse after vomiting, this indicates a Deficiency condition. The pulse is rapid and empty.

17. Bad breath indicates Heat in the Stomach.

18. If the patient always feels full and suffers from distention after eating, this indicates food retention. Food retention will also manifest with a thick and sticky tongue coating in the center of the tongue due to the accumulation of undigested food in the Stomach. A slippery pulse will also reflect food retention in the Stomach.

19. How is the patient's appetite?
    + Lack of appetite reflects a Spleen Qi Deficiency.
    + A ravenous appetite or always being hungry indicates Heat in the Stomach.

20. Ask the patient how his abdomen feels and look at the abdomen for signs of bloating or distention.
    + A feeling of bloating or distention in the abdomen indicates Qi Stagnation.
    + A feeling of fullness indicates food retention or fluid retention and Dampness.
    + A feeling of stuffiness indicates either Stomach Heat or a Stomach Qi Deficiency.
    + A feeling of oppression in the abdomen indicates a severe stagnation of Qi, Dampness, or Phlegm.

21. Ask about the patient's bowel movements. Diarrhea will reflect the strength of the Stomach and Spleen.
    + If Stomach Qi is not descending, it can lead to constipation.
    + If Spleen Qi is weak, Dampness may ensue and result in loose stools or diarrhea.

22. Palpate the abdomen.
    + If the abdomen feels worse with pressure, it indicates an Excess condition.
    + If it feels better with pressure, it indicates a Deficiency condition.
    The healthy abdomen should have a certain flexibility and buoyancy that is not too hard or too soft. Such an abdomen means that the Yuan Qi is adequate. It is often the case that the upper abdomen, the area below the

xiphoid, feels tense and hard. This area should feel softer than the other areas of the abdomen, pointing to a smooth flow of Lung and Heart Qi in the Upper Burner. Its tenseness is a reflection of the stress and emotions that are frequently trapped in the chest and which can obstruct the flow of Lung and Heart Qi.

The area of the abdomen below the navel should have more strength and solidity to it without being very hard. If it feels quite flaccid, it reflects a weakness of this area due to a weakness of Yuan Qi.

23. Palpate the abdomen for scar tissue, adhesions, or any masses, and to ascertain the health of the intestines.

   + Abdominal masses that move underneath your fingers may indicate Qi Stagnation, muscle spasms, or gas pockets.

   + If the masses feel very hard and do not move, they indicate Blood Stasis and may be symptomatic of a benign or malignant tumor. In such cases refer the patient to a physician.

ADDITIONAL TECHNIQUES

1. Manipulate down the sternum to the navel; this relieves fullness and heaviness in the chest due to dietary dysfunctions. It also helps to release the tension and stress commonly held in the "emotional center," the area of CV17. It assists in regulating the flow of Qi, Blood, and Fluids through the channels and organs in this area.

2. Manipulate the hypochondriac area with circular digital pressure in the intercostal spaces to disperse stagnated and obstructed Qi.

3. Apply circular thumb pressure on the inside of the costosternal break, on either side of the xiphoid process. This stimulates relaxation of the hypochondriac and epigastric regions and also helps to release gas that may be trapped in this area.

4. Massage of the abdominal area should proceed first with circular palmar pressure. This should be followed by circular digital pressure as the area relaxes and responds. Such massage is beneficial to assimilation and digestion in the gastrointestinal tract. Teh tah chu may be used in the treatment of the abdominal area.

5. Apply thumb stroking or circular thumb pressure to the Stomach Channel, from St36 to St38, and on the dorsum of the foot, between the second and third metatarsals. Use of the knuckles is permitted if thumb strength is lacking.

6. Stroke from the wrist distally to the end of the fifth metacarpal. The points SI3 and SI4, located in this area, help to treat Dampness affecting the chest and the Gall Bladder, and hypochondriac pain.

7. Circular thumb or circular digital pressure in the fleshy part under the arch of the foot helps to release trapped gas.

8. Extra attention should be given to Bl18, Bl19, Bl20, and Bl21.

9. Treat the midsection of the back using teh tah chu.

POINT LOCATION AND ACTION

1. CV17

Location: Midway between the nipples at the center of the sternum.

Pressure is activated with the pad of the middle finger gently pressing directly toward the table.

Action: This is a very important point for releasing stagnant emotional energy trapped in the chest and for dispelling sensations of fullness and hypochondriac constriction. It helps breathing by opening up the chest. It is also helpful for relaxing the diaphragm when there are spasms and pain and therefore can also be used to treat hiatal hernia.

Comment: CV17 is the Mu point for the Upper Burner and the Heart Envelope. It is an Influential point for tonifying Qi, especially of the Heart and Lung. It is also an Intersecting point with the Spleen, Small Intestine, Kidney, Triple Burner, and Heart Envelope.

2. TS-C2

Location: In a depression 1 tsun inferior and lateral to the costosternal break, on the edge of the costal cartilage.

Direct pressure with the edge of the thumbs to the edge of and slightly under the costal cartilage. This point may be pressed bilaterally.

Action: TS-C2 relaxes the hypochondria, disperses obstructed Qi, and relieves pain.

Comment: The deep pathway of the Stomach Channel passes through this area.

3. Co2

Location: On the radial side of the second finger, distal to the metacarpophalangeal joint at the junction of the red and white skin.

Grasp the patient's finger with your hand so that your thumb falls naturally on the joint. Apply pressure directly into the joint space with the thumb.

Action: This point clears Heat from the Colon. Use for Excess Heat patterns with fever, constipation, dry stools, abdominal distention, and pain.

Comment: This is the Spring and Water point of the Colon Channel.

4. CV14

Location: 6 tsun above the umbilicus, on the anterior midline of the body.

The point is activated with the thumb or third finger. Place one hand gently above CV14, palm down, to help stabilize the point pressure of the thumb or third finger of the opposite hand. Ask the patient to inhale, and to exhale slowly. As the patient exhales, apply pressure directly toward the table. Hold the point for 15–30 seconds and then slowly release. As you release your pressure, begin circling your finger.

Action: CV14 subdues Rebellious Stomach Qi (Stomach energy ascending instead of descending), and is particularly helpful for digestive problems that stem from emotionality. This point also helps clear Heart Fire and calms the Shen. It treats spasms of the diaphragm, vomiting, acid regurgitation, and stomachache.

Comment: This is the Mu point for the Heart.

5. CV13

Location: 5 tsun above the umbilicus, on the anterior midline of the body.

The point is activated with the thumb or third finger. Gently rest one hand above CV13, palm down, to help stabilize the point pressure of the thumb or third finger of the opposite hand. Ask the patient to inhale, and to exhale slowly. As the patient exhales, apply pressure directly toward the table. Hold the point for 15–30 seconds and then slowly release. As you release your pressure, begin circling your finger.

Action: CV13 calms Rebellious Stomach Qi with symptoms of nausea, belching, hiccuping, vomiting, and feelings of fullness in the epigastrium. It also helps to harmonize the Upper and Middle Burners. Its greatest effect is on Excess Stomach patterns. CV13 specifically treats the upper portion or the fundus of the stomach, and the esophagus.

Comment: This is an Intersecting point of the Stomach and Small Intestine channels with the Conception Vessel.

6. CV12

Location: Midway between the end of the sternum and the umbilicus, or 4 tsun above the umbilicus on the anterior midline of the body.

The point is activated with the thumb or third finger. Gently rest one hand above CV12, palm down, to help stabilize the point pressure of the thumb or third finger of the opposite hand. Ask the patient to inhale, and to exhale slowly. As the patient exhales, apply pressure directly toward the table until a slight pulsation is felt. Hold the point for 15–30 seconds and then slowly release. As you release your pressure, begin circling your finger.

Action: This is a major point for any digestive problem, since it tonifies both Stomach and Spleen Qi. It is particularly helpful for calming Rebellious Stomach Qi and for resolving Damp Spleen. It strengthens the Spleen's function of transforming and transporting Qi and Fluids and diminishes digestive stagnation. It helps to relieve epigastric pain, gastritis, abdominal distention and pain, constipation, diarrhea, borborygmus, and ulcers. It is also helpful for bringing emotional energy downward from the chest to the feet, and for opening up the chest. CV12 specifically treats the middle portion of the stomach and affects the stomach's digestion directly.

Comment: This is the Mu point for the Stomach as well as for the Middle Burner. As well, it is an Intersecting point of the Small Intestine, San Jiao, and Stomach channels. It is also the Influential point of the Yang Organs and is therefore an important point for digestion.

7. CV11

Location: 3 tsun above the umbilicus, on the anterior midline of the body.

The point is activated with the thumb or third finger. Gently rest one hand above CV11, palm down, to help stabilize the point pressure of the thumb or third finger of the opposite hand. Ask the patient to inhale, and to exhale slowly. As the patient exhales, apply pressure directly toward the table. Hold the point for 15–30 seconds and then slowly release. As you release your pressure, begin circling your finger.

Action: CV11 regulates the Stomach and the Spleen, activates the rotting and ripening of food in the Stomach, and catalyzes the descending of Stomach Qi. It treats abdominal pain and swelling due to food stagnation, indigestion, borborygmus, vomiting, and epigastric pain. This point is better for Excess conditions.

8. CV10

Location: 2 tsun above the umbilicus, on the anterior midline of the body.

The point is activated with the thumb or third finger. Rest one hand gently above CV10, palm down, to help stabilize the point pressure of the thumb or third finger of the opposite hand. Ask the patient to inhale, and to exhale slowly. As the patient exhales, apply pressure directly toward the table. Hold the point for 15–30 seconds and then slowly release. As you release your pressure, begin circling your finger.

Action: CV10 tonifies the Stomach and the Spleen. It stimulates the descending of Stomach Qi and thereby reduces digestive stagnation from food retention. This point directly treats the lower portion of the stomach, the pylorus, and the duodenum. It also treats abdominal pain and distention, duodenal ulcers, gastritis, epigastric pain, indigestion, borborygmus and sour regurgitation.

Comment: CV10 is an Intersecting point of the Spleen Channel and the Conception Vessel.

9. St20

Location: 2 tsun lateral to CV13, 3 tsun above the umbilicus.

This point may be manipulated bilaterally. Pressure is with the third fingers directly toward the table.

Action: St20 helps relieve stagnation of food in the stomach as well as abdominal distention.

10. St21

Location: 4 tsun above the umbilicus, 2 tsun lateral to CV12.

This point may be manipulated bilaterally. Pressure is with the third fingers directly toward the table and slightly lateral.

Action: A good local point for Stomach problems, pressure at St21 helps to strengthen both the Stomach and Spleen and to dispel Heat from the Middle Jiao, and is therefore helpful for burning pain in the epigastrium. It also reduces digestive stagnation. It is useful for dispelling Rebellious Stomach Qi and therefore can help with nausea and vomiting. It alleviates pain due to Qi obstruction in the hypochondrium, ulcers, gastritis, indigestion, food retention, and diarrhea. This point is used more for Excess conditions.

11. Liv14

Location: On the mammillary line, two ribs below the nipple in the sixth intercostal space.

Pressure is activated bilaterally with the third fingers, directly down into the intercostal space.

Action: Liv14 encourages the smooth flow of Liver Qi and aids the Stomach; it also expands and relaxes the chest. This point is used whenever Liver Qi stagnates in the Middle Jiao and invades the Stomach, resulting in indigestion, hypochondriac pain and distention, nausea, vomiting, belching, and acid regurgitation. It harmonizes the relationship between the Liver and Stomach.

Comment: This is the Mu point for the Liver and is also an Intersecting point of the Spleen and Liver channels.

12. St25

Location: 2 tsun lateral to the umbilicus.

This point may be manipulated bilaterally with the thumbs. Apply pressure directly toward the table.

Action: St25 regulates the Spleen, Stomach, Colon, and Small Intestine. It also relieves digestive stagnation and is especially indicated for alleviating diarrhea and pain. It serves to clear Heat from the Stomach, Colon, and Small Intestine and can therefore help with burning pain in the epigastrium and with constipation. It is also useful for hernia, ulcers, borborygmus, meteorism, and vomiting.

Comment: This is the Mu point for the Colon.

13. TS-Ab1

Location: On the midline of the body, midway between the navel and the pubic bone.

Pressure is activated with the thumb or third finger directly toward the table. The second finger may be placed on top of the third finger for added pressure.

Action: This point removes obstructions of Qi from the lower abdomen and helps to dispel pain and distention in this area.

14. St34

Location: 2 tsun proximal to the lateral superior border of the patella.

Pressure is applied with the thumb slightly medial and down toward the table.

Action: This point treats acute and Excess Stomach patterns. It calms Rebellious Stomach Qi with symptoms of belching, nausea, hiccuping, vomiting, and acid regurgitation.

Comment: This is the Hsi or Accumulation point of the Stomach Channel.

15. GB34

Location: In the depression anterior and inferior to the head of the fibula.

Pressure is activated with the thumb into the depression, toward the tibia.

Action: GB34 regulates the smooth flow of Liver Qi and removes stagnation, particularly in the hypochondriac region. It helps Stomach Qi to descend, and therefore treats nausea, vomiting, belching, and acid regurgitation. It also treats Damp Heat in the Liver and Gall Bladder.

Comment: This is the Influential point of the sinews. It is the Sea and Earth point of the Gall Bladder Channel.

16. St36

Location: 3 tsun below St35, 1 tsun lateral to the anterior crest of the tibia. (St35 is at the lateral foramen of the patella.)

Stand alongside the patient facing the patient's knee. Place the pad of the thumb of the hand closest to the patient's head on the point. Gently hold the foot with the other hand and tilt the leg toward your body as you press toward the tibia. This will give more pressure into the point. This point may be held for 15–30 seconds. Circle as you release your pressure.

Action: This point has a very strong regulating and tonifying effect on the Stomach, Spleen, Lung, Kidney, and Intestines when these Organs are deficient. It helps to remove digestive stagnation and is beneficial for loss of appetite and dull epigastric pain. It redirects Rebellious Stomach Qi downward and is useful for all Stomach disorders, such as indigestion, borborygmus, meteorism, ulcers, gastritis, stomachache, nausea, and vomiting.

Comment: This is the Sea and Earth point of the Stomach Channel.

17. St37

Location: 6 tsun below St35 (St35 is at the lateral foramen of the patella), 1 tsun from the anterior crest of the tibia.

Pressure is activated with the thumb toward the tibia.

Action: St37 regulates the functions of the Stomach and Large Intestine. It helps send Rebellious Stomach Qi downward. This point is useful for digestive disorders, such as indigestion, borborygmus, meteorism, and diarrhea caused by Damp Heat. It helps with food stagnation in the stomach.

Comment: This is the deep ending of the Colon Channel.

18. Sp6

Location: 3 tsun proximal to the vertex of the medial malleolus, just posterior to the tibial border.

Stand at the foot of the table. Grasp the patient's leg with your hand and place the pad of the thumb on the point. Gently press toward the tibia until you feel a sulcus in the bone. Hold the point for 15–30 seconds and then slowly release, circling as you lighten your pressure. This point can be pressed bilaterally.

Action: Sp6 tonifies and strengthens the Spleen, Liver, and Kidney. This point is particularly helpful in assisting the free flow of Liver Qi when it is stagnating in the Lower Burner, producing constipation and abdominal pain, distention and flatulence. In removing obstructions of Qi from the Liver Channel, it helps to calm negative emotions and relieve pain in the lower abdominal area. It relieves fatigue, loose stools, and poor appetite due to Spleen Qi Deficiency. It helps to dispel digestive stagnation; it helps Spleen Qi to ascend and therefore assists with prolapse and hernias.

Comment: This point has a definite action on the genitourinary system by helping to remove Damp from the Lower Burner. It also has a profound effect on Blood, nourishing it or removing Blood Stasis and Blood Heat. It is also used for insomnia due to a Spleen and Heart Blood Deficiency. It is the Intersecting point of the Liver and Kidney channels with the Spleen Channel.

19. Ki6

Location: On the medial aspect of the foot, 1 tsun distal to the lower border of the medial malleolus.

Pressure is with the pad of the thumb into the point.

Action: Ki6 helps calm the Shen, especially in cases of anxiety due to Yin Deficiency. It also eases abdominal pain.

20. Sp4

Location: Approximately 1 tsun proximal to Sp3, in the depression distal and inferior to the base of the first metatarsal bone at the border of the red and white skin. This point may be pressed bilaterally.

Standing at the foot of the table, grasp the dorsum of the patient's foot with your hand so that the thumbs naturally fall below the arch of the foot. Pressure is with the thumb toward the metatarsal bone.

Action: Sp4 tonifies the Stomach and Spleen. It is used to treat Excess patterns of the Stomach, such as food retention,

Heat in the Stomach, Rebellious Stomach Qi, Blood Stasis in the Stomach, and Dampness in the epigastrium. It also treats epigastric and abdominal pain.

Comment: This is the Luo point (Connecting point) for the Spleen, and is also a Confluent point of the Penetrating Vessel. (The Penetrating Vessel is one of the eight Extraordinary Vessels.) It is called the Sea of Blood or the Vital Vessel due to its profound effects on the uterus and menstruation. Because it is connected to the Stomach Channel via St30 and the Spleen Channel via a descending branch on the inner thigh and foot, it also has an influence on digestive problems.

21. St44

Location: Proximal to the margin of the web between the second and third toes, in the depression distal and lateral to the second metatarsophalangeal joint.

Pressure is with the thumb toward the second metatarsophalangeal joint.

Action: This point regulates Stomach Qi, stops pain, and clears Stomach Heat and Fire. St44 is used mostly for Excess conditions.

Comment: This is the Spring and Water point of the Stomach Channel.

22. Bl18

Location: 1.5 tsun lateral to the lower border of the spinous process of the ninth thoracic vertebra.

Pressure is applied bilaterally with the thumbs, straight down toward the table.

Action: Bl18 treats stagnation of Liver Qi or Damp Heat in the Liver and Gall Bladder. It is used to treat Stagnant Liver Qi in the epigastrium and hypochondrium with nausea and acid regurgitation.

Comment: This is the Yu point (Associated point) for the Liver.

23. Bl19

Location: 1.5 tsun lateral to the lower border of the spinous process of the tenth thoracic vertebra.

Pressure is applied bilaterally with the thumbs, straight down toward the table.

Action: Bl19 calms Rebellious Stomach Qi, thereby treating belching, vomiting, nausea, and hiccuping. It also treats Damp Heat in the Liver and Gall Bladder.

Comment: This is the Yu point (Associated point) for the Gall Bladder.

24. Bl20

Location: 1.5 tsun lateral to the lower border of the spinous process of the eleventh thoracic vertebra.

Pressure is applied bilaterally with the thumbs, straight down toward the table.

Action: Bl20 is a major point for tonifying the Stomach and Spleen and regulating the Middle Jiao. It helps the Spleen's transporting and transforming functions and reduces digestive stagnation. Bl20 treats all Spleen Qi Deficiency patterns with symptoms of abdominal distention, loss of appetite, fatigue, and loose stools. It treats indigestion, gastritis, ulcers, borborygmus, acute or chronic diarrhea, constipation, and stool with undigested food. It also stimulates the ascending of Spleen Qi.

Comment: This is the Yu point (Associated point) for the Spleen.

25. Bl21

Location: 1.5 tsun lateral to the lower border of the spinous process of the twelfth thoracic vertebra.

Pressure is applied bilaterally with the thumbs, straight down toward the table.

Action: Bl21 is a major point for tonifying both Stomach and Spleen Qi. It stimulates the descending of Stomach Qi and therefore treats Rebellious Stomach Qi symptoms of belching, regurgitation, vomiting, and nausea. Bl21 treats indigestion, borborygmus, abdominal distention, and flatulence. It relieves stagnation of food in the stomach and promotes the Spleen function of transforming and transporting Qi, Blood, and Fluids.

Comment: This is the Yu point (Associated point) for the Stomach.

CHAPTER
20

TREATMENT FOR CONSTIPATION

AMMA THERAPY ETIOLOGY

In the United States, one of the conditions for which self-medication is most frequently sought is constipation. Advertisers tout the problem of "irregularity," and Americans spend over two hundred million dollars annually on laxatives in an effort to regulate the movement of their bowels. How often a person should move his bowels depends on the individual. The range of the number of movements can vary even in healthy persons, with one movement a day considered the norm, and two to three times daily not uncommon. The medical definition of constipation is the failure to have a bowel movement after three days or more; however, bowel movements on a once-every-other-day schedule are generally not a healthy sign and can definitely lead to a toxemic condition. Unusually hard and dry stools, infrequent or difficult defecation, and sluggish bowels are conditions also referred to as constipation.

The colonic contents are propelled by what is known as mass peristalsis, a type of propulsion that consists of infrequent contractions en mass for considerable distances. Constipation that results from a weakness of the muscles of the colon and rectum is called atonic constipation.

Constipation in adults usually results from several factors, including improper eating habits, which usually includes a low-fiber diet; disregarding the urge to defecate; and as a side-effect of certain medications and emotions. Improper eating habits include eating the wrong foods, eating under stress, overeating, and eating shortly before bedtime. Ignoring the defecation reflex is usually due to one or more of the following factors: working under conditions of stress over long periods of time, worry, anxieties and fears, insufficient relaxation time to empty the bowels, eating when harried, irregular meals, and insufficient exercise. As a result of ignoring the needs of the bowels, a reconditioning of the reflex occurs, with the end result that rectal distention is no longer followed by an urge to defecate. Feces are then retained in the rectum, and colonic stasis ensues.

Many medications can cause constipation as a side-effect. If a patient is taking any drugs, the Amma practitioner should always check the patient's medication in the Physician's Desk Reference to discover the possible influence of the drug on the patient's condition. Emotions can also play a role in constipation. Anxiety and fear can cause the colon to tighten up and block the movement of feces. Excitement due to changes in lifestyle, for example, changing jobs or going on a trip, can often upset the colon's normal activities.

Some people are so obsessed with their bowel movements that they bombard the digestive system with all kinds of laxatives, cathartics, purgatives, enemas, and suppositories. This misuse of artificial stimulants to produce peristaltic action can easily lead to colon dependency and result in atonic constipation. In addition, those who suffer from hemorrhoids, anal fissures, and fistulas tend to avoid painful bowel movements and so develop or foster constipation.

Constipation particularly afflicts the elderly, those confined to bed, and invalids. In these cases, constipation can be related primarily to insufficient physical activity. When children are constipated it can often be traced to poor diet.

Some parents introduce their children to laxative use early in childhood, resulting in a lifelong obsession and extensive dependency on artificial stimulants to induce a bowel movement.

From a wholistic perspective the bowels should be moved every day. A healthy stool is one that does not have a foul odor, is light brown in color, and has a cylindrical shape that is a few inches in length. From a traditional Chinese medicine viewpoint, the functions of the Colon are to receive the dregs from the Small Intestine, to absorb Fluids, and to excrete feces. Diet naturally plays an important role as a cause of constipation. People who consume large quantities of hot and spicy foods can cause the Fluids of the Stomach, Colon, and the Small Intestine to dry up. Excessive consumption of hot foods—such as alcohol, lamb, beef—and dry foods—such as broiled or baked meats—can cause Internal Heat and Dryness, which results in constipation. These foods produce dry stools, and the lack of moisture prevents the Colon from moving the feces.

A depletion of Fluids in the Colon, which is usually concomitant with a Blood or Yin Deficiency, will lead to constipation. This type of dry constipation is often seen in the elderly, those with very thin bodies (indicative of a Yin Deficiency), and in women after giving birth, when there has been an excessive loss of blood that leads to overall depletion of body Fluids. In a hot and dry climate, the exogenous pathogenic factor, Dry Heat, can cause dry constipation. In addition, constipation often results from a febrile disease; the stimulation of a bowel movement is essential to alleviating the fever.

Although Spleen Qi normally is an ascending energy, and a dysfunction of the Spleen usually results in watery stools or diarrhea, a deficient Spleen can also result in constipation. The excessive consumption of cold and raw foods can weaken the Spleen's ability to transform and transport Fluids, thus preventing the feces from being moved down through the Colon. If the Spleen Qi is deficient there may simply not be enough energy to propel the colonic contents. Excessive physical work can also weaken the Spleen through the strain and weakening of the musculature. Conversely, lack of physical exercise can also cause constipation, for lack of exercise weakens the Spleen, also causing a Spleen Qi Deficiency. Exercise is a means of stimulating peristaltic movement; lack of exercise can lead to Liver Qi Stagnation, which can result in constipation as well. Chronic constipation can also develop after childbirth in women who already suffer from a Spleen Qi Deficiency. The stools from a Spleen Qi Deficiency are often long and thin in appearance.

Problems with the Stomach can also lead to constipation. The Stomach is considered to be the origin of Fluids; it likes "wet," as opposed to the Spleen, which likes "dry." Dry stools will result from deficient Stomach Fluids, a form of Yin Deficiency of the Stomach. This is not due to Heat but rather to an absence of Fluids. Poor eating habits—eating in a rush, eating late at night, eating erratically, eating under stress, and eating non-nutritious foods and foods laden with chemicals and pesticides—exhaust the Qi of the Stomach and, over time, the Yin of the Stomach as well. However, Heat in the Stomach also leads to constipation,

for Heat will burn up the Stomach Fluids. It can also cause blockages in the descending of Stomach energy, so that there is insufficient energy descending to foster excretion. Heat in the Stomach can be due to the excessive ingestion of hot foods or to smoking (tobacco is considered to be a "hot" energy). Deep-fried, greasy foods can lead to internal accumulations of Heat as well.

The Liver is another of the major Organs involved with constipation, for the smooth flow of Liver Qi is essential for a smooth bowel movement. If the Liver Qi stagnates in the Lower Burner, the Colon will be affected and the stool will stagnate as well, resulting in small, pebble-size stools.

In addition to the involvement of the Colon, Stomach, Spleen, and Liver in creating the conditions for constipation, the Kidney also influences bowel movements since it controls the two lower outlets or orifices, the anus and the urethra. Both Kidney Yin and Kidney Yang Deficiencies will affect the Colon—Deficient Kidney Yin through Fluid Deficiency, resulting in a lack of Fluids to moisten the feces so they cannot move smoothly downward; and Deficient Kidney Yang when there is not enough Qi to move the stools. If Kidney Yang remains deficient over a long period of time, the resulting Cold in the Lower Burner will also prevent the movement of stools. The difficulty here is not due to lack of moisture but rather to obstruction by the Cold, making defecation very difficult to perform and resulting in straining in order to move the bowels. If a person works extremely long hours over a long period of time under great stress, Kidney Yin and/or Yang energies may be depleted and result in constipation from Dryness or from Cold. A sudden onset of an exogenous invasion of External Cold can produce Internal Cold in the Colon. Constipation due to Cold usually manifests with acute abdominal pain.

As with all illness, emotions can play a major role as a cause of constipation. The Colon is the Yang partner of the Lung (which is a Yin Organ); it is therefore affected by the same emotions as the Lung—worry, depression, and sadness. These emotions deplete Lung Qi, which in turn affects the descending function of the Lung, the energy that normally helps to send Qi to the Colon. The Colon, receiving insufficient Qi from the Lung, can no longer perform its functions adequately. Qi becomes stagnant and obstructs the Colon, resulting in constipation and hard, small stools, sometimes alternating with diarrhea.

Long-standing anger, resentment, and other negative emotions can cause stagnation of Liver Qi in the Lower Burner, which can lead to constipation and pain, as this is an Excess condition. When negative emotions persist over long periods of time, they invariably lead to internal accumulations of Heat, with the Stomach being the Organ most easily affected, as its Fluids will dry up. Mental overwork—too much cerebrating, ruminating, and worry—will deplete Spleen Qi, interfering with the Spleen's ability to transform and transport Fluids and resulting in Dryness in the Colon and constipation due to deficiency.

In addition to regular Amma therapy treatments, a balanced diet and regular exercise are recommended for the relief of constipation. Increasing fiber and water intake also helps, however care

should be taken not to drink excessively, as excess water intake can be damaging to the kidneys. Fiber improves the bulk of the stool and helps with moving the contents through the intestines. Fruits, vegetables, whole grains, and legumes are rich in fiber. Water-soluble fiber, considered the superior form because it binds to fats and toxins and removes them from the system, is found in oats, apples, and seaweed. Fiber can also be provided through supplements. Bowel movements may be regulated by developing the habit of attempting bowel movements at the same time each day.

Supervised fasting and detoxification diets, in conjunction with cleansing enemas, should be used occasionally to help remove toxic debris accumulations from the body and colon. Specific digestive enzymes, such as bromelain and papain, and/or herbs may be used to help promote better digestion and elimination. Natural herbal laxatives can be used to replace chemical stimulants. The patient should be taught abdominal self-massage, which is to be done daily by massaging the abdomen up the ascending colon on the right side, across the transverse colon, and then down the descending colon. This is very helpful to promote digestion if it is done after meals and prior to defecation. Frequent massage to the abdomen can help allay abdominal distention and treat constipation. The use of a small footstool on which to place the feet while the patient defecates will help ease the process.

The following treatment is very effective for alleviating constipation. While there is direct manipulation of the colon area through local points, which stimulate and facilitate peristaltic movement, there is also stimulation of more distal points, which are known to affect proximal areas and help to free obstructed Qi.

AMMA THERAPY TREATMENT

The therapist will first thoroughly review the patient's medical history, diet, exercise regimen, lifestyle, and stress factors from the entrance case history before beginning the rest of the assessment. This information is important in determining the types of recommendations that will be made. It is important to note the onset of the condition and whether the condition is relatively new or is chronic. Patients who have suffered with chronic constipation and who have become addicted to laxatives, purgatives, and cathartics will be more difficult to treat and must understand that the rehabilitation of the colon will take some time and require dietary changes, proper exercise, and, in some cases, changes in lifestyle as well.

Many of the points utilized in the following treatment are used not only for their systemic actions but for their local effect on the muscles and organs located in the abdominal cavity. Manipulation of these points help to release muscle spasms, move trapped gas, and stimulate peristaltic movement.

AMMA THERAPY ASSESSMENT

1. How frequent are the patient's bowel movements? This will help determine the severity of the condition.

2. What is the shape of the patient's stools?
   + A normal stool is light brown in color, several inches long, and has a cylindrical shape.
   + Constipation with small, pebble-like stools indicates Liver Qi Stagnation and Heat in the Large Intestine.
   + Long and skinny stools indicate a Spleen Qi Deficiency.

3. Are the stools very dry?
   + Dry stools can be an indication of Excess Heat or of a Yin Deficiency.
   + If the stools are dry due to Excess Heat, usually of the Stomach or Colon, there will be additional Heat signs, such as thirst, a dry yellow coating on the tongue, and a desire to drink cold liquids.
   + If the dry stools are due to a Yin Deficiency, usually of the Stomach or Kidney, the patient's mouth will be dry but the desire will be to sip fluids.

4. If the patient's stools are not dry but there is difficulty in defecation, this points to stagnation of Liver Qi. This can also refer to an atonic rectum and/or an atonic anal sphincter.

5. Stools that suddenly burst forth and scatter about are an indication of Dampness, either Damp Cold or Damp Heat. In the latter case, the stools will have a yellow cast.

6. If the patient suffers from alternating constipation and diarrhea, this means that Stagnant Liver Qi has invaded the Spleen. This is often a sign of irritable bowel syndrome.

7. What is the color of the patient's stools?

✦ Dark stools indicate Heat.

✦ Pale stools indicate Dampness, usually of the Gall Bladder.

✦ If the stools are light or clay-colored, an inflammation or obstruction of the bile ducts is indicated. In this case there may be a serious underlying disease and the patient should be referred to a physician.

✦ Green stools in children are an indication of Cold.

✦ Blood in the stool, which is an indication of Heat, may also point to more serious conditions, such as bleeding ulcers, hemorrhoids, or tumors. Black stools indicate occult blood in the stool, usually a result of bleeding in the upper intestinal tract. In these cases, refer the patient to a physician for diagnostic tests.

8. Does the patient have any pain?

✦ If the patient suffers with constipation and abdominal pain, this indicates stagnation of Liver Qi or Internal Cold and Yang Deficiency.

✦ Pain due to Cold is a much more severe pain.

✦ Pain from Liver Qi Stagnation often occurs with abdominal distention.

9. How does the patient feel after defecation?

✦ If the patient must strain to achieve defecation, this indicates a Qi or Yang Deficiency.

✦ If the condition feels worse after a bowel movement, this also indicates a Deficiency condition, either Qi or Yang.

✦ If the patient feels better after defecation, this indicates he is suffering from an Excess condition.

✦ If he suffers with cramps after defecation, this means he is suffering from an Internal Cold condition or stagnation of Qi.

10. Does the patient's stool smell? If the stools have a penetrating, foul smell, that is an indication of Heat.

11. Check the tongue and the pulses.

✦ Excess Heat will manifest with a yellow, thick, and sometimes greasy coating. The pulse will be full and rapid.

✦ Internal Cold will manifest with a pale tongue and a moist, thick, white coating. The pulse will be slow and tight.

✦ If Liver Qi has invaded the Spleen, causing alternation of constipation and diarrhea, the tongue will be red on the sides or pale, and the Spleen pulse will be weak while the Liver pulse will be wiry.

✦ If the patient is suffering from a Blood Deficiency, the tongue will be pale or normal looking and dry, and the pulse will be thin or weak.

✦ In a Yang Deficiency condition, the tongue will be pale and wet with a deep and weak pulse.

✦ In Yin Deficiency conditions, the tongue will be peeled with cracks and the pulse will be empty and floating. This condition is most prevalent in elderly patients suffering from Kidney Yin Deficiency.

12. Look at the abdomen for swelling and distention. Palpate the abdomen from

side to side using the heel of the palm and then the palmar aspect of the fingers of one hand alternating with the heel of the palm and the palmar aspect of the fingers of the other hand.

+ If the patient is constipated, pain will be experienced upon palpation.
+ If the abdomen feels worse with pressure, it indicates an Excess condition.
+ If it feels better with pressure, this indicates a Deficiency condition. The healthy abdomen should have a certain flexibility and buoyancy that is not too hard or too soft.

13. Resting the palm of one hand on the transverse colon, palpate the ascending colon with the other hand. In male patients suffering with prostate problems, pain can be experienced when pressure is applied at the beginning of the ascending colon.

14. Palpate the abdomen for scar tissue, adhesions, or any masses and to ascertain the health of the intestines.

+ Abdominal masses that move underneath your fingers may indicate Qi stagnation, muscle spasms, or gas pockets.
+ Masses that feel very hard and do not move indicate Blood Stasis, and may be symptomatic of a benign or malignant tumor. In such cases refer the patient to a physician.

ADDITIONAL TECHNIQUES

1. Manipulate the hypochondriac area with circular digital pressure in the intercostal spaces to disperse stagnated and obstructed Qi.

2. Apply circular thumb pressure on the inside of the costosternal break, on either side of the xiphoid process. This stimulates relaxation of the hypochondriac and epigastric regions and helps to release trapped gas in these areas.

3. Massage of the abdominal area should proceed first with circular palmar pressure, to be followed by circular digital pressure as the area relaxes and responds to pressure. This is beneficial to assimilation and digestion in the gastrointestinal tract. Teh tah chu may be used in the treatment of the abdominal area. Focus should be directed to the massage of the colon area, up the ascending colon on the right side of the patient's body; across the transverse colon, approximately 2 inches above the navel; and down the descending colon on the left side of the body. The treatment may begin lightly with this approach, after which the therapist will then move to the patient's head and begin the basic Amma treatment.

The therapist will return to the manipulation of the colon several times within the course of the treatment, applying increasing pressure when appropriate. The patient should also be taught this technique as a form of daily self-massage.

4. If the transverse colon feels lumpy upon palpation and the therapist hears borborygmi, kneed the colon using circular palmar and circular digital pressure.

5. Moxibustion may be performed on

the colon, following the same direction as the massage to the colon in cases of Internal Cold or Yang Deficiency. A vulnerary should be applied prior to moxibustion to prevent injury to the skin. Moxibustion may be done with a moxa stick or with ginger moxa. The patient may also be instructed to perform moxibustion on himself daily.

6. Moxibustion may also be done to points St36, St44, and Liv2 in cases of Internal Cold or Yang Deficiency.

7. The following sequence is for advanced Amma therapists for the treatment of chronic constipation.

Place both palms on the abdomen with fingers lying inside the costosternal break, pointing toward the sternum. Begin manipulating with a slight alternating pumping action, maintaining pressure without digging the fingertips into the patient's abdomen. Continuing this pumping motion, move straight down to the level of CV12. Then press CV12 as taught in previous treatments. Continue by manipulating the following points in sequence: TS-Ab2, TS-Ab3, and TS-Ab4. Manipulate these three points bilaterally. Then press CV10 and St25 bilaterally. Finish this abdominal manipulation sequence by pressing in 1-tsun increments along the Stomach Channel, from St25 down to the pubic bone.

8. When the patient is lying prone, concentration should be given to circular palmar and circular digital pressure of the lower lumbar and sacral areas. Circular digital pressure is also applied to the sacral area, to stimulate points that regulate the Lower Burner and points that are specific to the treatment of hemorrhoids.

9. If the patient is suffering from lower back pain due to chronic constipation, utilize the techniques taught in the treatment for lower back pain.

POINT LOCATION AND ACTION

1. Co4

Location: In the center of the flesh between the first and second metacarpal bones, closer to the second metacarpal bone.

Grasp the patient's thumb so that the second and third fingers fall on the palmar aspect of the patient's hand. Gently push up on the palmar aspect of the web that lies between the thumb and index finger. Using the thumb of the opposite hand, place its lateral side on the radial edge of the second metacarpal bone, then roll the lateral edge of the thumb into the depression on the second metacarpal bone. Pressure is toward the second metacarpal bone.

Action: This major point has a wide range of functions. Relative to the Colon, it clears Heat in the Large Intestine and regulates and moistens the Colon. It harmonizes ascending and descending energies, thus balancing the energies of the Stomach and Spleen. It will also treat pain in the Intestines.

Comment: This point is the Organ point for the Colon.

2. Co2

Location: On the radial side of the second finger, distal to the metacarpophalangeal joint at the junction of the red and white skin.

Grasp the patient's finger with your hand so that your thumb falls naturally to the joint. Pressure is directly into the joint space with the thumb.

Action: Co2 clears Heat from the Colon. Use this point for Excess Heat patterns with fever, constipation, dry stools, and abdominal distention and pain.

Comment: This is the Spring and Water point of the Colon Channel.

3. Co11

Location: In the depression at the lateral end of the transverse cubital crease, midway between Lu5 and the lateral epicondyle of the humerus when the elbow is half-flexed.

Bend the patient's elbow and place your thumb on the point. Gently open the arm and press. The force is straight into the joint.

Action: Co11 clears Heat from any Organ in the body; it therefore clears Heat from the Colon and Small Intestine and is useful for constipation due to Excess Heat. This point also treats febrile disease and the constipation that results from fever.

Comment: This is the Sea and Earth point of the Colon Channel.

4. SJ5

Location: 2 tsun proximal to SJ4, between the ulna and the radius. (SJ4 is located with the palm facing downward, at the junction of the ulna and carpal bones in the depression lateral to the tendon of the extensor digitorum muscle).

Pressure is activated with the pad of the thumb down into the point.

Action: St5 treats abdominal pain and

constipation and clears Heat from the Colon.

Comment: This is the Luo point for the San Jiao Channel. This point may be pressed at the same time as HE6, using the thumb and third fingers.

5. HE6 (P6)

Location: 2 tsun proximal to the transverse crease of the wrist, between the tendons of the palmaris longus and flexor carpi radialis.

With the pad of the thumb, activate pressure down into the point. When used with SJ5, pronate the forearm while the thumb presses downward into SJ5 and the third finger presses upward, activating HE6.

Action: This point calms the Shen. It treats Stomach pain and Heat in the Colon.

Comment: This is the Luo point for the Heart Envelope (Pericardium) Channel.

6. CV14

Location: 6 tsun above the umbilicus, on the anterior midline of the body.

The point is activated with the thumb or third finger. Gently rest one hand above CV14, palm down, to help stabilize the point pressure of the thumb or third finger of the opposite hand. Ask the patient to inhale, and to exhale slowly. As the patient exhales, apply pressure directly toward the table. Hold the point for 15–30 seconds and then slowly release. As you release your pressure, begin circling your finger.

Action: This point regulates both the Heart and the Stomach. It helps to calm the Spirit of the Heart (Shen) and is therefore useful for digestive disturbances that are emotionally based. It assists in moving energy down out of the chest and toward the Lower Burner.

Comment: This is the Mu point for the Heart.

7. CV12

Location: Midway between the end of the sternum and the umbilicus, or 4 tsun above the umbilicus on the anterior midline of the body. The point is activated with the thumb or third finger.

Gently rest one hand above CV12, palm down, to help stabilize the point pressure of the thumb or third finger of the opposite hand. Ask the patient to inhale, and to exhale slowly. As the pa-tient exhales, apply pressure directly toward the table until a slight pulsation is felt. Hold the point for 15–30 seconds and then slowly release. As you release your pressure, begin circling your finger.

Action: This is a major point for any digestive problem, since it tonifies both Stomach and Spleen Qi. It strengthens the Spleen's function of transforming and transportating Qi and Fluids, and diminishes digestive stagnation. It helps to relieve epigastric pain, gastritis, abdominal distention and pain, constipation, diarrhea, borborygmus, and ulcers. It is also helpful for bringing the emotional energy down from the chest toward the feet and for opening up the chest. CV12 specifically treats the middle portion of the Stomach, and affects the Stomach digestion directly.

Comment: This is the Mu point for the Stomach as well as for the Middle Burner. It is an Intersecting point of the Small Intestine, San Jiao, and Stomach channels. It is also the Influential point of the

Yang Organs and is therefore an important point for digestion.

8. CV10

Location: 2 tsun above the umbilicus, on the anterior midline of the body. The point is activated with the thumb or third finger.

Gently rest one hand above CV10, palm down, to help stabilize the point pressure of the thumb or third finger of the opposite hand. Ask the patient to inhale, and to exhale slowly. As the patient exhales, apply pressure directly toward the table. Hold the point for 15–30 seconds and then slowly release. As you release your pressure, begin circling your finger.

Action: CV10 tonifies the Stomach and the Spleen. It stimulates the descending of Stomach Qi and thereby reduces digestive stagnation from food retention. CV10 directly treats the lower portion of the Stomach, the pylorus, and the duodenum. It helps to harmonize the Middle and Lower Burners by encouraging the food to move from the stomach to the intestines.

Comment: This is the Intersecting point of the Spleen Channel and the Conception Vessel.

9. TS-Ab2

Location: 4 tsun above the umbilicus and 1 tsun lateral to CV12.

This point may be pressed bilaterally. Pressure is applied with the third fingers directed straight down toward the table.

Action: This point regulates and strengthens the Stomach and the Middle Burner.

10. St19

Location: 6 tsun above the umbilicus, 2 tsun lateral to CV14.

Pressure is toward the rib cage with the pads of the thumb.

Action: St19 regulates Stomach Qi, helps descend the energy of the Stomach Channel, and removes digestive stagnation.

11. St21

Location: 4 tsun above the umbilicus, 2 tsun lateral to CV12.

This point may be pressed bilaterally. Pressure is with the third fingers directly toward the table and slightly lateral.

Action: St21 regulates and strengthens the Stomach and the Middle Burner, clears Heat from the Middle Burner, and reduces digestive stagnation. This point alleviates pain due to Qi obstruction in the hypochondrium; it also alleviates ulcers, gastritis, indigestion, and food retention. St21 is used more for Excess conditions of the Stomach.

12. TS-Ab3

Location: 1.5 tsun below CV12 and 1 tsun lateral to the Conception Vessel.

This point may be pressed bilaterally. Pressure is applied with the third fingers directed straight down toward the table.

Action: TS-Ab3 harmonizes the Stomach and the Middle Burner.

13. TS-Ab4

Location: 1.5 tsun inferior and lateral to TS-Ab3, on a 45 degree angle.

This point may be pressed bilaterally. Pressure is applied with the third fingers directed straight down toward the table.

Action: TS-Ab4 harmonizes the Stomach and the Intestines.

14. St25

Location: 2 tsun lateral to the umbilicus.

This point may be pressed bilaterally with the thumbs. Pressure is directly toward the table.

Action: St25 regulates the Spleen, Stomach, and Middle and Lower Burners, and moistens and regulates the Colon. It clears Heat from the Stomach, Colon, and Small Intestine and therefore helps with burning pain in the epigastrium and constipation.

Comment: This is the Mu point for the Colon.

15. Sp15

Location: 4 tsun lateral to the center of the umbilicus.

This point may be pressed bilaterally with the thumbs. Pressure is directly toward the table.

Action: This point is very useful for constipation due to Spleen Qi Deficiency. It activates the Spleen function of transforming and transporting Qi, Blood, and Fluids, particularly to promote peristalsis. It also treats chronic constipation due to Spleen Qi Deficiency.

16. TS-Ab5

Location: 1 tsun lateral to the navel.

This point may be pressed bilaterally with the thumbs. Pressure is directly toward the table.

Action: TS-Ab5 is a local point used to remove obstructions from the Colon and reduce digestive stagnation.

17. CV7

Location: 1 tsun inferior to the navel, on the midline of the body.

Pressure is with the pad of the third

finger or thumb directly toward the table.

Action: CV7 nourishes Yin and Blood and regulates the Lower Burner.

Comment: The Penetrating Vessel intersects with the Conception Vessel at this point.

18. CV6

Location: On the midline of the abdomen, 1.5 tsun below the umbilicus.

Pressure is with the pad of the third finger or thumb directly toward the table.

Action: CV6 helps to move stagnant Qi and relieve pain in the Lower Burner.

19. TS-Ab1

Location: Half the distance measured between the pubic bone and the umbilicus, on the midline of the body.

Pressure is with the pad of the third finger or thumb directly toward the table.

Action: TS-Ab1 is a local point for regulating the Lower Burner. It removes obstructions in the Colon and helps to relieve pain in this area.

20. TS-Ab6

Location: 1.5 tsun lateral and 0.5 tsun above TS-Ab1.

Pressure is with the pad of the third finger or thumb directly toward the table.

Action: This point regulates the Lower Burner and removes obstructions of Qi in the Lower Burner.

21. St36

Location: 3 tsun below St35, 1 tsun lateral to the anterior crest of the tibia. (St35 is at the lateral foramen of the patella.)

Stand alongside the patient facing the patient's knee. Place the pad of the thumb of the hand closest to the patient's head on the point. Gently hold the foot with the other hand and tilt the leg toward your body as you press toward the tibia. This will give more pressure into the point. This point may be held for 15–30 seconds. Circle as you release your pressure.

Action: This point has a very strong regulating and tonifying effect on the Stomach, Spleen, Lung, Kidney, Colon, and Small Intestine when there is constipation due to deficiency. This point also tonifies Qi and Blood.

Comment: This is the Sea and Earth point of the Stomach Channel.

22. St37

Location: 6 tsun below St35 (at the lateral foramen of the patella), 1 tsun from the anterior crest of the tibia.

Pressure is directed with the thumb toward the tibia.

Action: St37 regulates the functions of the Stomach, Colon, and Small Intestine.

Comment: This is the deep ending of the Colon Channel. Note that an extra point is located between St36 and St37, 2 tsun below St36. This point is called "appendix," as sensitivity in this area indicates inflammation of the appendix.

23. GB34

Location: In the depression anterior and inferior to the head of the fibula.

Pressure is activated with the thumb in the depression, toward the tibia.

Action: GB34 regulates the smooth flow of Liver Qi and removes stagnation, particularly in the hypochondriac region but also in the Lower Burner.

Comment: This is the Influential point of the sinews. It is the Sea and Earth point of the Gall Bladder Channel.

24. Sp6

Location: 3 tsun proximal to the vertex of the medial malleolus, just posterior to the tibial border.

Stand at the foot of the table. Grasp the patient's leg with your hand and place the pad of the thumb on the point. Gently press toward the tibia until you feel a sulcus in the bone. Hold the point for 15–30 seconds and then slowly release, circling as you lighten your pressure. This point can be pressed bilaterally.

Action: Sp6 tonifies and strengthens the Spleen, Liver, and Kidney. It is particularly helpful in assisting the free flow of Liver Qi when it is stagnating in the Lower Burner, producing constipation and abdominal pain, distention, and flatulence. In removing obstructions of Qi from the Liver Channel, it helps to calm negative emotions and relieve pain in the lower abdominal area. Sp6 nourishes Blood and Yin and can be used to treat both Blood and Yin Deficiency. This point also treats lower abdominal pain due to its action of promoting the smooth flow of Liver Qi.

Comment: This point is the Intersecting point of the three Yin channels of the leg.

25. Liv5

Location: 5 tsun proximal to the vertex of the medial malleolus, in a depression on the medial aspect of the tibia.

Pressure is applied with the pad of the thumb directly into the depression.

Action: Liv5 treats Liver Qi Stagnation in the Middle and Lower Burners. It also treats lower abdominal pain and distention.

Comment: This is the Luo point for the Liver Channel.

26. St44

Location: Proximal to the margin of the web between the second and third toes in the depression distal and lateral to the second metatarsophalangeal joint.

Pressure is with the thumb toward the second metatarsophalangeal joint.

Action: St44 regulates the Stomach Qi, stops pain, and clears Stomach Heat and Fire. It is used mostly for Excess conditions.

Comment: This is the Spring and Water point of the Stomach Channel.

27. Liv2

Location: 0.5 tsun proximal to the margin of the web between the first and second toes.

Grasp the patient's toe with your hand and press into the lateral joint space with your thumb. Angle your thumb to fit into the joint space. This point may be more tender than others; it should be pressed gently at first and then with increasing pressure. Hold for 15–30 seconds and then slowly release, circling as you lighten your pressure.

Action: Liv2 helps to treat constipation affected by Rising Liver Fire. It also sedates Liver Yang.

Comment: This is the Spring and Fire point of the Liver Channel.

28. Sp21

Location: On the midaxillary line, 6 tsun below the axilla and midway between the axilla and the free end of the eleventh rib.

This point can be manipulated bilaterally, with the patient in either the supine or prone position. The point is activated with the pads of the third fingers pressing directly into the intercostal space.

Action: Sp21 is one of the major points of Oriental medicine. It is the Great Luo (Connecting) point of the Spleen. This point helps to regulate Qi and Blood via its connection to the minute Blood Luo channels throughout the body, and is therefore used as a general tonification point.

29. Bl20

Location: 1.5 tsun lateral to the lower border of the spinous process of the eleventh thoracic vertebra.

Pressure is applied bilaterally with the thumbs, straight down toward the table.

Action: Bl20 is a major point for tonifying the Stomach and the Spleen and regulating the Middle Jiao. It helps the Spleen's transporting and transforming functions and reduces digestive stagnation. Bl20 treats all Spleen Qi Deficiency patterns with symptoms of abdominal distention, lack of appetite, fatigue, and loose stools. It also treats indigestion, gastritis, ulcers, borborygmus, acute or chronic diarrhea, constipation, and stool with undigested food. Bl20 also stimulates the ascending of Spleen Qi.

Comment: This is the Yu point (Associated point) for the Spleen.

30. Bl21

Location: 1.5 tsun lateral to the lower border of the spinous process of the twelfth thoracic vertebra.

Pressure is applied bilaterally with the thumbs, straight down toward the table.

Action: Bl21 is major point used for tonifying both Stomach Qi and Spleen Qi. It stimulates the descending of Stomach Qi and therefore treats Rebellious Stomach Qi symptoms of belching, regurgitation,

vomiting, and nausea. Bl21 treats indigestion, borborygmus, abdominal distention, and flatulence. It relieves stagnation of food in the Stomach and promotes the Spleen function of transforming and transporting Qi, Blood, and Fluids.

Comment: This is the Yu point (Associated point) for the Stomach.

31. Bl23

Location: 1.5 tsun lateral to the lower border of the spinous process of the second lumbar vertebra.

This point may be manipulated bilaterally with the thumbs. Pressure is directly toward the table. Pull the muscle slightly upward while maintaining pressure downward.

Action: Bl23 tonifies both Kidney Yin and Kidney Yang. It promotes the formation of Blood in Blood Deficiency conditions. Bl23 treats constipation due to Blood Deficiency, Kidney Yin Deficiency, or Kidney Yang Deficiency. It also treats low back pain due to constipation.

Comment: This is the Yu point (Associated point) for the Kidney.

32. Bl25

Location: 1.5 tsun lateral to the lower border of the spinous process of the fourth lumbar vertebra, approximately at the level of the upper border of the iliac crest.

Pressure is applied bilaterally with the thumbs, straight down toward the table.

Action: Bl25 activates the excreting function of the Colon. It is very good for treating chronic constipation and low back pain resulting from constipation.

Comment: This is the Yu point (Associated point) for the Colon.

21

TREATMENT FOR DIARRHEA

AMMA THERAPY ETIOLOGY

Patients frequently present with complaints of diarrhea. According to Western medicine, diarrhea is defined as watery stool with increased stool volume. It is usually associated with frequent bowel movements, that is, more than three bowel movements a day. Diarrhea results from one or more of the following imbalances: poor absorption of solutes, altered intestinal motility, and alterations in cellular form and structure of the intestinal wall. Diarrhea may be acute or chronic. The many causes of diarrhea reflect the sources of imbalance in the homeodynamic model of health.

A common cause of acute diarrhea is food poisoning resulting from the ingestion of contaminated foods. The primary contaminants of foods are strains of staphylococcus, *Escherichia coli,* or salmonella bacteria. Eggs and processed meats, chicken, and seafood are often contaminated as a result of unsanitary conditions in handling as well as insufficient cooking at high enough temperatures to kill all the bacteria. The toxins produced by the bacteria that have been introduced into the gastrointestinal tract directly attack the mucous membranes and interfere with the functioning of the intestines. In response to the toxins, the mucous membranes begin to secrete more liquid and mucus while absorbing less water from the content of the bowel. Watery stools or diarrhea result. The symptoms of cramps, nausea, vomiting, and diarrhea usually last between twelve and twenty-four hours.

Another common but acute type of diarrhea is viral gastroenteritis, a contagious condition that frequently manifests during the fall and winter. In this condition the virus enters into absorptive epithelial cells on the tip of the villus, causing them to slough off and be destroyed. These functioning cells are replaced by immature cells, resulting in decreased absorption. The symptoms include diarrhea, nausea, vomiting, headache, low-grade fever, abdominal cramps, malaise, and hyperactive bowel sounds. The incubation period is generally between forty-eight and seventy-two hours, and the symptoms should be alleviated within twenty-four to forty-eight hours after acute onset.

Acute diarrhea can also be catalyzed by noninfectious causes. Many medications produce diarrhea as a side-effect. For example, antibiotics, which are among the most frequently prescribed medications, and chemotherapy agents often cause diarrhea.

An example of diarrhea resulting from an accumulation of nonabsorbed solutes is osmotic diarrhea. This condition exists when food is not being digested properly, thus leaving certain food compounds or solutes in the intestines. These solutes in turn cause water and salts to be retained within the intestinal lumen, resulting in diarrhea. This is usually a chronic type of condition, and is seen in people who experience an intolerance to substances such as lactose, glucose, and fats.

Chronic diarrhea that alternates with constipation can be an indication of a condition called irritable bowel syndrome, a condition that is also called spastic colon. This condition is associated with altered intestinal motility. It is accompanied by symptoms of abdominal distention (bloating), abdominal pain, and nausea. Stress, worry, and anxiety are known to be major factors in this condition. Irritable bowel syndrome is difficult to control through diet and treatment alone, since it often has a strong emotional component that must be addressed, as is true for many Organ dysfunctions. Often the patient will have little recognition of the emotional component and blame his bowels as the cause of pain and discomfort. However, testing through sigmoidoscopy or colonoscopy produces no observable inflammation of the intestines or other abnormalities. Irritable bowel syndrome is perhaps the most common gastrointestinal problem. The small intestine and the colon are both involved in this syndrome of disturbed and irregular motility.

Ulcerative colitis is a condition of the intestines affecting the colon and sometimes the lower ileum as well. In this condition there is ulceration of the intestinal mucosa and chronic inflammation of the colon and rectum. The major symptoms of ulcerative colitis are bloody diarrhea and abdominal pain. Severe cases manifest with diarrhea containing blood and mucus that may occur ten to twenty times a day.

Crohn's disease, also called regional ileitis or enteritis, is an inflammation of the intestines that can affect all layers of the bowel wall. It is most often seen in the terminal ileum and jejunum of the small intestine, and in the colon. There are intermittent attacks of diarrhea accompanied by abdominal pain, usually on the right side. The patient may also suffer from loss of weight and a consistent low-grade fever.

From the homeodynamic perspective, acute diarrhea is due to an invasion by exogenous pathogens, namely Cold,

Damp or Summer Heat. Exogenous Cold and Damp can enter directly into the Large Intestine through the Lower Burner. While this can occur in cold weather, often it occurs in the summer and fall. The exogenous pathogens of Cold and Damp can directly invade the Colon through exposure to unseasonably cold weather when one is inadequately dressed. Damp Cold can penetrate into the Lower Burner from the ground, entering into the channels of the legs and flowing up the legs to the Spleen, interfering with the transformation and transportation of Fluids and resulting in diarrhea. Damp Cold can also enter directly into the orifices of the Lower Burner, for example, by entering the body while sitting on a damp, cold bench at a sports event or remaining in a cold and wet bathing suit. Both of these situations would allow Cold to invade the Large Intestine through the Lower Burner.

When exogenous Damp enters the Colon it blocks the absorption of Fluids; they then accumulate and diarrhea ensues, characterized by an acute attack of loose stools and abdominal pain and distention. Summer Heat also directly invades the Large Intestine and is a common cause of acute diarrhea in the summertime. The person may also have accompanying symptoms of fever and aversion to cold.

Acute diarrhea may also be due to diet. Eating contaminated food or excessive amounts of cold and raw foods or greasy and hot foods can all catalyze sudden attacks of loose bowels or diarrhea.

Chronic diarrhea is often due to several factors. Chronic exposure to exogenous pathogens, particularly Dampness, can lead to chronic diarrhea. While we tend to associate diarrhea with the Colon, we must look past the Colon to disharmonies of the Spleen for the source of this problem. The Organ most affected in this condition is the Spleen. While the Spleen can be negatively affected by invasions of exogenous Damp as stated above, resulting in acute attacks of diarrhea, chronic diarrhea can also be due to long-term exogenous invasions. Living in a damp house or climate or working in a wet environment over a long period of time are other ways that Damp can enter the body and cause injury to the Spleen. Since the Spleen controls the entire digestive process through its transformation and transportation of food essences and Fluids, disharmonies of the Spleen will always affect the digestive process and result in symptoms of abdominal bloating, poor appetite, and loose stools or diarrhea. When the transformation and transportation of the food essences and Fluids is impaired, unabsorbed food particles remain in the bowels with the accompanying retention of water.

Diet obviously plays a major role in the health of the Spleen. The Spleen is adversely affected by excessive consumption of greasy foods, sweets, and cold foods, including ice-cold drinks, fruits, and raw vegetables. These all disrupt the harmony of the Spleen and give rise to an interior Damp condition, which then results in loose stools or diarrhea. Greasy and hot food can also give rise to Internal Damp Heat in the Colon, which can also produce diarrhea, along with blood and mucus in the stool. Eating under stress or worry, eating excessively or insufficiently, eating on the run, or simply continual overeating all contribute to a weakening of Spleen energies.

Chronic deficiency of the Spleen, Colon, and Stomach can result in a sinking of Spleen Qi. This can cause hemorrhoids and, more significantly, the prolapse of the anus. Sinking of Spleen Qi results in chronic diarrhea accompanied by loss of appetite, chronic fatigue, a desire to drink warm liquids, and a desire to have the abdomen massaged.

The functions of the Spleen do not exist in isolation from other Organs; the Spleen is therefore influenced by other Organ disharmonies, particularly those of the Kidney and the Liver. The Spleen works with and assists the Kidney in the transportation of Fluids throughout the body. When the Kidney Yang energy is weak, the Spleen will not get the warmth, nourishment, and support it needs from the Kidney to transform and transport Fluids. They will first accumulate, causing Internal Dampness, and then when the Spleen can no longer contain them, it will deposit them into the Colon, resulting in diarrhea. A Yang Deficiency will often lead first to a Spleen Yang Deficiency and then evolve into a Kidney Yang Deficiency. Working under stressful conditions, insufficient rest, and an irregular diet all contribute to a weakening of both the Kidney and Spleen energies.

The Liver influences the Spleen, and disharmonies between them are commonly seen in the clinical setting. Liver Qi assists the Spleen in its transformation and transportation functions through its role of making sure there is an uninterrupted flow of Qi, Blood, and Fluids to all parts of the body. In addition, it aids digestion through the smooth secretion of bile. By providing for the smooth flow of Qi, Blood, and Fluids throughout the entire body, the Liver helps Spleen Qi

ascend and Stomach Qi descend, their normal directions of flow. When the Liver Qi is disrupted it often becomes blocked and begins to stagnate. This will in turn affect the Spleen, impairing its ability to transform and transport food essences and Fluids. In addition, the normal flow of Spleen Qi, which is upward, is blocked, and the result is that Spleen Qi begins to descend instead of ascend, thus producing diarrhea. In Five Element theory, this is referred to as the Liver overcontrolling the Spleen.

In looking at these disturbances we must remember the influence of emotions as major contributors to Colon, Spleen, Kidney, and Liver dysfunctions, all of which can result in diarrhea. While Western medicine is belatedly coming to recognize the influence of emotions on the disease process, TCM and wholistic medicine have long acknowledged the role that long-standing emotions play in the cause of disease. Emotions play a major role in digestive disorders.

The word *stress* is a broad term that often does not provide a detailed recognition of the specific emotions involved or their influence in the onset and progression of a disease. We know that the Colon is paired with the Lung as a Yin/Yang couple and, as a result, it can also be affected by sadness and worry. These emotions deplete the Lung Qi, which then fails to cause Qi, Blood, and Fluids to descend to the Colon. This can result in a stagnation in the Colon and spasticity, which can produce alternating constipation and diarrhea. Worry, fretting, and dwelling on negative feelings affect the Spleen (also the Lung), causing a weakening of all Spleen functions. Worry is a fact of life in our fast-paced society: people worry about finances, family, and employment. Excessive mental work can also deplete the Spleen's energies.

Depression or long-term frustration (anger) can upset the Liver's spreading function and result in disharmony between the Liver and the Stomach and/or Spleen. Anger can misdirect Liver Qi to invade the Spleen, causing the rebellion of Qi in the Stomach and Spleen. In this situation Stomach Qi ascends instead of descends, causing burping, regurgitation, and perhaps even vomiting, and Spleen Qi descends instead of ascends, resulting in diarrhea. Fear and anxiety can deplete the Kidney Yang energies. When this happens, the Spleen fails to get the warmth it needs from the Kidney, producing an Interior Cold condition that results in loose stools. A Kidney and Spleen Yang Deficiency occurring together will result in chronic diarrhea.

In addition to regular Amma therapy treatments, a balanced diet and regular exercise are recommended for the relief of diarrhea. Drinking green clay or chamomile tea is often beneficial.

Specific digestive enzymes can be beneficial for promoting proper digestion and absorption of nutrients, as can the addition of good bacteria, such as acidophilus, to repopulate the colon. The assistance of a certified herbalist in conjunction with regular Amma therapy treatments can be very helpful.

The following is a basic treatment for both acute and chronic diarrhea. It is necessary to emphasize once more that this treatment is not done in isolation from dietary changes, and that emotional work with a qualified psychologist for persons suffering from chronic conditions may be a necessary recommendation to supplement regular Amma therapy treatments.

AMMA THERAPY TREATMENT

The first concern of the Amma therapist is to assess the severity of the patient's condition, since the acuteness and chronicity as well as the severity of the illness will determine the treatment plan. The therapist will want to rule out any kind of immediate danger to the bioenergetic system. Once the Amma therapist has established the severity of the condition through study of the patient's medical history and by asking the appropriate questions, he will then continue the assessment through pulse and tongue diagnosis; by looking at the patient's general demeanor, the color of the face, and the body type; by assessing the emotional state and whether the patient is malnourished; and through palpation of the abdominal area. All of this information is integrated into the treatment plan.

AMMA THERAPY ASSESSMENT

1. Question the patient as to whether this is an acute or chronic condition. Acute diarrhea has a sudden onset and will usually be accompanied by fever and aversion to cold. This indicates an invasion by Damp Cold or Damp Heat. This could be the result of food poisoning or viral gastroenteritis.

2. What is the frequency of the patient's bowel movements? Frequent diarrhea with watery stools indicates a chronic Spleen and Stomach Deficiency.

3. Does the diarrhea occur at a particular time of day?
   + Diarrhea that occurs in the early morning (sometimes called "fifth-watch diarrhea") indicates a Kidney Yang Deficiency.
   + Diarrhea that occurs directly after eating is usually due to Spleen and Stomach Qi Deficiency.

4. Does the patient feel better or worse after passing diarrhea?
   + If the patient feels relief after diarrhea, this indicates an Excess condition. This would be the case in diarrhea due to overeating. Diarrhea due to overeating is accompanied by fetid smelling stool, abdominal pain and distention, fullness in the epigastrium, foul belching, a feeling of relief after defecation, and a dirty tongue coating with a slippery pulse.
   + If the patient feels worse after diarrhea, this indicates a Deficiency condition.

5. Does the stool smell?
   + A putrid smell to the stool indicates Heat.
   + The absence of smell indicates the presence of Cold due to Spleen Yang Deficiency.

6. What is the color of the stools?
   + Dark stools indicate Heat.
   + Watery stools are a sign of Cold.
   + Pale yellow stools are a sign of Liver and Gall Bladder Damp Heat.
   + Black stools or very dark stools are a sign of Blood Stasis.

7. Does the stool burn when it passes? A burning feeling in the anus during a loose bowel movement indicates the presence of Heat. Ask the patient if he has recently eaten hot and spicy foods, as this can sometimes account for burning in the anus. However, chronic burning in this area may be an indication of irritable bowel syndrome or colitis.

8. Is there undigested food in the stools? This indicates a Spleen Qi Deficiency.

9. If the patient does not have diarrhea and the stools are only a little bit loose but he has trouble controlling the urge to defecate, this points to a Middle Burner Deficiency and a sinking of Spleen Qi.

10. Does bright red blood precede the stools? This is a sign of Damp Heat in the Colon, the Heat scorching the blood vessels of the Large Intestine.

11. Do watery stools precede the Blood? This is a sign of Spleen Qi Deficiency; the Spleen is not keeping the Blood in the vessels.

12. Is there mucus in the stools? This is a sign of Dampness in the Colon.

13. Does the patient experience any pain?
    + Diarrhea with pain indicates Heat or interference from the Liver (Liver Qi Stagnation).
    + Diarrhea with abdominal pain and borborygmi is a sign of Interior Cold in the Large Intestine and is similar to a Spleen Yang Deficiency.

- ✦ A fixed, stabbing abdominal pain indicates Blood Stasis or an abscess or swelling.
- ✦ A pain without a fixed location and that is difficult to locate is usually due to Qi Stagnation, usually in the channels.

14. Is the diarrhea accompanied by borborygmi?
    - ✦ This is a sign of a Spleen Qi Deficiency.
    - ✦ Borborygmi accompanied by abdominal distention without loose stools points to Liver Qi Stagnation.

15. Does the patient suffer from flatulence? Flatulence is usually a sign of Liver Qi Stagnation.
    - ✦ An offensive smell indicates Damp Heat in the Colon or Heat in the Stomach.
    - ✦ No smell indicates Interior Cold due to Spleen Yang Deficiency.

16. Chronic diarrhea accompanied by abdominal pain and distention, flatulence, and negative emotions indicates that Liver Qi has invaded the Spleen.

17. Diarrhea that alternates with constipation, commonly referred to in Western medicine as irritable bowel syndrome, accompanied by heartburn and belching indicates Stagnant Liver Qi invading the Spleen.

18. Look at the patient's tongue.
    - ✦ If the patient is suffering from Damp Heat in the Colon, he will have a red tongue with a sticky or greasy yellow coating and a rapid and slippery pulse.
    - ✦ If the patient is suffering from exogenous Cold invading the Colon, his tongue will have a thick white coating and he will have a deep and wiry pulse.
    - ✦ If the patient is suffering from Interior Cold in the Colon or Spleen Yang Deficiency, he will have a pale tongue that is swollen and wet with a deep and slow pulse.

19. When a patient suffers from Collapse of Colon Qi the symptoms are chronic diarrhea; prolapse of the anus; hemorrhoids; fatigue and loss of appetite; pale tongue; and a thin, deep, and weak pulse.

20. A patient suffering from a Spleen Qi Deficiency will manifest loose stools, fatigue, lack of appetite, and a sallow complexion. His tongue will be pale or normal looking; sometimes the sides will be swollen and the pulse will feel weak or empty. This is commonly seen in the clinical situation.

21. Look at the abdomen for swelling and distention. A normal abdomen should not be distended, nor should it be concave. If it is distended, this could be due to gas, bloating, water, or mucus. If it is concave, that can be due to long-standing diarrhea resulting from a nutritional deficiency.

22. When there is a very thin abdominal wall or very active peristaltic movement, you can actually look at the abdomen and see it fluctuating, indicating the peristaltic movement.

23. Using a stethoscope, listen for bowel sounds over all four quadrants. This should be done before any palpation. More than thirty bowel sounds per minute indicates gas, diarrhea, or hyperactive peristalsis.

24. Palpate the abdomen to evaluate for an Excess or Deficient condition. The

healthy abdomen should have a certain flexibility and buoyancy that is not too hard or too soft.

+ If the abdomen feels worse with pressure, it indicates an Excess condition.

+ If it feels better with pressure, this indicates a Deficiency condition.

25. Palpate the abdomen for scar tissue, adhesions, or any masses and to ascertain the health of the intestines.

+ Abdominal masses that move underneath your fingers may indicate Qi Stagnation, muscle spasms, or gas pockets.

+ If the masses feel very hard and do not move, they indicate Blood Stasis and may be symptomatic of a benign or malignant tumor. In such cases refer the patient to a physician.

ADDITIONAL TECHNIQUES

1. When there is tenderness in the abdominal area, teh tah chu can be applied. Focus should be directed to the massage of the colon area—up the descending, across the transverse, and down the ascending colon.

2. If the patient is suffering from diarrhea due to overeating, knead the abdomen gently to help remove food stasis. Drinking green clay or some form of chlorophyll may be very helpful in resolving this problem.

3. Apply circular digital pressure to the Liv13 area. Liv13 is located below the free end of the eleventh floating rib. This point treats diarrhea and food stagnation. Liv13 is the Mu point for the Spleen and is used when Liver Qi invades the Middle Burner, interfering with the normal direction of Spleen Qi and resulting in diarrhea. This area helps to harmonize the functions of the Liver and Spleen.

4. When the patient is suffering from borborygmus and, upon palpation, large areas of gas can be felt as palpable masses, this gas must be dispersed. If this is felt in the epigastrium, use teh tah chu and concentrate your manipulation on the area just below the xyphoid process. Use circular digital pressure until you feel the gas disperse.

5. If there is borborygmus and large areas of gas in the lower abdomen, use teh tah chu and manipulate the area until you feel the gas disperse.

6. When the patient is lying prone, concentration should be given to circular palmar and circular digital pressure of the lower lumbar and sacral areas. Circular digital pressure is also applied to the sacral area to stimulate points that regulate the Lower Burner and points that are specific to the treatment of hemorrhoids.

POINT LOCATION AND ACTION

1. Co4

Location: In the center of the flesh between the first and second metacarpal bones, closer to the second metacarpal bone.

Grasp the patient's thumb so that the second and third fingers fall on the palmar aspect of the patient's hand. Gently push up on the palmar aspect of the web that lies between the thumb and index finger. Using the thumb of the opposite hand, place its lateral side on the radial edge of the second metacarpal bone, then roll the lateral edge of the thumb into the depression on the second metacarpal bone. Pressure is toward the second metacarpal bone.

Action: This major point has a wide range of functions. Relative to the Colon, it clears Heat in the Large Intestine and will treat diarrhea due to Damp Heat. It harmonizes ascending and descending energies, thus balancing the energies of the Stomach and Spleen. It will also treat pain in the Large Intestine.

Comment: This is the Organ point for the Colon.

2. CV12

Location: Midway between the end of the sternum and the umbilicus, or 4 tsun above the umbilicus on the anterior midline of the body.

The point is activated with the thumb or third finger. Gently rest one hand above CV12, palm down, to help stabilize the point pressure of the thumb or third finger of the opposite hand. Ask the patient to inhale, and to exhale slowly. As the patient exhales, apply pressure directly toward the table until a slight pulsation is felt. Hold the point for 15–30 seconds and then slowly release. As you release your pressure, begin circling your finger.

Action: CV12 is a major point for any digestive problem since it tonifies both Stomach and Spleen Qi. It strengthens the Spleen's function of transforming and transporting Qi and Fluids, thereby help-

ing to resolve Dampness. It helps to relieve epigastric pain, gastritis, abdominal distention and pain, constipation, diarrhea, borborygmus, and ulcers. It is also helpful for bringing the emotional energy down from the chest toward the feet, and opening up the chest.

Comment: This is the Mu point for the Stomach as well as for the Middle Burner. It is an Intersecting point of the Small Intestine, San Jiao, and Stomach channels. It is also the Influential point of the Yang Organs and is therefore an important point for digestion.

3. CV10

Location: 2 tsun above the umbilicus, on the anterior midline of the body.

The point is activated with the thumb or third finger. Gently rest one hand above CV10, palm down, to help stabilize the point pressure of the thumb or third finger of the opposite hand. Ask the patient to inhale, and to exhale slowly. As the patient exhales, apply pressure directly toward the table. Hold the point for 15–30 seconds and then slowly release. As you release your pressure, begin circling your finger.

Action: CV10 tonifies the Stomach and Spleen. It stimulates the descending of Stomach Qi and thereby reduces digestive stagnation from food retention. It directly treats the lower portion of the stomach, the pylorus, and the duodenum. CV10 also helps to harmonize the Middle and Lower Burners by encouraging the food to move from the stomach to the small intestines, which is helpful for patients who suffer from loose stools or diarrhea due to overeating and retention of food in the digestive system. This point transforms Dampness and Damp Heat conditions.

Comment: This is the Intersecting point of the Spleen Channel and the Conception Vessel.

4. Co11

Location: In the depression at the lateral end of the transverse cubital crease. Midway between Lu5 and the lateral epicondyle of the humerus, when the elbow is half-flexed.

Bend the patient's elbow and place your thumb on the point. Gently open the arm and press. The force is straight into the joint.

Action: This point clears Heat from any Organ in the body; it therefore clears Heat from the Large Intestine and is useful for diarrhea due to Heat or Damp Heat.

Comment: This is the Sea and Earth point of the Colon Channel.

5. St21

Location: 4 tsun above the umbilicus, 2 tsun lateral to CV12.

This point may be pressed bilaterally. Pressure is with the third fingers directed toward the table and slightly lateral.

Action: St21 regulates and strengthens the Stomach and the Middle Burner. It clears heat from the Middle Burner and reduces digestive stagnation due to retention of food. St21 also strengthens the Spleen's ability to transform and transport digestive substances.

6. St25

Location: 2 tsun lateral to the umbilicus.

This point may be pressed bilaterally with the thumbs. Pressure is directed toward the table.

Action: St25 regulates the Spleen, Stomach, and Middle and Lower Burners, regulates the Colon, and transforms Intestinal Dampness and Damp Heat. This point also treats abdominal pain and diarrhea.

Comment: This is the Mu point for the Colon.

7. CV6

Location: On the midline of the abdomen, 1.5 tsun below the umbilicus.

Pressure is with the pad of the third finger or thumb directed toward the table.

Action: CV6 helps to move stagnant Qi and relieve pain in the Lower Burner. It transforms Dampness in the Lower Burner and tonifies the Spleen.

8. Sp9

Location: On the lower border of the medial condyle of the tibia, in the depression between the posterior border of the tibia and the gastrocnemius muscle, at the depression at the end of the crease when the knee is flexed.

Pressure is with the pad of the thumb into the depression.

Action: Sp9 harmonizes the Spleen and transforms Dampness and Damp Heat. It treats diarrhea with undigested food or mucus in the stool.

Comment: This is the Sea and Water point of the Spleen Channel.

9. St36

Location: 3 tsun below St35, 1 tsun lateral to the anterior crest of the tibia. (St35 is at the lateral foramen of the patella).

Stand alongside the patient facing the patient's knee. Place the pad of the thumb of the hand closest to the patient's head on the point. Gently hold the foot with the other hand and tilt the leg toward your body as you press toward the tibia. This will direct more pressure into the point. This point may be held for 15–30 seconds. Circle as you release your pressure.

Action: This point has a very strong regulating and tonifying effect on the Stomach, Spleen, Lung, Kidney, Colon, and Small Intestine when these Organs are deficient. It helps to remove digestive stagnation and is beneficial for loss of appetite and dull epigastric pain. It redirects Rebellious Stomach Qi downward and is useful for all Stomach disorders, such as indigestion, diarrhea, borborygmus, meteorism, ulcers, gastritis, stomachache, nausea, and vomiting.

Comment: This is the Sea and Earth point of the Stomach Channel.

10. St37

Location: 6 tsun below St35 (St35 is at the lateral foramen of the patella), 1 tsun from the anterior crest of the tibia.

Pressure is directed with the thumb toward the tibia.

Action: St37 regulates the functions of the Stomach and Large Intestine and thereby helps treat chronic diarrhea.

Comment: This is the deep ending of the Colon Channel. Note that an extra point is located between St36 and St37, 2 tsun below St36. This point is called "appendix," as sensitivity in this area indicates inflammation of the appendix.

11. St39

Location: One finger's breadth lateral to the anterior crest of the tibia, 3 tsun below St37 or 1 tsun below St38.

Pressure is directed by the thumb toward the tibia.

Action: St39 regulates the function of the Stomach and the Small Intestine, clears Heat, and transforms Damp, stops lower abdominal pain, and treats diarrhea and borborygmi.

Comment: This is the deep ending of the Small Intestine Channel.

12. Sp6

Location: 3 tsun proximal to the vertex of the medial malleolus, just posterior to the tibial border.

Stand at the foot of the table. Grasp the patient's leg with your hand and place the pad of the thumb on the point. Gently press toward the tibia until you feel a sulcus in the bone. Hold the point for 15–30 seconds and then slowly release, circling as you lighten your pressure. This point can be pressed bilaterally.

Action: Sp6 tonifies and strengthens the Stomach, Spleen, Liver, and Kidney. It is utilized in Spleen Deficiency patterns that manifest with loose stools, lack of appetite, and fatigue. This point also treats Dampness regardless of whether it is Cold or Heat, especially in the Lower Burner, and thus can treat mucus in the stools. It is particularly helpful in assisting the free flow of Liver Qi when Liver Qi has been stagnating in the Lower Burner, producing Dampness, abdominal pain, distention, and flatulence. In removing obstructions of Qi from the Liver Channel, it also helps to calm negative emotions.

Comment: This point is the Intersecting point of the three Yin channels of the leg.

13. Sp4

Location: Approximately 1 tsun proximal to Sp3, in the depression distal and inferior to the base of the first metatarsal bone at the border of the red and white skin. This point may be pressed bilaterally.

Standing at the foot of the table, grasp the dorsum of the patient's foot with your hand so that the thumbs naturally fall below the arch of the foot. Pressure is with the thumb toward the metatarsal bone.

Action: Sp4 tonifies the Stomach and Spleen. It is used to treat Excess patterns of the Stomach, such as food retention and Dampness in the epigastrium. It also treats epigastric and abdominal pain.

Comment: This is the Luo point (Connecting point) for the Spleen, and is also a Confluent point of the Penetrating Vessel.

14. Sp3

Location: At the medial aspect of the foot, proximal and inferior to the head of the first metatarsal bone, at the junction of the red and white skin.

Stand at the foot of the table. Grasp the patient's foot with your hand so that your thumb rests in the depression proximal to the head of the first metatarsal bone. Pressure is with the pad of the thumb directly into the depression by the bone.

Action: Sp3 tonifies, regulates, and strengthens the Spleen; it also regulates the Stomach and the Colon. This point relieves digestive stagnation; eliminates and transforms Dampness in the Middle and Lower Jiao; treats diarrhea, hemorrhoids, and fistulas; and treats borborygmi, undigested food, and abdominal distention.

Comment: This is the Organ point of the Spleen. It is the Stream and Earth point of the Spleen Channel.

15. St44

Location: Proximal to the margin of the web between the second and third toes, in the depression distal and lateral to the second metatarsophalangeal joint.

Pressure is with the thumb toward the second metatarsophalangeal joint.

Action: St44 regulates Stomach Qi, stops pain, and clears Stomach Heat and Fire. This point is used mostly for Excess conditions; it promotes digestion and is especially good for fullness due to retention of food.

Comment: This is the Spring and Water point of the Stomach Channel.

16. Ki7

Location: 2 tsun above Ki3, on the anterior border of the Achilles tendon. The point Ki3 is located in the depression between the medial malleolus and the Achilles tendon, level with the vertex of the medial malleolus.

Pressure is directed with the thumbs or third finger toward the Achilles tendon. This area may be generally manipulated using circular digital pressure.

Action: This point tonifies Kidney Yang, helps to disinhibit Damp in the Lower Burner, and treats diarrhea and borborygmus.

Comment: This is the River and Metal point of the Kidney Channel.

17. Liv3

Location: In the depression distal to the junction of the first and second metatarsal bones.

Pressure is applied with the pads of the thumbs and directed toward the first metatarsal.

Action: Liv3 sedates Liver Yang, calms

the Shen, and promotes the smooth flow of Liver Qi.

Comment: This is the Organ point for the Liver. It is also the Stream and Earth point of the Liver Channel.

18. Liv2

Location: Between the first and second toe, 0.5 tsun proximal to the margin of the web.

Grasp the patient's toe with your hand and press into the lateral joint space with your thumb. Angle your thumb to fit into the joint space. As this point may be more tender than others, it should be pressed gently at first and then with increasing pressure. Hold for 15–30 seconds and then slowly release, circling as you lighten your pressure.

Action: Liv2 drains Liver Fire, clears Heat, calms the Shen, transforms Damp Heat in the Lower Burner, and treats diarrhea due to Damp Heat.

Comment: This is the Spring and Fire point of the Liver Channel.

19. TS-B1

Location: Halfway between the inferior angle of the scapula and the spine.

Pressure is bilateral using the pads of the thumbs or third fingers and is directed down and angled to the opposite shoulder.

Action: This point harmonizes the Colon and treats chronic diarrhea.

Comment: This point is also useful in the treatment of cough, asthma, and bronchitis due to allergies and colds. In these cases the pressure is directed straight down toward the table.

20. TS-B2

Location: 0.5 tsun lateral to TS-B1.

Pressure is bilateral using the pads of the thumbs or third fingers, and is directed down and angled to the opposite shoulder.

Action: This point harmonizes the Colon and treats chronic diarrhea.

Comment: TS-B2 is also useful in the treatment of cough, asthma, and bronchitis due to allergies and colds. In these cases the pressure is directed straight down toward the table.

21. Bl18

Location: 1.5 tsun lateral to the lower border of the spinous process of the ninth thoracic vertebra.

Pressure is applied bilaterally with the thumbs, straight down toward the table.

Action: Bl18 regulates and tonifies the Liver and treats Stagnant Liver Qi or Damp Heat in the Liver and Gall Bladder. This point is used to treat Stagnant Liver Qi in the epigastrium and hypochondrium and abdominal pain. It subdues Liver Yang.

Comment: This is the Yu point (Associated point) for the Liver.

22. Bl20

Location: 1.5 tsun lateral to the lower border of the spinous process of the eleventh thoracic vertebra.

Pressure is applied bilaterally with the thumbs, straight down toward the table.

Action: Bl20 is a major point for tonifying the Stomach and Spleen and regulating the Middle Jiao. It helps the Spleen's transporting and transforming functions and reduces digestive stagnation. Bl20 treats all Spleen Qi Deficiency patterns with symptoms of abdominal distention, lack of appetite, fatigue, and loose stools.

It treats indigestion, gastritis, ulcers, borborygmus, acute or chronic diarrhea, constipation, and stool with undigested food. It also stimulates the ascending of Spleen Qi.

Comment: This is the Yu point (Associated point) for the Spleen.

23. Bl21

Location: 1.5 tsun lateral to the lower border of the spinous process of the twelfth thoracic vertebra.

Pressure is applied bilaterally with the thumbs, straight down toward the table.

Action: Bl21 is a major point for tonifying both Stomach Qi and Spleen Qi. It stimulates the descending of Stomach Qi and therefore treats Rebellious Stomach Qi symptoms of belching, regurgitation, vomiting, and nausea. It also treats indigestion, borborygmus, abdominal distention, and flatulence. Bl21 relieves stagnation of food in the stomach and promotes the Spleen function of transforming and transporting Qi, Blood, and Fluids.

Comment: This is the Yu point (Associated point) for the Stomach.

24. Bl22

Location: 1.5 tsun lateral to the lower border of the spinous process of the first lumbar vertebra.

Pressure is applied bilaterally with the thumbs, straight down toward the table.

Action: Bl22 helps to transform and transport Fluids in the Lower Burner; it also helps to transform Dampness and disperse stagnation. This point treats diarrhea, borborygmi, undigested food, and rectal prolapse.

Comment: This is the Yu point (Associated point) for the San Jiao.

25. Bl23

Location: 1.5 tsun lateral to the lower border of the spinous process of the second lumbar vertebra.

This point may be manipulated bilaterally with the thumbs. Press directly toward the table and, while maintaining the pressure downward, pull the muscle slightly upward.

Action: Bl23 tonifies the Kidney, resolves Dampness in the Lower Burner, and treats diarrhea with undigested food and Cold diarrhea (diarrhea that comes directly after eating).

Comment: This is the Yu point (Associated point) for the Kidney.

26. Bl25

Location: 1.5 tsun lateral to the lower border of the spinous process of the fourth lumbar vertebra.

Pressure is applied bilaterally with the thumbs, straight down toward the table.

Action: Bl25 benefits the Colon functions; resolves Damp Heat in the Colon; and treats constipation or diarrhea, prolapse of the rectum, and hemorrhoids.

Comment: This is the Yu point (Associated point) for the Colon.

27. Bl57

Location: Inferior to the belly of the gastrocnemius muscle on the line connecting Bl40 and the calcaneal tendon, approximately 8 tsun below Bl40. Pressure is straight down with the thumb or the third finger.

This point can be very sensitive, so

carefully palpate the calf muscles first. If they are very tight, gently manipulate the area with circular digital pressure and do not press the point.

Action: Bl57 helps to harmonize and regulate the Colon and transform Damp Heat. It treats prolapse of the anus, diarrhea, abdominal pain, and hemorrhoids.

28. Bl67

Location: On the lateral side of the small toe, approximately 0.1 tsun proximal to the corner of the nail.

Using the corner of the knuckle of the index finger, manipulate the point.

Action: Bl67 helps to relieve diarrhea in women due to ovulation and premenstrual symptoms. It also relaxes the groin. This point is helpful in the treatment of chronic conditions when used over the long term.

Comment: This is the Well and Metal point of the Bladder Channel.

TREATMENT FOR HEADACHES

AMMA THERAPY ETIOLOGY

Headache, or cephalalgia in medical terms, is one of the most common patient complaints. Millions of dollars are spent yearly on aspirins and other analgesic remedies for headache. While a headache can be a symptom of a more serious disease, few headaches characterize grave problems.

A headache can range in severity from mild to agonizing. It can be specific to a particular area of the head or it can be generalized. It can be infrequent, recurrent, radiating, throbbing, or penetrating. From the Western medical viewpoint, two of the more common categories of headaches are tension headaches and vascular headaches. The category of tension headache includes the common headache from stress or mental overwork, headaches from temporomandibular joint dysfunction, and headaches characterized by atypical facial pain. The category of vascular headache includes migraines, cluster headaches, exertional headaches, hypertensive headaches, and toxic headaches. All headaches can further be categorized as acute or chronic. These categories are by no means all-inclusive and, with sinus headaches, are the most common types seen in the clinical setting.

Tension headaches are also called muscle-contraction headaches. They are the most common form of headache, and result from sustained muscle spasms of the cervical, frontal, temporalis, and masseter muscles. Tension headaches usually begin bilaterally at the occiput, frontal, or temporal areas, with steady pain often more pronounced at the posterior neck and occipital regions. The pain may move, becoming generalized over the top of the head or at the temporal areas. It may also be experienced in the orbit of the eyes or confined to one side of the head, although unilateral pain is more commonly seen in migraine headaches. The pain arises with a steady pressing or throbbing ache that can be quite severe, sometimes almost unbearable, but is more often sustained, persistent, and dull. These headaches can be acute or chronic, and are described as the feeling of having one's head in a vise or feeling a tight band squeezing the head. Tension headaches often occur daily, and are unique because the pain may be consistently present for days, weeks, or months.

Tension headaches are more common among people who are chronically tense and anxious; those who suffer from cervical misalignment, poor posture, or postural defects; and those whose occupations require a posture with sustained contractions of the cervical, frontal, or temporal muscles. They can result from muscle and eye strain after long periods of driving or reading, bookkeeping, studying, or computer work. The improper lifting of heavy weight can cause severe headaches and neck pain when it results in pulling or tearing of the cervical muscles and ligaments. Headaches due to muscle spasms and misalignments of the spine may also result from a trauma, such as whiplash or a head injury. Such headaches are called posttraumatic headaches and, when not treated appropriately, can leave the patient with dull, generalized pains in the head that come and go, sometimes lasting for years. The initial head pains that follow the injury can evolve into chronic headaches due to the prolonged and habitual muscle spasms and contractions.

Tension headaches may be accompanied by some dizziness, tinnitus, or blurry vision. Sometimes nausea or vomiting may occur, but this is more common in the migraine type of headache. Some of the symptoms of tension headaches are similar to the symptoms of migraine headaches; many patients are afflicted with both occurring at the same time or with tension headaches occurring in between migraine attacks.

Temporomandibular joint syndrome is closely related to muscle-contraction headaches. The pain involves the masseter and temporalis muscles, which may be tender and in spasm and can involve associated muscles of the neck. The patient complains of either unilateral or bilateral pain at the jaw and temporal regions, often radiating into the ear. Associated symptoms include limited ability to completely open the mouth, bruxism, and malocclusion. The simple act of chewing food can aggravate this condition. Dental assistance in the form of a biteplate or mouthpiece during sleep to prevent bruxism can sometimes help.

Atypical facial pain or atypical facial neuralgia is a syndrome characterized by consistent, aching, unilateral facial pain, usually at the lower orbit of the eyes, the maxillary area, or the jaw. The pain begins without provocation and may involve the neck and head, sometimes lasting for hours or days. This condition commonly affects middle-aged women. Patients often manifest accompanying symptoms of anxiety and chronic depression. Western physicians are not in agreement as to whether such headaches should be categorized as migraine or tension headaches. Extensive medical testing rarely finds any pathology and medications are usually not helpful.

A contraceptive headache can mimic a tension headache, and must not be overlooked if the patient is on birth control pills. Such headaches feel as if the head were circumvented with a tight band. They may also evolve into a migraine headache, and can range in severity from rather mild to extreme. There may be additional symptoms of depression, and the patient may be ill-tempered. Such patients should be advised to consult their physicians about these side-effects, and they should consider stopping the contraceptive to avoid more severe symptoms in the future. Many women are also prone to headaches during menstruation and menopause.

The term *vascular headache* is applied to a group of syndromes, etiology unknown, in which pain results from the dilation of one or more branches of the carotid artery which in turn stimulates the nerve endings that innervate that artery. The most common form of vascular headache is the migraine headache, a type of headache that affects women more than men. There is a strong inheritance factor with migraines—65 percent of all people who suffer with migraines have a family history of migraines. Some patients first begin to suffer with migraines during their teens. While many personality studies have been conducted to determine whether a particular type of individual is prone to migraines, it has not been conclusively decided that any one type has a propensity toward this type of headache. Migraine headaches are frequently unilateral.

There is no conclusive research as to the cause of migraine headaches. Some studies support the view that these headaches are vascular in origin and involve the intracranial and extracranial arteries of the head. Some studies have shown that there is vasoconstriction and a decreased flow of blood during the prodromal or aural phase, followed by the headache phase, which is characterized by vasodilation and increased blood flow. Still other studies point to a neuronal imbalance, which results in spasms of the blood vessels that lead to headaches.

Migraines are generally classified into two types: the common migraine and the classic migraine. The common migraine occurs most frequently. Its prodrome phase is not clearly defined; it may arise as gastrointestinal problems and visual disturbances that occur from several hours to several days before the actual onset of the headache. The classic migraine actually only occurs in 10 percent of all migraines. It has a clearly defined prodrome which begins ten to thirty minutes before the onset of the headache. The symptoms are paroxysmal attacks of pain, visual field problems, paresthesia, weakness, dizziness, sweating, vomiting, confusion, paralysis in some cases, and even loss of consciousness. The classic prodrome symptom is seeing zig-zags of light in one quadrant of the visual field, a symptom called scintillating scotomata. This type of migraine can last from one hour to several hours.

Symptoms common to both types of migraines are irritability, nausea, vomiting, pale complexion, sweating, and generalized edema. People with migraines usually seek to rest during the acute phase of the attack in a quiet and darkened room, away from noise and lights.

They may feel exhausted and generally weak for several hours or days following the headache. The frequency of attacks can vary from several times a week to a couple of times a year.

Cluster headaches are sometimes associated with migraines because they are believed to have a vascular cause; however, their etiology also remains unknown. They occur less often than migraines and are more common in men between the ages of thirty and sixty years of age. The onset is acute without a prodrome, occurring with intense, throbbing pain behind the nostril and one eye, causing lacrimation of the eye and nasal congestion on the side of the pain. The pupil of the eye may become constricted and the eyelid may droop (ptosis) on the affected side. The headache peaks in five minutes and usually does not last more than two hours. It can occur after awakening from a nap or a night's sleep or can sometimes awaken the person during the night. It can occur several times during a night over a period of weeks and then not recur for months. A person suffering from cluster headaches does not experience the symptoms of nausea, vomiting, or visual disturbances, as does the migraine sufferer.

Other types of vascular headaches include exertional headaches that occur during exercise; hypertensive headaches that occur in patients with severe hypertension, characterized by early morning occipital headaches; and toxic headaches. Toxic headaches can result from exposure to a toxic environment or breathing noxious fumes, such as household cleaners, turpentine, gasoline, paints and dyes, formaldehyde, pesticides, stale air, or second-hand smoke, in a place without adequate ventilation. Toxic headaches can also be triggered by ingesting chemicals, such as alcohol (brandy, bourbon, red wine); coloring and flavoring agents (tartrazine); and food additives such as nitrites, sulfites, and monosodium glutamate (MSG).

There are also some kinds of common headaches that fall outside the categories of tension and vascular headaches. These are often short-term headaches that accompany the common cold, flu, or infections of the ears, eyes, and throat. Acute headaches can also result from a high fever. The common sinus headache is due to an inflammation of the sinuses resulting from repeated colds, influenza virus, allergies, and the overuse of antibiotics. It can be discriminated from other types of headaches by the localization of pain in any of the maxillary, frontal, and ethmoidal sinuses, with the additional symptoms of nasal congestion, post-nasal drip, and sometimes purulent discharge from the nose.

Most people self-medicate for headaches with over-the-counter analgesics, such as aspirin or acetaminophen. When these fail to relieve the symptoms, a physician will generally prescribe muscle relaxants, tranquilizers, or codeine. Many of these drugs have potentially dangerous side-effects. Long-term use of aspirin can cause gastric bleeding; long-term use of analgesic combinations such as Fiorinal can be addictive, since it contains a barbiturate. Drugs containing acetaminophen, such as Tylenol, are toxic to the liver with chronic use. Narcotics and antidepressants can be addictive.

Drug treatment for migraines uses ergotamine tartrate, a powerful vasoconstrictor that aims to prevent the painful dilation of the cranial blood vessels. However, long-term use of this drug can produce side-effects, and also may make the headaches more frequent, since vaso-constriction is always followed by vasodilation, which can trigger another headache. Other drugs used for migraine treatment are propranolol, serotonin antagonists, calcium channel blockers and antidepressants, clonidine, thiazides, and other antihypertensive drugs, all of which have known side-effects. Treatment of cluster headaches is more difficult, but again ergotamine tartrate and serotonin antagonists are sometimes used, as well as lithium and steroids such as prednisone.

In looking at headaches from the homeodynamic perspective we see that emotions are a major component of the disease process. Anger is most often a cause of headaches, since anger generates Heat and Heat naturally rises. Headaches due to Ascendant Liver Yang or Liver Fire frequently manifest in the Gall Bladder Channel in the temple area of the head. Like the Liver, the Gall Bladder is affected by these negative emotions. The obstruction of the free flow of Liver Qi due to negative emotions also affects the sinews, causing weakness and contraction of the tendons, ligaments, and muscles of the head, neck, and shoulders. The person whose Yang energy of the Liver is rising is very prone to headaches and outbursts of irritability and anger. Additional symptoms can be dizziness, tinnitus, and insomnia. Headaches that move from the neck and shoot painfully into the eyes are usually due to Excess Fire in the Gall Bladder Channel. Headaches that center primarily in the eyes are considered to be more of a

migraine type of headache that is due to Liver Fire. Headaches can also result from Liver Qi Stagnation when the Liver energy invades the Middle Burner and obstructs the descending energy of the Stomach, causing food to be retained in the stomach. These types of headaches are also due to emotions, and usually occur on the forehead or at the temple area. They are accompanied by hypochondriac pain, digestive problems, abdominal bloating, and belching.

Worry can also catalyze a headache by affecting Heart and Lung Qi. Energy from the Upper Burner should meet the rising Liver energy and helps the Liver Qi to spread out in the hypochondrium. When Lung and Heart Qi are weak, Liver energy will continue to rise to the head, thus precipitating headaches. Headaches due to worry often occur on the forehead or the very top of the head and have a dull quality to them.

Fear is another emotion that can cause headaches, either through depletion of Kidney Qi, which will affect the entire head, or through promoting the rising of Liver energy due to Kidney Deficiency.

Another cause of headaches is stress and overwork. Overwork may be due to too much mental strain resulting from sedentary occupations where too much time is spent in long hours of concentration. Coupled with worry about job performance or grades in school, this can lead to frequent headaches and even migraines. Children who obsess about grades or who are pushed by their parents to excel may begin to get these headaches in childhood.

Any profession where the person works long hours without sufficient rest will weaken the Spleen and the Kidney. Kidney Yin Deficiency can cause a headache throughout the entire head, or lead to Liver Yang or Liver Fire Rising, which can cause blockages in the Gall Bladder Channel on one side of the head, the equivalent of a migraine headache.

Of course, diet plays a major role in the development of headaches. Malnutrition, which is often caused by various forms of dieting, as well as certain forms of vegetarianism, can cause Blood and Qi Deficiencies resulting in headaches at the top of the head. Conversely, people who overeat and stuff themselves can cause Stomach Qi dysfunctions resulting in headaches on the forehead. Ingesting too many hot and warm energy foods, such as spicy foods and alcohol, will produce Internal Heat, affecting the Liver and Stomach. Liver Fire will produce temporal headaches, while Stomach Fire will produce frontal headaches. Other factors that can negatively influence the Stomach are irregular eating patterns, eating foods without any nutritional value, eating late at night, and eating under stress. All of these can cause Stomach Yin Deficiency and result in frontal headaches that are sharply painful.

Depletion of Kidney Essence is another cause of headaches. In men, depletion of Kidney Essence can be due to excess sexual activity, where there is a loss of Jing and insufficient time in between activity to restore the Essence with rest and nutrition. For women, the activity of giving birth successively in a short period of time can weaken the Uterus, the Liver, and the Kidney Essence, as the body does not have sufficient time to replenish itself between

births. Frequent miscarriages can produce this same effect.

A diet that includes an excessive intake of salt can result in a Kidney Deficiency, causing a dull pain throughout the entire head or the occiput. Too many sour foods, such as vinegar, grapefruits, and pickles, will also affect the Liver. Too many hot and spicy foods, alcohol, fried foods, or simply overeating can create Stomach Heat, which can cause intense frontal headaches, accompanied by a desire for cold drinks, constipation, a slippery pulse, and a tongue with a thick yellow coating.

Finally, when looking at diet we must take into account the high level of chemicals present in the food, such as MSG, food colorings and additives, aspartamine, sulfites, and preservatives, many of which can cause headaches. Certain foods, such as chocolate and caffeine, are known to trigger migraine headaches in some people. In particular, sweets can artificially induce emotional highs and lows that foster stress. As always, the therapist must conduct a thorough examination of the patient's dietary regimen.

Our constitutional inheritance can play a formidable role in the propensity toward headaches. When headaches begin to occur and recur in childhood, a weak constitution can be suspected. The parents' health at the time of conception, their age, the circumstances under which conception takes place, and factors such as diet and stress are all significant, as is the health of the mother during pregnancy and any medications or abusive substances she may have taken during that period of time. Emotional upsets during pregnancy can result in Heart weakness; the use of drugs or alcohol can affect the Liver, Kidney, or

Heart; if the mother smokes during pregnancy, the Lung can be affected. All of these can weaken the child's constitution and increase the chance of headaches and other dysfunctions.

Trauma can also cause headaches through Blood Stasis, and the effects of an accident or fall may not be felt for years. Sometimes falls in childhood, where there is injury to the head or to the coccyx, can result in chronic headaches years later. Upon questioning and prodding, patients will often recall concussions or injuries as children, or they will recall accidents that occurred many years earlier to the exact site of the pain of their current headache. When the pain always occurs in exactly the same spot, Blood Stasis from an earlier trauma should be suspected.

Blood Stasis can also result from prolonged Liver Qi Stagnation and is often seen in chronic headaches. These headaches, resulting from Blood Deficiencies, are usually very painful and are more common in elderly people and women. Blood Deficiency in the elderly is due to Kidney Essence decline; Blood Deficiency in women is due to menses. When Blood Stasis is present the tongue will have a purplish hue and the pulse will be wiry, hesitant, or choppy.

From the perspective of the Amma therapist, headaches that begin at the occipital area are not necessarily due to muscle spasms or tension, but can also be due an invasion by exogenous influences, particularly Wind Cold or Wind Heat. When these pathogens enter the body, the onset of symptoms is rapid. The entryway is generally through the back of the neck, since this is where the Yang Channels, the more superficial channels, converge. The circulation of Wei Qi is obstructed and this causes the pain and stiffness at the occipital area.

Occipital pain and stiffness are often the very first sign of the onset of an exterior condition, such as a cold or flu. Treated early, these conditions can be alleviated very quickly. Once patients are taught to recognize the symptoms of an attack by exogenous influences, they become very skilled at seeking treatment early and taking the proper herbal remedies. In these cases the illness never goes beyond minor discomfort that is easily resolved in a day or two.

Exogenous Dampness can indirectly affect the head through an invasion of the Lower and Middle Burners, and can block the rising of Yang energy to the head, resulting in headaches. All of the Yang channels either begin or end in the head. With the exception of the Liver and Heart channels, both of which have internal pathways that reach the head, the rest of the Yin channels only reach the head through linking up with their Yang partners' divergent pathways. Consequently, the blocking of Yang energy by Dampness to the head can be a cause of headaches. Symptoms include a feeling of heaviness in the head and problems with concentration and thinking. Such headaches are worse in rainy or damp weather and are accompanied by other signs of exogenous invasion.

Internal Dampness can also be a cause of headaches. The head feels heavy and blocked up. In such cases there will be additional signs of Dampness or Phlegm, such as a slippery pulse, a phlegmy cough, or feeling full in the hypochondriac region or epigastrium. Internal Dampness is due to failure of the Spleen to transform and transport Qi,

Blood, and Fluids, or can result from an exogenous invasion of Damp that was not treated properly and that has remained in the system for a prolonged period of time.

Since all the channels' energies connect to the head in one fashion or another, energy blockages in any of the primary channels can result in a headache. These blockages also disrupt the functional orb of the pertaining organ, and that can result in headaches. For example, blockages of Qi in the descending and dispersing function of the Lungs can cause stagnation of Qi in the sinus and face, giving rise to a sinus headache or headache due to cold or flu; Rebellious Qi of the Stomach can produce a headache as well as dizziness, nausea, and vomiting; obstructions in the Colon Channel can result in chronic constipation, leading to a toxic accumulation in the body that can result in a headache; obstructions in the Bladder Channel can produce headaches in the eyes; obstructions and stagnation of Spleen energy can produce chest pains and neck pains; Heat from the Small Intestine or San Jiao can rise and stagnate at GV14, causing a headache.

From an Amma perspective, the subject of headaches is quite complex. Its proper treatment depends on the ability of the therapist to correctly assess the problem and treat accordingly.

AMMA THERAPY TREATMENT

The first order of business of the Amma therapist is to alleviate the acute and urgent pain of the headache. Attention can then be directed to the appropriate Organs and channels in cases where the headache condition is chronic. Clearly, if the root of the dysfunction is not addressed, the problem will be sure to return. The therapist must determine what type of headache the patient has.

After reviewing the medical records and utilizing pulse and tongue diagnosis, the therapist must inquire as to exactly where the pain is located, what is the intensity of the pain, how long the patient has had the pain, what were the specific circumstances as to the onset of the headache, if this is a chronic condition, and how often there are exacerbations. The therapist is also interested in the quality of the pain—is it throbbing, dull, stabbing, hot? Are there associated symptoms, such as nausea, dizziness, impaired vision, or occipital pain and stiffness? The therapist will want to question whether there is a certain time of the day, week, or month that the headache begins, or worsens, in the case of chronic headaches. After eliciting this information, the therapist begins palpatory assessment.

While Western medicine considers headaches to be difficult to treat, assessing tension and muscle spasms is an easy process for the Amma therapist. The therapist must check the cervical region for muscular spasms and vertebral misalignment. Basic palpation of the muscles of the neck, head, and upper back, as well as the temporal and masseter muscles, will reveal spasms and significantly tight, sensitive, and painful areas that can then be treated through manipulation of the musculature and the use of appropriate points. The therapist must also consider where the pain is localized and which channels move through that area. Muscular spasms and subluxations can obstruct the movement of Qi in the channels that pass through those areas. On the other hand, headaches are frequently caused by obstructions of Qi and Blood along a particular energetic pathway that may subsequently result in muscle contractions. Manipulation of the points locally and distally on that pathway can free obstructed energy. Areas that may be considered as sources of pain if the pain does not follow a channel's pathway are the neck and shoulder area, ear, temporomandibular joint, eye, nose, and mouth (dental) areas.

Therapists should also note that headaches can manifest in different areas of the head at different times due to the fact that many patients suffer from more than one pattern or syndrome at the same time. Headaches due to deficiency include Qi and Blood Deficiency, Liver Blood Deficiency, and Kidney Deficiency. Excess conditions include Stomach Heat, Blood Stasis, Phlegm, Liver Yang Rising, Liver Fire Rising, or Liver Wind. Many patients will have already taken medications to no avail. In those cases the therapist must consider the possible iatrogenic effects of the medications on the bioenergy system.

Many patients respond very well to Amma therapy and can successfully be taught self-massage techniques and the use of teh tah chu. Often adjunctive therapies such as biofeedback, chiropractic, and acupuncture are helpful. Any patient whose headaches do not improve but instead get progressively worse, becoming more frequent and constant, should be referred to a physician. This problem can be a sign of a serious condition, such as a brain tumor or other brain lesions. Since the stress level of modern America is fairly high, it can often be assumed that stress is either causing or contributing to a headache. The therapist must address the emotional component of the illness on some level, as well as treat the acute distress, if more permanent relief is to be provided and the headache is to be prevented from recurring. Psychological counseling may be recommended.

The following treatment contains numerous points for the alleviation of various types of headaches. It is the responsibility of the therapist to properly assess the patient and to extrapolate those points that would best treat the headache pattern.

AMMA THERAPY ASSESSMENT

1. Ask the patient where the pain is located. Is the pain localized behind one eye? Pain behind one eye is a sign of migraines.
   + If it is a dull pain, it is resultant from a Liver Blood Deficiency.
   + If it is a sharp pain, it is resultant from Liver Yang Rising.
2. Does the patient have a headache on the sides of the head? Check the temple area and the sides of the head to see if there are any distended veins. This indicates Qi and Blood Stagnation. Headaches on the sides of the head, or one side only, correspond to the Gall Bladder Channel, and pain in this area is due to Liver Yang or Liver Fire invading the Gall Bladder Channel.

3. Does the patient have a headache at the vertex of the head?
   + Headaches at the vertex of the head are often due to Liver Blood Deficiency, with insufficient Blood reaching the top of the head. A deep branch of the Liver Channel moves up the forehead to join the Governing Vessel at the vertex. The patient will feel better if he lies down and the headache is dull in nature.
   + In some cases a headache at the vertex may be very sharp and painful, in which case it is due to Liver Yang Rising.

4. Does the patient have a frontal headache?
   + Sharp pain in the forehead is usually due to Stomach Heat.
   + Dull pain in the forehead is usually due to Stomach Deficiency.
   + Frontal headaches can also be due to Phlegm or Dampness in the head, in which case the patient will complain of being unable to think clearly and of feeling foggy or blocked in his head. He may also complain of dizziness and blurred vision.
   + Frontal headaches may also be experienced when patients suffer from a frontal sinus condition.

5. Does the patient have a headache stemming from the occipital region?
   + Acute headaches at the occiput are usually due to exogenous invasions of Wind Cold or Wind Heat, in which case other signs and symptoms will be present as indicated in the treatment for colds.

+ Bladder patterns, such as a Bladder infection, can cause obstruction in the energy of the channel. In this case the pain can be acute.
+ Chronic occipital headaches or headaches that radiate from the occiput over the top of the head are usually due to Kidney Deficiency affecting the flow of energy in the Bladder Channel.

6. Does the patient complain of the entire head hurting? When the whole head is affected, it is important to ascertain whether the pain is dull or acute. Acute headaches are usually due to exogenous invasions, which are always Excess conditions. Headaches due to Excess conditions are more painful than those due to Deficiency conditions.
   + Sharp pain is indicative of an Excess condition.
   + Dull headaches usually are due to a Deficiency of Kidney Essence.

7. Is the onset of the headache acute or gradual?
   + An acute onset usually means there as been an exogenous invasion.
   + A gradual onset means it is an interior condition.

8. What is the character of the patient's pain?
   + A fixed, stabbing pain that occurs in chronic headaches is due to Blood Stasis.
   + A throbbing or pulsating pain, or a pounding headache that is felt on the sides of the head or temples along the Gall Bladder Channel or behind the eyes and

where the patient is also experiencing nausea or vomiting and/or visual problems, such as flashing lights or auras (symptoms we associate with a migraine headache), are due to Liver Yang Rising.

+ Liver Fire Rising would have these same signs, and also include Heat signs, such as constipation, scanty dark urine, thirst, and a red tongue with a yellow coating. Liver Fire is an Excess condition, while Liver Yang is due to both Excess and Deficiency patterns. The tongue may therefore be pale in Liver Yang syndromes.

+ A feeling of heaviness in the head accompanied by complaints of difficulty in concentrating or focusing indicates either Dampness or Phlegm. Other symptoms like dizziness and blurry vision will often also be present.

9. Does the patient suffer with a stiff neck?

+ Acute stiff neck alleviated by warmth indicates exogenous invasion of Wind Cold.

+ Chronic stiff neck with headache usually reflects Liver Yang Rising.

10. Does the headache worsen when the patient is emotional? A headache that worsens when the patient is angry or emotional is generally due to Ascendant Liver Yang or Liver Fire Rising.

11. Is the headache related to the patient's menses?

+ Headaches that occur before the onset of the menses are generally due to Ascendant Liver Yang.

+ A headache that gets worse during the menses could be the result of Blood Stasis, Liver Qi Stagnation, or Liver Fire Rising.

+ A headache that occurs at the end of the period is due to Blood Deficiency.

12. Is the headache related to eating?

+ A headache that improves with eating indicates a Blood or Qi Deficiency.

+ A headache that worsens from eating sour foods, such as vinegar or grapefruit, is caused by Ascendant Liver Yang.

+ A headache that worsens after eating or from overeating may indicate that food is being retained in the stomach, in which case the patient will also suffer from nausea, belching, and sour regurgitation, Stomach Yin Deficiency, Heat or Fire in the Stomach, or Dampness or Phlegm in the Middle Burner.

13. Does the patient feel better when lying down?

+ It is a sign of Deficiency if the patient feels better when lying down.

+ It is a sign of Excess if the patient feels worse when lying down and better when sitting up.

14. Does the headache improve with exercise?

+ In general, a headache that improves with exercise is a sign of Ascendant Liver Yang or Phlegm.

+ A headache that worsens with exercise and feels better with relaxation and rest is due to Blood or Qi Deficiency.

15. Does the nature of the headache change with the weather?

+ Headaches that worsen in hot weather can be due to Ascendant Liver Yang or Liver Fire Rising.

+ A headache that worsens in cold weather may indicate a Yang Deficiency.

+ A headache that worsens in rainy weather indicates that Dampness is the cause.

16. Does the nature of the headache change with the time of day?

+ Chronic headaches that worsen at night can point to a Blood or Yin Deficiency.

+ Headaches that are more painful during the day can indicate Yang Deficiency, Dampness, or Qi Deficiency.

17. Palpate the head for tenderness, temperature, bumps, swellings, masses or scar tissue.

+ As in all assessments, if pressure to the affected area relieves pain and discomfort, the condition is a Deficiency condition.

+ If pressure causes more pain and discomfort, it is a sign of an Excess condition.

18. Assess the neck as presented in the treatment for stiff neck with shoulder pain to determine whether muscle spasms and/or misalignment are causing or influencing the headaches.

19. Check to see if the legs are the same length. Poor posture or postural defects can contribute to headaches. When one leg is longer due to spasms of the gluteal muscles, the ensuing pelvic tilt can put a strain on the spinal column, resulting in a subluxation of the cervical spine which can produce a headache.

Have the patient lie supine, with his legs straight. The ankles should be aligned so that they are touching. The two ankles should be observed relative to each other. Differences in leg length will be visible if the ankles are not proportionally aligned. Gluteal spasms always occur on the side of the longer leg. More attention must be paid to the gluteal region during treatment, if this is the case, and chiropractic care may be necessary as well.

ADDITIONAL TECHNIQUES

1. If the patient complains of a temporal headache or a headache on the sides of the head and you palpate a slight swelling over the area, a good beginning technique is to cup the palms over both sides of the head and gently hold the area for approximately one minute. While doing this technique the therapist should concentrate on drawing the negative energy out of the temples into his palms, and shaking out his hands afterward to expel the energy.

2. If the patient complains of a frontal headache, use firm thumb stroking over the forehead to disperse the Qi.

3. If the patient complains of a sinus headache, use thumb stroking over the maxilla in conjunction with the appropriate sinus points.

4. If the patient complains of an occipital headache, use the additional techniques from the treatment for stiff neck with shoulder pain, such as traction to the back of the neck using GB12 and GB20.

5. If the therapist feels tightness in the temple area, particularly the area adjacent with the outer canthus of the eye, ask the patient when he last had his eyes examined and if he has been noticing any eyestrain or any other problems with his eyes, such as allergies. Use circular digital pressure to the area in very small increments and end by pressing TS-H4 for the eyes. A cold washcloth can be applied to alleviate swelling in the temple area.

6. If the headache is isolated to the top of the head, manipulate from GV23 back past GV20 using circular digital pressure in very small increments. This movement stimulates two extra points, the first 1 tsun anterior to GV20, the second 1 tsun posterior to GV20.

7. If the headache is at the top of the head but rises up from the occiput, focus your attention on releasing the tension in the neck muscles.

8. In the case of migraine headaches, if the patient comes in for treatment while in an acute situation, vigorous treatment to the head and neck must be avoided, as this will exacerbate the patient's pain. Minimal manipulation of these areas should be used, and the focus of the treatment should be on distal areas and points.

9. Using circular digital pressure, manipulate below and lateral to the inion, and follow with circular digital pressure along the occiput.

10. Apply circular digital pressure around the ears, following the pathway of the Gall Bladder Channel. During this treatment the therapist can return to using circular digital pressure to the temples, around the ears, and on the sides of the head.

11. Apply thumb stroking on GV20, laterally to the ears. Alternate thumb stroking on GV20; the direction is posterior toward the occiput. These movements stimulate three extra points, 1 tsun posterior to GV20 and 1 tsun bilateral to GV20.

12. The following pattern may be used by advanced Amma therapists in the treatment of acute headaches. Begin with extra point yu yao in the center of the eyebrow. Press TS-H3, directly above yu yao, with the pad of the third finger. Then press GB14. Continue to move up toward the hairline in 0.5-tsun increments. Next, place the pads of the third fingers on TS-H2 and press. Continue to move up to the hairline in 0.5-tsun increments. Then press GB1 and SJ23. Move from SJ23 in 0.5-tsun increments to St8. End the sequence with extra point yin tang, located midway between the medial ends of the eyebrows.

POINT LOCATION AND ACTION

1. Extra point (yin tang)

Location: Located on the midline between the medial ends of the two eyebrows.

Use the pad of the third finger to press this point. Relax the hand and rest the second and fourth fingers on Bl2.

Action: This point calms the Spirit, dispels Wind, and clears Heat. It treats frontal headaches, sinus headaches, and eye pain.

2. GB1

Location: 0.5 tsun lateral to the outer canthus of the eye, in the depression on the lateral side of the orbit.

Palpate for a slight sulcus at the outer orbit of the eye. Pressure is with the pad of the third finger angled into the sulcus.

Action: GB1 is a local point for eye disorders and headaches, particularly those in which the pain is in, around, or behind the eye. This point opens and brightens the eyes.

Comment: This is an Intersecting point of the Small Intestine, Gall Bladder, and San Jiao channels.

3. Bl2

Location: In the depression proximal to the medial end of the eyebrow, directly above the inner canthus.

In the treatment of headaches, use the pads of the third fingers and hook under the supraorbital ridge. The pressure is straight back toward the head. End by stroking the point several times. This point may be pressed bilaterally.

Action: This is a good local point for the eyes. Since the eyes are the sense organ of the Liver, this point helps to balance the Liver Qi that nourishes the eyes, smoothing the flow of Liver Qi to the area and thus helping to remove obstructed Qi. It treats frontal headaches and pain in, around, and behind the eyes. This point is beneficial for all eye disorders.

4. TS-H2

Location: 0.5 tsun superior to Bl2.

Using the pad of the third finger, press straight down toward the table. This point may be pressed bilaterally.

Action: This local point treats frontal and sinus headaches, and helps to open and brighten the eyes.

5. Extra point (yu yao)

Location: In the middle of the eyebrow, on the supraorbital ridge.

Rest the palm on the patient's forehead, so that the pad of the third finger is on top of the midpoint of the eyebrow and the first half of the pad extends slightly over the supraorbital ridge. Apply pressure into the depression in the bone by bending the first joint of the middle finger. This point may be pressed bilaterally.

Action: This local point treats frontal and sinus headaches, all eye disorders, and opens and brightens the eyes. It is helpful for Liver Yang and Liver Blood Deficiency conditions that affect the eyes.

6. TS-H3

Location: 0.5 tsun superior to yu yao.

Using the pads of the third fingers, press straight down toward the table. This point may be pressed bilaterally.

Action: This local point treats frontal and sinus headaches and helps to open and brighten the eyes.

7. GB14

Location: 1 tsun above the midpoint of the eyebrow, directly above the pupil.

Pressure is with the pad of the index or third finger, directly downward.

Action: GB14 is a local point for frontal headaches and sinus headaches and all eye disorders. It opens and brightens the eyes. This point is also used to treat facial paralysis.

Comment: GB14 is an Intersecting point between the Stomach and Gall Bladder channels.

8. TS-H4

Location: 1 tsun superior to SJ23.

Pressure is with the top of the pad of the third finger directly into the point.

Action: This point treats unilateral headache, treats trigeminal neuralgia and facial paralysis, and dispels Liver Wind.

9. Extra point (tai yang)

Location: In the depression about 1 tsun posterior to the midpoint between the lateral end of the eyebrow and the outer canthus.

Support the patient's head with one hand while exerting pressure with the pad of the third finger of the other hand directly into the depression.

Action: This point brightens the eyes and clears Heat. It also treats headaches due to Wind Heat and Ascendant Liver Yang, Liver Fire, and Liver Wind.

10. GB4

Location: Within the hairline of the temporal area, one-quarter of the distance between St8 and GB7. (GB7 is located anterior and superior to the auricle. A space can be felt when the jaw is moved.)

Support the patient's head with one hand while exerting pressure with the pad of the third finger of the other hand directly into the depression.

Action: GB4 is a local point for migraine

headaches on the sides of the head due to Ascendant Liver Yang, Liver Fire, or Liver Wind.

Comment: This is an Intersecting point of the San Jiao and Stomach channels with the Gall Bladder Channel.

11. GB5

Location: Within the hairline of the temporal area, midway between St8 and GB7.

Support the patient's head with one hand while exerting pressure with the pad of the third finger of the other hand directly into the depression.

Action: GB5 is a local point for migraine headaches on the sides of the head due to Ascendant Liver Yang, Liver Fire, or Liver Wind.

Comment: This is an Intersecting point of the Gall Bladder, Stomach, and San Jiao channels.

12. GB6

Location: Within the hairline of the temporal area, midway between GB5 and GB7.

Support the patient's head with one hand while exerting pressure with the pad of the third finger of the other hand directly into the depression.

Action: GB6 is a local point for migraine headaches on the sides of the head due to Ascendant Liver Yang, Liver Fire, or Liver Wind.

Comment: This is an Intersecting point for the Gall Bladder, San Jiao, and Stomach channels.

13. St8

Location: 0.5 tsun within the anterior hairline at the corner of the forehead, 4.5 tsun lateral to the Governing Vessel.

Pressure is with the pad of the third finger angled toward the Governing Vessel.

Action: St8 dispels Wind and treats frontal headaches, dizziness, vertigo, and blurry vision.

Comment: This is an Intersecting point of the Gall Bladder Channel with the Stomach Channel.

14. St1

Location: Directly inferior to the center of the pupil, on the midpoint of the infraorbital ridge.

Ask the patient to close his eyes. While sitting at the head of the table, take the thumb of one hand and gently pull the skin down away from the infraorbital ridge. Then, using the thumb of the other hand, lean the lateral edge onto the top of the infraorbital ridge and roll the thumb into the depression.

Action: This point treats all eye disorders and headaches related to eyestrain.

Comment: This is an Intersecting point of the Conception Vessel with the Stomach Channel.

15. TS-H5

Location: 1 tsun posterior to St8.

Pressure is with the pad of the third finger angled toward the Governing Vessel.

Action: This point dispels Wind and treats frontal headaches, dizziness, vertigo, and blurry vision.

16. GV 20

Location: On the midline of the head halfway between the frontal hairline and the vertex of the external occipital protuberance, or 7 tsun from the posterior hairline and 5 tsun behind the anterior hairline.

Pressure is with the third finger or the thumb directly toward the feet. Hold the point for 15–30 seconds before slowly circling and releasing.

Action: This point calms the Shen, clears the brain, subdues Liver Yang and Wind, and helps spread Liver Qi. It also treats depression and helps the Yang energies ascend to the head to clear the mind.

Comment: This is the Intersecting point of the Six Yang channels, either directly or through their other branches with the Governing Vessel.

17. GV24

Location: On the midline of the head, 0.5 tsun within the anterior hairline.

Pressure is with the pad of the third finger in an inferior direction.

Action: GV24 calms the Liver and the Spirit. It treats anxiety and is a local point for frontal and vertex headaches.

Comment: GV24 is an Intersecting point of the Bladder and Stomach channels with the Governing Vessel.

18. Bl10

Location: 1.3 tsun lateral to GV15, on the lateral side of the trapezius muscle. (GV15 is located at the nape of the neck, 0.5 tsun above the hairline, on the posterior midline between the spinous processes of the first and second vertebrae).

Pressure is with the pad of the third finger hooking up toward the occiput.

Action: This is a local point for any type of occipital headache, headache pain traveling over the top of the head, and frontal headaches. It is useful for neck pain and injuries. Bl10 helps to open and brighten the eyes.

Comment: This point can also be used as a distal point for lower back pain.

19. GB20

Location: In the depression between the sternocleidomastoid and the trapezius muscles.

This point can also be accessed bilaterally whether the patient is in the supine or prone position, by pressing the third finger up toward the occiput. If the third finger is not strong enough by itself, it may be combined with the second finger, and the two fingers together hook up under the occiput.

Action: This point treats occipital headaches, especially those due to both Interior Wind, such as in Liver Fire Rising conditions, and Exterior Wind, such as Wind Cold or Wind Heat conditions. It relaxes the sinews and treats stiff and painful neck problems; it also treats all eye disorders and headaches that involve the eyes.

Comment: This is an Intersecting point of the San Jiao and Gall Bladder channels.

20. GB21

Location: Midway between GV14 and the acromion, at the highest point of the shoulder.

This point is pressed bilaterally from the supine or prone position, using the thumbs. The force is slightly medial and down toward the feet.

Action: GB21 treats neck and shoulder pain, relaxes the sinews, helps the Liver Qi to move smoothly, and releases tension in the neck and shoulders.

Comment: This is an Intersecting point of the San Jiao and Gall Bladder channels.

21. Lu5

Location: With the elbow slightly bent, this point can be found lateral to the biceps tendon at the cubital crease.

Wrap the patient's elbow with your hand, placing the top of your thumb at the cubital crease next to the lateral side of the biceps tendon, in alignment with the Lung Channel, and press gently with the pad of the thumb straight down toward the table. Hold the point for 15–30 seconds and then gently release, circling as your pressure lightens.

Action: This point clears Heat from the Upper Burner.

Comment: This is the Sea and Water point of the Lung Channel.

22. Lu7

Location: In a slight depression at the origin of the styloid process of the radius, 1.5 tsun above the transverse crease of the wrist.

Grasp the patient's hand and, using your thumb, press into the depression between the tendon and the bone.

Action: This point tonifies the Lung when Lung Qi Deficiency is allowing Liver Yang to ascend to the head. It is also good for expelling exogenous influences from the head.

Comment: This is the Luo point for the Lung and a Confluent point for the Conception Vessel.

23. Ht3

Location: Between the medial end of the transverse cubital crease and the medial epicondyle of the humerus with the elbow bent.

Grasp the elbow with your hand that is closest to the patient's body. Using the pad of your thumb, press laterally directly toward the joint space of the medial epicondyle of the humerus. Hold the point for approximately 15 seconds or longer, depending on the emotional condition of the patient.

Action: Ht3 is a major point for calming the Shen, and therefore the emotions. It helps to clear Heat or Fire from the Heart and regulates the flow of Blood and Qi. Ht3 can also be used locally for elbow pain.

Comment: This is the Sea and Water point of the Heart Channel.

24. HE6 (P6)

Location: On the anterior aspect of the forearm, 2 tsun proximal to the transverse crease of the wrist, between the tendons of the palmaris longus and flexor carpi radialis.

Pressure is activated with the pad of the thumb. When used with SJ5, pronate the forearm while the thumb presses downward into SJ5 and the third finger presses upward, activating HE6.

Action: This point calms the Spirit; regulates Liver Qi and helps it to flow smoothly; treats migraine headaches with nausea, hypochondriac pain, and vomiting; and directs Rebellious Qi downward.

Comment: Luo point of the Heart Envelope Channel.

25. SJ5

Location: 2 tsun proximal to SJ4, between the ulna and the radius. (SJ4 is located with the palm facing downward, at the junction of the ulna and carpal bones in the depression lateral to the tendon of the extensor digitorum muscle).

Pressure is activated with the pad of the thumb.

Action: This point subdues Liver Yang and treats the sides of the head, helping

to remove obstructions from the channels. It treats unilateral, temporal, or occipital headaches, trigeminal neuralgia, and painful obstruction of the neck and shoulders.

Comment: This is the Luo point of the San Jiao Channel. This point may be used simultaneously with HE6.

26. Ht8

Location: On the palmar surface between the fourth and fifth metacarpal bones, proximal to the metacarpophalangeal joint. When a fist is made the point will be found where the tip of the little finger rests.

Pressure is with the pad of the thumb directly into the point.

Action: This point calms the Shen and helps to clear Heat or Fire from the Heart.

Comment: This is the Spring and Fire point of the Heart Channel.

27. Co4

Location: In the center of the flesh between the first and second metacarpal bones, closer to the second metacarpal bone.

Grasp the patient's thumb so that the second and third fingers fall on the palmar aspect of the patient's hand. Gently push up on the palmar aspect of the web that lies between the thumb and index finger. Using the thumb of the opposite hand, place its lateral side on the radial edge of the second metacarpal bone, then roll the lateral edge of the thumb into the depression on the second metacarpal bone. Pressure is toward the second metacarpal bone.

Action: This point treats the face and

head and relieves Wind Heat from the head. It is used as a distal point for treating the head and face, particularly when treating frontal headaches.

Comment: This is the Organ point for the Colon.

28. CV17

Location: Midway between the nipples at the center of the sternum.

Pressure is activated with the pad of the middle finger gently pressing directly toward the table.

Action: This is a very important point for releasing stagnating emotional energy trapped in the chest and for tonifying the Qi of the chest, which relates to the Heart and the Lung, the Upper Burner. CV17 helps breathing by opening up the chest and redirecting Rebellious Qi.

Comment: This is the Mu point for the Upper Burner, Mu point for the Heart Envelope, and Influential point of the Qi. It is also an Intersecting point for the Spleen, Kidney, Small Intestine, San Jiao, and Heart Envelope channels.

29. CV12

Location: Midway between the end of the sternum and the umbilicus, or 4 tsun above the umbilicus on the anterior midline of the body.

The point is activated with the thumb or third finger. Rest one hand gently above CV12, palm down, to help stabilize the point pressure of the thumb or third finger of the opposite hand. Ask the patient to inhale, and to exhale slowly. As the patient exhales, pressure is applied directly toward the table until a slight pulsation is felt. The point is held for 15–30 seconds and then slowly released. As you release your pressure, begin cir-

cling your finger.

Action: CV12 harmonizes the Middle Burner and regulates the Yin of the Stomach, reducing digestive stagnation. This point is also helpful for bringing emotional energy down from the chest toward the feet and opening up the chest.

Comment: This is the Mu point for the Stomach as well as for the Middle Burner. It is also an Intersecting point of the Small Intestine, San Jiao, and Stomach channels, as well as the Influential point of the Yang Organs.

30. CV6

Location: 1.5 tsun inferior to the umbilicus on the midline of the anterior body.

Pressure is with the pad of the third finger or thumb directly toward the table.

Action: CV6 tonifies the Kidney, the Spleen, Qi, Yang, and Blood for the entire body.

31. Liv8

Location: On the medial side of the knee joint. When the knee is flexed the point is found proximal to the medial end of the transverse popliteal crease, between the upper border of the medial epicondyle of the femur and the tendon of the semimembranosus muscle.

Pressure is with the pad of the third finger into the depression.

Action: This point nourishes Liver Blood and moves the Blood. It is used for Liver Blood Deficiency patterns and Blood Stasis patterns.

Comment: This is the Sea and Water point of the Liver Channel.

32. St36

Location: 3 tsun below St35, 1 tsun lateral to the anterior crest of the tibia. (St35 is at the lateral foramen of the patella).

Stand alongside the patient, facing the patient's knee. Place the pad of the thumb of the hand closest to the patient's head on the point. Gently hold the foot with the other hand and tilt the leg toward your body as you press toward the tibia. This will give more pressure into the point. This point may be held from 15–30 seconds. Circle as you release your pressure.

Action: This point tonifies Blood and Qi in Deficiency syndromes and tonifies the Stomach, Spleen, Wei Qi, and Nutrient Qi.

Comment: This is the Sea and Earth point of the Stomach Channel.

33. Liv5

Location: 5 tsun proximal to the vertex of the medial malleolus, in a depression on the medial aspect of the tibia.

Pressure is applied with the pad of the thumb directly into the depression.

Action: This point regulates the flow of Liver Qi and helps to remove obstructions from the channel.

Comment: This is the Luo point for the Liver Channel.

34. Sp6

Location: 3 tsun proximal to the vertex of the medial malleolus, just posterior to the tibial border.

Stand at the foot of the table. Grasp the patient's leg with your hand and place the pad of the thumb on the point. Gently press toward the tibia until you feel a sulcus in the bone. Hold the point for 15–30 seconds and then slowly release, circling as you lighten your pressure. This point can be pressed bilaterally.

Action: Sp6 tonifies the Spleen, Liver, and Kidney; promotes the smooth flow of Liver Qi; nourishes the Blood and Yin; moves the Blood and helps eliminate Blood Stasis; and calms the Shen.

Comment: This point is the Intersecting point of the three Yin channels of the leg.

35. Liv3

Location: In the depression distal to the junction of the first and second metatarsal bones.

Pressure is with the pads of the thumbs toward the first metatarsal.

Action: This point tonifies the Liver, regulates the flow of Liver Qi and Blood, subdues Liver Yang and Wind, clears Liver Fire, and redirects Rebellious Liver Qi downward.

Comment: This is the Organ, Stream, and Earth point of the Liver Channel.

36. Liv2

Location: 0.5 tsun proximal to the margin of the web between the first and second toes.

Grasp the patient's toe with your hand and press into the lateral joint space with your thumb. Angle your thumb to fit into the joint space. This point may be more tender than others and should be pressed gently at first and then with increasing pressure. Hold for 15–30 seconds and then slowly release, circling as you lighten your pressure.

Action: Liv2 helps to sedate Rising Liver Fire and Wind, releases stress, and calms the Spirit. It also treats headaches due to Excess Liver Fire or Wind.

Comment: This point can be used in combination with Co4 to sedate the Liver

Qi. It is the Spring and Fire point of the Liver Channel.

37. GB43

Location: Between the fourth and fifth toes proximal to the margin of the web.

Pressure is with the thumb angled toward the lateral foot.

Action: This point regulates the Gall Bladder and subdues Liver Yang and Wind. It removes obstructions in the Gall Bladder Channel and affects the opposite end of the channel, that is, the temple and eye regions. It is a distal point for headaches.

Comment: This is the Spring and Water point of the Gall Bladder Channel.

38. St44

Location: Proximal to the margin of the web between the second and third toes, in the depression distal and lateral to the second metatarsalphalangeal joint.

Pressure is with the thumb toward the second metatarsalphalangeal joint.

Action: St44 clears Heat from the Stomach and helps remove Wind from the face. It is a distal point for headaches.

Comment: This is the Spring and Water point of the Stomach Channel.

39. Bl60

Location: In the depression between the lateral malleolus and the calcaneal tendon, level with the vertex of the lateral malleolus.

Pressure is with the pad of the third finger while supporting the foot with the opposite hand or, while the patient is prone, grasping the calcaneal tendon, with the thumb and index finger so that the thumb is on Bl60, pressing with the pad of the thumb toward the index finger.

Action: This is a distal point for occipital headaches due to exogenous or endogenous factors. It is also used for headaches due to Kidney Deficiency.

Comment: This is the River and Fire point of the Bladder Channel.

40. Bl64

Location: On the lateral side of the dorsum of the foot, proximal to the tuberosity of the fifth metatarsal bone, at the border of the dorsal and plantar skins.

With the patient in the supine position, grasp the foot with the opposite hand and hook the thumb into the depression proximal to the tuberosity. Pressure is directly into the depression.

Action: This is a distal point for headaches. It also calms the Spirit and eliminates Wind and Heat.

Comment: This is the Organ point for the Bladder Channel.

41. Bl18

Location: 1.5 tsun lateral to the lower border of the spinous process of the ninth thoracic vertebra.

Pressure is applied bilaterally with the thumbs, straight down toward the table.

Action: This point regulates and tonifies the Liver and treats Stagnant Liver Qi. It also subdues Liver Yang and Liver Fire.

Comment: This is the Yu point (Associated point) for the Liver.

42. Bl20

Location: 1.5 tsun lateral to the lower border of the spinous process of the eleventh thoracic vertebra.

Pressure is applied bilaterally with the thumbs, straight down toward the table.

Action: Bl20 is a major point for tonifying the Stomach and the Spleen and regulate the Middle Jiao. It helps the Spleen's transporting and transforming functions and reduces digestive stagnation.

Comment: This is the Yu point (Associated point) for the Spleen.

43. Bl21

Location: 1.5 tsun lateral to the lower border of the spinous process of the twelfth thoracic vertebra.

Pressure is applied bilaterally with the thumbs, straight down toward the table.

Action: This is a major point for tonifying both Stomach and Spleen Qi. It stimulates the descending of Stomach Qi, relieves stagnation of food in the stomach, and promotes the Spleen function of transforming and transporting Qi, Blood, and Fluids.

Comment: This is the Yu point (Associated point) for the Stomach.

44. Bl23

Location: 1.5 tsun lateral to the lower border of the spinous process of the second lumbar vertebra.

This point may be manipulated bilaterally with the thumbs. Press directly toward the table and, while maintaining the pressure downward, pull the muscle slightly upward.

Action: Bl23 tonifies the Kidney and nourishes Kidney Essence. It also nourishes the Blood and strengthens the Brain.

Comment: This is the Yu point (Associated point) for the Kidney.

TREATMENT FOR PREMENSTRUAL SYNDROME

AMMA THERAPY ETIOLOGY

Premenstrual syndrome (PMS) is the name given to a range of physical and psychological symptoms that begin one to two weeks before the onset of menstruation and subside once the menstrual flow begins. Emotional symptoms of PMS can include anxiety, irritability, anger, depression, sadness, feeling "blue," and mood swings. Physical symptoms include abdominal distention and cramping, swelling and discomfort of the breasts, peripheral edema, cravings for sweets, weight gain, mild to severe headaches, and insomnia. The PMS syndrome can occur anytime between menarche and menopause, however the majority of women who seek treatment for PMS are between thirty and forty years of age. It has been estimated that approximately one-third to two-thirds of all menstruating women are affected by PMS.

From the Western perspective, there is no evidence that conclusively indicates any one etiological factor as the cause of PMS; hormonal imbalances, hypoglycemia, deficiencies of vitamin B and magnesium, changes in endorphin activity, and psychological dysfunctions have all been implicated as the primary precipitating factor. While there is documentation to support each of these as the major culprit in triggering PMS symptoms, none has been able to completely explain the PMS phenomena.

The Western approach to dealing with PMS emphasizes a low-salt and low-sugar diet, abstinence from caffeine, sufficient exercise, therapeutic counseling, and stress-management practices, combined with the use of drugs, such as painkillers, diuretics, synthetic hormones, oral contraceptives, tranquilizers, sedatives, and antidepressants.

Premenstrual syndrome is better understood from the TCM perspective. Problems with the menses are very much related to the functions of the Liver, the Penetrating Vessel (which enters the Uterus), and the Conception Vessel. The Penetrating Vessel is one of the eight Extraordinary Vessels. It is called the Sea of Blood because it helps to regulate menstruation by removing obstructions of Qi and Blood. It has its origin in the Kidney and travels with the Kidney Channel from Ki11 to Ki21. For a normal period to occur the Blood must be abundant and free-flowing, that is, able to move adequately. The proper movement of Blood is dependent upon the free flow of Liver Qi. The influence of the Liver on the menses is felt through its influence on the volume of blood circulating in the body, which regulates the amount through storage and release, depending on the body's needs. The smooth flow of Liver Qi and Blood has a direct effect on the uterus, thus affecting menstruation. The Liver not only provides for the smooth flow of Qi, Blood, and Fluids throughout the body, but it also provides for a calm emotional life through that same smooth flow. If the flow of Liver Qi is interrupted or stagnates, the effect on one's emotional life will be felt as anger, depression, and irritability.

Factors that can lead to premenstrual syndrome are significant emotional fluctuations, diet, stress, and overwork.

Emotions such as anger and frustration that are not properly dealt with in a constructive manner can lead to stagnation of Liver Qi, which is a major factor in the symptoms of irritability, mood swings, dietary bingeing, breast swelling and discomfort, abdominal distention, and depression. Conversely, when Liver Qi stagnates and does not flow in a free and uninterrupted manner, it can cause negative emotional states, such as anger, irritation, and frustration. When this situation is long-standing it can lead to ongoing states of depression and a negative outlook on life. Long-standing negative emotions can turn into Liver Fire, which in turn can create Blood Heat.

From a dietary standpoint, the excessive consumption of hot, fatty, and greasy or fried foods can also produce Liver Fire. From the TCM perspective, "hot" foods include lamb, beef, alcohol, deep-fried foods, and foods that are extremely spicy. Excessive consumption of dairy products and fried foods produces mucus, which congeals into Phlegm. When Phlegm combines with Liver Fire, produced either through diet or through stagnation of Liver Qi, the result is Phlegm Fire. This Phlegm Fire can gather in the breasts, resulting in cystic formations or lumps. It can also accumulate in the chest and "mist the mind," resulting in severe mental disturbances.

Insufficient consumption of animal protein can lead to a Blood Deficiency, which in turn can cause a Liver Blood Deficiency. This is more prevalent in women who need a sufficient supply of Blood-producing foods to replace the Blood that is lost during menses. Liver Blood Deficiency often leads to Liver Qi Stagnation.

Other factors involved in PMS are stress and overwork, which can weaken the Yin of both the Liver and the Kidney. Deficiency of these Organs can also result in Stagnant Liver Qi, which interferes with the movement of Blood in the Conception and Penetrating Vessels. This in turn affects the Uterus, the result of which is premenstrual tension, breast swelling and discomfort, and difficult and painful periods and/or irregular menstruation. Overwork and chronic illness also lead to a deficiency of Qi and Blood of the Stomach and Spleen, which in turn leads to malnourishment of the Penetrating and Conception Vessels, and to stagnation.

Excessive sexual activity and the act of childbirth can both affect the menses. When the Liver and Kidney are weakened by excessive sexual activity or by successive births in a short period of time, a deficiency of the Liver and Kidney is induced. This in turn affects the Penetrating Vessel, which becomes deficient in Qi and Blood.

A Spleen and Kidney Yang Deficiency can also lead to PMS symptoms, with an accumulation of Cold and Dampness involving the lower abdomen and lower back and accompanied by diarrhea or loose stools and frequent and pale urination. Cold contracts, causing Blood Stasis in the Uterus and subsequent painful periods. Women are more prone to invasion of Cold when the Uterus and the Blood are in a weakened state.

Thus there are basically two types of conditions when looking at PMS: Excess conditions, consisting of either Liver Qi Stagnation or Phlegm Fire impeding and obstructing the flow of energy in the chest and mind; or Deficiency conditions, consisting of Liver Qi and Blood Deficiency, Liver and Kidney Yin Deficiency, or Spleen and Kidney Yang Deficiency.

Amma therapy is extremely beneficial for the treatment of premenstrual syndrome, and produces excellent results. However, it is important that the patient be treated several days before the onset of her menstrual period. In addition to treatment, dietary changes, proper supplementation, and exercise make PMS a relatively easy problem to resolve.

AMMA THERAPY TREATMENT

The Amma therapist questions the regularity or irregularity of the patient's menstrual cycle and the date of her last menses. If the patient experiences severe PMS, one treatment directly before the onset of the period will not be sufficient; the patient may require weekly treatments at first, simultaneous to instituting dietary changes. In thoroughly studying the patient's medical history, the Amma therapist will want to know how long the patient has suffered with this problem and if she engaged in any type of excessive exercise during puberty, as this is often a factor in the development of PMS later in life. Other factors frequently associated with PMS are the recent cessation of oral contraceptives; a history of amenorrhea, miscarriages, or abortion; or a recent pregnancy or tubal ligation. Premenopausal women are often beset by symptoms of PMS.

The assessment will include pulse and

tongue diagnosis; checking the patient's general demeanor, the color of the face, the body type and emotional state; palpation of the breasts for any tenderness, distention, cysts, or lumps; and palpation of the abdominal area. When inquiring about menstrual history the therapist is looking for information on the length of the menstrual period, as well as the color and consistency of the flow. If the patient is on oral contraceptives or using some other type of internal contraceptive device, her answers to the practitioner's inquiries will be of limited value in the assessment. Special attention must be given to women on oral contraceptives. Considering the numerous side-effects that these medications have on women—including edema, weight gain, change in menstrual flow, skin rashes, itching, hives, headaches, nervous tension, irritability, migraine headaches, nausea and vomiting, bloating, breast enlargement, and reduced tolerance to contact lenses—it can be said that oral contraceptives induce iatrogenic effects through causing stagnation, generally of Liver Qi.

AMMA THERAPY ASSESSMENT

1. What is the frequency of the patient's menses?
   + If the patient's period is generally early and has an abundant red flow, it is an indication of Blood Heat or a Qi Deficiency.
   + If the periods are generally late with a scanty, light-colored flow, it indicates either Blood Deficiency, Blood Stasis, or Internal Cold.
   + Irregular periods can indicate Liver Qi Stagnation, Liver Blood Stagnation, or Spleen Deficiency.

2. What is the consistency and color of the menstrual flow?
   + If the flow is scanty, clotted with a purplish-red color, and the patient suffers from pain and swelling of the breasts, it indicates Liver Qi or Liver Blood Stagnation.
   + If the flow is pale and heavy, it indicates Spleen Deficiency.
   + If the Kidney is deficient then the flow will be pale and scanty.
   + A very heavy period that is dark red or bright red in color indicates Heat in the Blood.
   + A very heavy period that is pale in color indicates Blood Deficiency.
   + Purplish blood indicates Blood Stasis or Internal Cold.
   + Purple, clotted blood indicates Blood Stasis.
   + Thin blood indicates Blood or Yin Deficiency.
   + Turbid blood indicates Blood Heat or stagnation due to Cold.

3. Does the patient experience any pain?
   + Pain before the onset of the period indicates Qi or Blood Stagnation.
   + Pain that occurs during the period indicates Blood Heat or Stagnation due to Internal Cold.
   + Pain that occurs after the period is completed indicates a Blood Deficiency.

◆ If the pain feels better after passing blood, it indicates Blood Stasis.

◆ Pain with abdominal distention indicates stagnation of Qi.

◆ A burning pain indicates Blood Heat.

◆ A cramping pain indicates Cold in the Uterus.

◆ Stabbing pain or pulling pain indicates Blood Stasis, as does a bearing-down pain before the onset of the period.

◆ A bearing-down pain after the period is over indicates a Kidney Deficiency.

4. Look at the abdomen for signs of swelling and distention.

5. Palpate the abdomen to determine the extent of swelling and distention.

◆ If the abdomen feels worse with pressure, it indicates an Excess condition.

◆ If it feels better with pressure, a Deficiency condition is indicated.

6. Ask the patient's permission to palpate the breast tissue. Examine the breasts for swelling, tenderness, cystic masses, or lumps.

7. If the patient complains of swelling and painful breasts before the onset of her menses, abdominal bloating, depression, being short-tempered, a feeling of distention in the hypochondrium, borborygmus, and her tongue has a relatively normal body color but she has a wiry pulse, especially at the Liver position on the left wrist, Liver Qi Stagnation is indicated.

8. If the patient complains of extreme mood swings, dizziness, agitated behavior alternating with depression, mental restlessness, insomnia, un-controllable behavior and palpitations, and her tongue presents with a red body color and a yellow, sticky coating with a very red tip and she has a slippery and rapid pulse, the patient is suffering from Phlegm Fire harassing the upper body.

9. Liver Blood Deficiency is characterized by depression and crying spells before the period, breast and abdominal swelling, scanty periods, fatigue, dizziness, insomnia, numbness of the limbs, pale complexion, weak musculature, pale lips, muscle spasms, cramping and brittle nails. The tongue appears pale or paler on the sides and is dry; the pulse is thin and hesitant or choppy.

10. If the patient is suffering from a Liver and Kidney Yin Deficiency, there will be some breast swelling; irritability before the onset of the period that sometimes continues through the menstrual period and after it is finished; low back pain; dizziness; insomnia; five-palm heat (sweating from the palms, soles of the feet, and center of the chest); blurry vision; headaches; malar flush; dry eyes; tinnitus; night sweating; scanty menstruation or irregular menstruation; and numbness of the limbs. The tongue will be red and peeled and the pulse will be floating and weak or choppy.

11. If the patient is suffering from a Spleen and Kidney Yang Deficiency, her symptoms will be depression and crying before the onset of her period; some abdominal and breast swelling; fatigue; low back pain; cold limbs; frequent and pale urination; poor appetite; watery stools or diarrhea; borborygmus; and edema in the legs.

Pain is alleviated by pressure or the application of warmth. Her tongue will be pale and swollen and the pulse will be slow, deep, and weak.

ADDITIONAL TECHNIQUES

1. When there is tenderness in the abdominal area, teh tah chu can be applied to remove stagnation and increase the flow of Qi and Blood. Special attention should be given to the manipulation of Conception Vessel points and Stomach points in the Lower Burner.

2. If the patient is suffering from lower abdominal cramping and pain, focus should be directed to the downward manipulation of the inguinal area using circular digital and circular palmar pressure on top of the inguinal ligaments with teh tah chu. The leg may be gently moved outward to open up the inguinal area. Manipulation of this area will release stagnant Qi and Blood and restore proper circulation to the Liver Channel.

3. If the inguinal ligaments are very tight, loosen the area with circular palmar and circular digital pressure. Then press St25 followed by direct thumb pressure applied with the pads of the thumbs to the inguinal ligaments. Place the thumbs on top of the inguinal ligament, resting the hands on and over the ASIS. This may be done bilaterally, with pressure applied in 1-tsun increments directed laterally toward the hip bones, starting at the top of the ligaments and coming down to the pubic bone. This may also be done using teh tah chu. This technique treats chronic irregular menstruation. Consistent treatment over a three-month period will help to regulate the menses.

4. For painful and swollen breasts, teh tah chu may be applied directly to the breast tissue with gentle, circular digital and palmar pressure. Ask the patient's permission before applying the liniment. Support the breast with one hand while applying the liniment with the other. The patient may be instructed to soak some gauze in the liniment and apply it to her breasts overnight. She may want to wear an old shirt or brassiere to bed so that the area stays moist throughout the night and the liniment does not stain the bedding.

5. Special attention should be paid to the manipulation of the Liver Channel on the inside of the thigh and leg, in order to stimulate the smooth flow of Liver energy.

6. Manipulate the small of the back and the sacral area with teh tah chu. Pain in this area usually indicates a Kidney Deficiency.

7. Manipulate the Ki1 area. Ki1 helps to calm the Shen and tonify the Yin of the body.

POINT LOCATION AND ACTION

1. St8

Location: On the superior aspect of the head, in a depression 0.5 tsun within the anterior hairline at the corner of the forehead.

Pressure is with the pad of the third finger into the depression.

Action: St8 helps resolve Phlegm in the head and subsequently clears the head and difficulty in thinking.

Comment: This is the Intersecting point of the Stomach and Gall Bladder channels.

2. Lu1

Location: On the lateral aspect of the chest in the intercostal space between the first and second ribs, 6 tsun lateral to the midline of the chest.

Press down using the pad of the index finger, third finger, or thumb. Direct the pressure toward the center of the chest.

Action: Lu1 regulates the Lung, catalyzes the descending function of the Lung, opens up the chest, and calms the patient.

Comment: This point is the Mu point for the Lung and is used to treat acute conditions. It is also the Intersecting point of the Lung and Spleen channels.

3. Sp20

Location: In the second intercostal space directly below Lu1, 6 tsun lateral to the Conception Vessel.

Press down using the pad of the index finger, third finger, or thumb. Direct the pressure toward the table.

Action: Sp20 relaxes and opens up the chest and calms the patient.

4. CV17

Location: Midway between the nipples at the center of the sternum.

Pressure is activated with the pad of the middle finger gently pressing directly toward the table.

Action: This is an important point for releasing stagnating emotional energy trapped in the chest and for tonifying the energy of the Upper Burner, which relates to the Heart and the Lung. This point helps breathing by opening up the chest, and releases emotional stress, tension, and pain in the chest.

Comment: This is the Mu point for both the Upper Burner and the Heart Envelope; it is also the Influential point of the Qi and is often referred to as the Upper Sea of Qi. It is an Intersecting point with the Spleen, Small Intestine, Kidney, San Jiao, and Heart Envelope channels.

5. CV12

Location: Midway between the end of the sternum and the umbilicus, or 4 tsun above the umbilicus on the anterior midline of the body. The point is activated with the thumb or third finger.

Rest one hand gently palm down above CV12 to help stabilize the point pressure of the thumb or third finger of the opposite hand. Ask the patient to inhale, and to exhale slowly. As the patient exhales, apply pressure directly toward the table until a slight pulsation is felt. Hold the point for 15–30 seconds and then slowly release. As you release your pressure, begin circling your finger.

Action: CV12 harmonizes the Middle Burner, reverses the flow of Rebellious Qi, strengthens the Spleen, and treats abdominal distention and pain. This point is also helpful for bringing emotional energy down from the chest toward the feet and opening up the chest.

Comment: This is the Mu point for both the Stomach and the Middle Burner. It is an Intersecting point of the Small

Intestine, San Jiao, and Stomach channels and is an Influential point of the Yang Organs.

6. Co11

Location: In the depression at the lateral end of the transverse cubital crease, midway between Lu5 and the lateral epicondyle of the humerus when the elbow is half-flexed.

Bend the patient's elbow and place your thumb on the point. Gently open the arm and press. The force is straight into the joint.

Action: Co11 clears Heat from any Organ in the body, and is therefore useful when Phlegm Fire is causing negative emotional behavior.

Comment: This is the Sea and Earth point of the Colon Channel.

7. SJ6

Location: 3 tsun proximal to SJ4, between the ulna and the radius. (With the palm facing downward, SJ4 is located at the junction of the ulna and carpal bones, in the depression lateral to the tendon of the extensor digitorum muscle.)

Pressure is activated with the pad of the thumb down into the point.

Action: SJ6 transforms Phlegm, clears Fire and Heat, and expands and relaxes the chest. This point regulates Qi and Qi flow, particularly in the hypochondriac region and the sides of the ribs, where pain can be due to Stagnant Liver Qi and Blood.

Comment: This is the River and Fire point of the Triple Burner Channel.

8. HE6 (P6)

Location: On the anterior aspect of the forearm, 2 tsun proximal to the transverse crease of the wrist on the line connecting HE3 and HE7, between the tendons of the palmaris longus and flexor carpi radialis muscles.

Pressure is activated with the pad of the thumb.

Action: HE6 calms the Spirit; helps resolve Phlegm in the Heart; helps regulate and promote the smooth flow of Liver Qi, particularly in the chest and breasts; clears Fire and Heat; and helps move the Blood.

Comment: This is the Luo point for the Heart Envelope.

9. HE7 (P7)

Location: At the midpoint of the transverse crease of the wrist, located in the depression between the tendons of the palmaris longus and flexor carpi radialis muscles.

Pressure is activated with the pad of the thumb.

Action: HE7 calms the Spirit and clears the Brain; clears Heart Fire and helps to alleviate anxiety and mental restlessness; and helps to expand and relax the chest.

Comment: This is the Organ, Stream, and Earth point of the Heart Envelope Channel.

10. Lu7

Location: In a slight depression at the origin of the styloid process of the radius, 1.5 tsun above the transverse crease of the wrist.

Grasp the patient's hand and use your thumb to press into the depression between the tendon and the bone.

Action: Lu7 regulates the Conception Vessel and helps regulate the Uterus and menstruation.

Comment: This is the Luo point for the Lung and a Confluent point for the Conception Vessel.

11. CV6

Location: On the midline of the abdomen, 1.5 tsun below the umbilicus.

Pressure is with the pad of the third finger or thumb directly toward the table.

Action: CV6 helps to move Stagnant Qi and relieve pain in the Lower Burner. It tonifies Qi and Blood and regulates the Conception Vessel and menstruation.

12. TS-Ab1

Location: Midway between the navel and the pubic bone.

Pressure is activated with the thumb or third finger directly toward the table.

Action: This point removes obstructions of Qi from the lower abdomen and helps to dispel pain and distention in this area.

13. CV4

Location: On the midline of the abdomen, 3 tsun below the umbilicus.

Pressure is with the pad of the third finger or thumb directly toward the table.

Action: CV4 helps regulate the Lower Burner and menstruation, tonifies Blood and Yin in Blood Deficiency patterns, and helps calm the Shen by rooting Qi into the Lower Burner.

Comment: This is the Intersecting point of the Kidney, Spleen, and Liver channels with the Conception Vessel. It is also the Mu point for the Small Intestine.

14. CV2

Location: On the anterior midline of the body, 5 tsun below the umbilicus in a depression just above the pubic symphysis.

Gently hook the pad of the third finger into the depression on top of the pubic symphysis and press.

Action: CV2 regulates the menses and treats lower abdominal cramping and pain.

Comment: This is the Intersecting point with the Liver Channel.

15. St28

Location: 2 tsun lateral to CV4, 3 tsun below the umbilicus.

Pressure is with the pad of the third finger or thumb directly toward the table.

Action: St28 helps regulate Qi in the lower abdomen and helps regulate menstruation. It also relieves pain in the Lower Burner and treats lower abdominal distention.

16. St29

Location: 2 tsun lateral to CV3, 4 tsun below the umbilicus.

Pressure is with the pad of the third finger or thumb directly toward the table.

Action: St29 regulates menstruation. It helps to eliminate stagnation of Blood in the Uterus and is therefore used for menstrual problems due to Blood Stasis.

17. St30

Location: 2 tsun lateral to CV2, on the superior ridge of the pubic tubercle.

Pressure is with the pad of the third finger or thumb on the superior ridge of the pubic tubercle.

Action: St30 helps to regulate Qi and Blood in the lower abdomen, regulates menstruation, and helps encourage free flow of Liver Qi.

Comment: This is a Confluent point for

the Penetrating Vessel.

18. GB34

Location: In the depression anterior and inferior to the head of the fibula.

Use the pad of your thumb or third finger to press into the depression, toward the tibia.

Action: GB34 helps regulate and tonify the Liver and helps the Liver Qi to move freely and smoothly. It also helpful for stagnation of Liver Qi, particularly in the hypochondriac region.

Comment: This is the Influential point of the sinews. It is also the Sea and Earth point of the Gall Bladder Channel.

19. St36

Location: 3 tsun below St35, 1 tsun lateral to the anterior crest of the tibia. (St35 is at the lateral foramen of the patella).

Stand alongside the patient facing the patient's knee. Place the pad of the thumb of the hand closest to the patient's head on the point. Gently hold the foot with the other hand and tilt the leg toward your body as you press toward the tibia. This will give more pressure into the point. This point may be held for 15–30 seconds. Circle as you release your pressure.

Action: This is a major point for tonifying Qi and Blood in the channels, and is used to treat Deficiency patterns.

Comment: This point has been used since ancient times to strengthen the body's overall health by building up the Wei Qi and Nutrient Qi, thus increasing resistance to invasion by exogenous pathogens. It is the Sea and Earth point of the Stomach Channel.

20. Sp10

Location: With the knee flexed, this point is located on the anteromedial aspect of the thigh, 2 tsun superior to the medial superior ridge of the patella, in the prominence of the vastus medialis muscle.

Pressure is with the pad of the thumb or third finger into the prominence of the muscle.

Action: Sp10 regulates the Spleen and menstruation, regulates and tonifies the Blood, invigorates the Blood and helps Blood flow, and helps clear Blood Stasis.

21. Liv8

Location: With the knee flexed, this point is located in the depression on the medial end of the transverse popliteal crease between the upper border of the medial epicondyle of the femur and the tendon of the semimembranosus muscle.

Pressure is with the pad of the third finger into the depression.

Action: This point regulates and tonifies the Qi and Blood of the Liver. It helps encourage free flow of Liver Qi and tonifies Liver Blood, regulates menstruation, and moves Blood Stasis.

Comment: This is the Sea and Water point of the Liver Channel.

22. St40

Location: 8 tsun below St35 and 2 tsun lateral to the anterior crest of the tibia.

Pressure is with the pad of the thumb toward the tibia.

Action: St40 calms the Spirit and transforms Phlegm and Dampness in all parts of the body. It also regulates the menses.

Comment: This is the Luo point of the Stomach Channel.

23. Sp6

Location: 3 tsun proximal to the vertex of the medial malleolus, just posterior to the tibial border.

Stand at the foot of the table. Grasp the patient's leg with your hand and place the pad of the thumb on the point. Gently press toward the tibia until you feel a sulcus in the bone. Hold the point for 15–30 seconds and then slowly release, circling as you lighten your pressure. This point can be pressed bilaterally.

Action: This is a major point for gynecological problems. It tonifies Blood and Qi, nourishes Blood, and encourages the smooth flow of Blood. It is particularly helpful in assisting the free flow of Liver Qi when Liver Qi has been stagnating in the Lower Burner. This point also regulates the Uterus and menstruation, helps relieve pain in the Lower Burner, remove obstructions of Qi from the Liver channel, and calm negative emotions.

Comment: This point is the Intersecting point of the three Yin channels of the leg.

24. GB41

Location: In the depression distal to the junction of the fourth and fifth metatarsal bones.

Pressure is with the pad of the third finger directly into the depression.

Action: GB41 regulates the Liver, helps encourage free flow of Liver Qi, treats intercostal and hypochondriac pain, and treats painful breast swelling due to menstruation.

Comment: This is the Stream and Wood point of the Gall Bladder Channel.

25. Sp4

Location: Approximately 1 tsun proximal to Sp3, in the depression distal and inferior to the base of the first metatarsal bone at the border of the red and white skin.

This point may be pressed bilaterally. Standing at the foot of the table, grasp the dorsum of the patient's foot with your hand so that the thumbs naturally fall below the arch of the foot. Pressure is with the thumb toward the metatarsal bone.

Action: This point activates and regulates the Penetrating Vessel, and thereby regulates menstruation. It invigorates the Blood and helps remove Blood Stasis, calms the Spirit, and clears the Brain.

Comment: This is the Luo point (Connecting Point) for the Spleen and also a Confluent Point for the Penetrating Vessel.

26. Liv3

Location: In the depression distal to the junction of the first and second metatarsal bones.

Pressure is with the pads of the thumbs toward the first metatarsal.

Action: This point sedates Liver Yang, calms the Shen, and promotes the smooth flow of Liver Qi.

Comment: This is the Organ, Stream, and Earth point for the Liver Channel.

27. Ki6

Location: On the medial aspect of the foot, 1 tsun inferior to the lower border of the medial malleolus.

Pressure is with the pad of the thumb into the point.

Action: Ki6 regulates menstruation, helps the function of the Uterus, nourishes Kidney Yin, and helps calm the Shen, especially in cases of anxiety due to Yin Deficiency.

28. Ki3

Location: In the depression between the medial malleolus and the calcaneal tendon, level with the vertex of the medial malleolus.

Pressure is with the pad of the thumb or third finger into the depression.

Action: Ki3 regulates menstruation and the Uterus. It also tonifies the Essence of the Kidney.

Comment: This is the Organ, Stream, and Earth point for the Kidney Channel.

29. Bl18

Location: 1.5 tsun lateral to the lower border of the spinous process of the ninth thoracic vertebra.

Pressure is applied bilaterally with the thumbs, directed straight down toward the table.

Action: Bl18 regulates and tonifies the Liver and treats Liver Qi Stagnation or Damp Heat in the Liver and Gall Bladder. It is used to treat Stagnant Liver Qi in the epigastrium and hypochondrium. It also regulates menstruation and nourishes Liver Blood.

Comment: This is the Yu point (Associated point) for the Liver.

30. Bl20

Location: 1.5 tsun lateral to the lower border of the spinous process of the eleventh thoracic vertebra.

Pressure is applied bilaterally with the thumbs, directed straight down toward the table.

Action: Bl20 is a major point for tonifying the Stomach and the Spleen and regulating the Middle Jiao. It nourishes the Blood, as the Spleen is the Source of Blood, and tonifies Qi and Blood.

Comment: This is the Yu point (Associated point) for the Spleen.

31. Bl23

Location: 1.5 tsun lateral to the lower border of the spinous process of the second lumbar vertebra.

This point may be manipulated bilaterally with the thumbs. Press directly toward the table and, while maintaining the pressure downward, pull the muscle slightly upward.

Action: Bl23 tonifies the Kidney. It promotes the formation of Blood in Blood Deficiency, since the Kidney helps to produce the Blood through the formation of Marrow.

Comment: This is the Yu point (Associated point) for the Kidney.

32. Bl31–34

Location: Located within the four sacral foramen.

Pressure is applied bilaterally, using the pads of the thumbs or third fingers directly into the sacral foramen.

Action: Bl31–34 regulate the Lower Burner and menstruation, enliven the Blood, and treat pain and stiffness of the lower back.

CHAPTER
24

TREATMENT FOR HYPERTENSION

AMMA THERAPY ETIOLOGY

An estimated 60 million Americans have hypertension, or high blood pressure (HBP). Forty-five percent of persons over sixty-five years of age are hypertensive. High blood pressure is a sustained elevated mean arterial pressure. The condition directly contributes to more than thirty thousand deaths per year, primarily through stroke and cardiac failure. High blood pressure is a major risk factor in the development of coronary artery disease. Indirectly, hypertension is a contributing factor in many other diseases. Hypertension plays a role in about 70 percent of first heart attacks and 75 percent of first strokes. The condition is a primary risk factor for kidney failure and, if left unchecked, can cause vision loss and blindness.

Ninety-five percent of all hypertension is considered essential or idiopathic. Secondary hypertension is caused by some other systemic condition, such as an endocrine disorder, renal disease, and certain autoimmune diseases like scleroderma. Secondary hypertension accounts for only 5 percent of all cases. The onset of essential hypertension usually occurs between thirty and fifty years of age. People at particular risk include those with a family history of hypertension, middle-aged persons, the elderly, African-Americans, the obese, heavy drinkers, people who do little or no exercise, women who use oral contraceptives, and people who consume excessive amounts of saturated fats, cholesterol, and sodium. Medications such as prednisone and other immunosuppressants produce hypertension as a side effect. Smokers are at particular risk. Smoking can cause a fifteen to twenty point rise in blood pressure. While initially causing dilation of the blood vessels, nicotine subsequently causes vasoconstriction, which raises blood pressure. The constant vasoconstriction induced by heavy smoking cuts off the flow of oxygen and blood, causing degeneration of the blood vessels and lack of nourishment to the areas of the body they supply.

An associated condition of hypertension is atherosclerosis, a form of arteriosclerosis. Arteriosclerosis is the general term for three patterns of vascular disease, all of which cause thickening of the arteries and thus affect their elasticity. The major pattern is atherosclerosis where there is a deposition of atheromatous plaques containing cholesterol, fibrous tissue, and calcium on the innermost layer of the walls of large- and medium-sized arteries. It is usually a chronic disease in which thickening, hardening, and loss of elasticity of the arterial walls reduces the size of the lumen and leads to impaired blood circulation. This leads to increased vascular resistance and results in elevated blood pressure. Atherosclerotic changes are major contributing factors to high blood pressure in the elderly.

The American Heart Association and other authoritative sources estimate that half the people who have hypertension do not know that they have it—hence its reputation as the "silent killer." Because hypertension is often asymptomatic, many times the patient does not seek treatment until the disease is in its advanced stages.

The standard method of measuring blood pressure is with a sphygmomanometer (a blood pressure cuff). From a Western medical viewpoint the diagnosis of hypertension should be made after three successive readings taken on three different days. The blood pressure reading is a measurement of the force of the blood exerted on the walls of the arteries during the ventricular contraction phase (systole), and the pressure remaining in the arteries in the ventricular relaxation phase (diastole) of the heart. In addition to the blood pressure readings, a physical examination, blood and urine tests, and an electrocardiograph should be done to completely assess a patient's condition.

Normal systolic pressure should be 100–140 mm Hg. Normal diastolic pressure should be 60–90 mm Hg. Mild high blood pressure is considered to be 140–159/90–104. Severe high blood pressure is considered to be 160+/115+.

There are at least three systems involved in the regulation of blood pressure—the sympathetic nervous system, the renal system, and the endocrine system. The sympathetic nervous system responds rapidly to a decrease in cardiac output, which is the amount of blood pumped from one ventricle per beat (approximately seventy milliliters). The activation of the sympathetic nervous system also results in the acceleration of the heart rate and the force of the ventricular contraction.

Baroreceptors are specialized nerve receptors located in the carotid arteries and arch of the aorta. When the blood pressure rises above normal levels, the baroreceptors are stimulated to send inhibitory impulses to the sympathetic vasomotor center in the brain, which stimulates the vagus nerve, resulting in the dilatation of peripheral arterioles, a reduced heart rate, and a diminished contractility of the ventricles.

The renal system plays a role in the

regulation of blood pressure by controlling sodium and extracellular fluid volume. Increased water retention results from the retention of sodium, thus increasing extracellular volume. Increased extracellular volume in turn increases the venous return to the heart. This increases stroke volume (cardiac output), which then elevates the blood pressure. Another important mechanism related to the renal system is the renin-angiotensin mechanism. Renin, a protein-digesting enzyme, is released in response to sympathetic stimulation or to decreased blood flow through the kidneys. Renin activates the production of angiotensin II, a very potent vasoconstrictor. Angiotensin II elevates blood pressure by stimulating the secretion of aldosterone, which causes sodium retention by the kidneys. Increased sodium levels result in increased blood volume and subsequent increased cardiac output.

The endocrine system plays a role in the regulation of blood pressure via the hormone aldosterone as well as the antidiuretic hormone (ADH). ADH increases extracellular volume by stimulating the kidneys to retain water, thereby elevating blood pressure.

The regulation of blood pressure through traditional Western medical treatment is via pharmacological management. When fluid is retained in the extracellular tissues the medications most often prescribed are diuretics. A group of diuretics called thiazides can increase total cholesterol and serum blood sugar levels as well as increase uric acid levels, thereby contributing to kidney failure in those patients who already have an underlying renal pathology. When the blood pressure results from

increased heart rate, beta-blockers are the medication of choice. Once patients start these medications, they generally remain on them for years. These medications can have iatrogenic effects. Beta-blockers, such as Corgard, Inderal, or Tenormin, can give rise to bronchospasms, bradycardia, impotence, and increased cholesterol and triglycerides. Angiotensin-converting enzyme inhibitors, such as Capoten and Vasotec, are used when there is an imbalance in the renal system. They inhibit angiotensin-converting enzymes and lower the systemic vascular resistance (SVR) to prevent the retention of water by decreasing aldosterone secretion. Commonly experienced adverse reactions are cough, loss of taste, and, in more severe cases, nephrotic syndrome.

Adrenergic inhibitors affect the sympathetic nervous system, lowering the blood pressure by decreasing cardiac output. Side-effects that are associated with this group of medications are bronchospasm, bradycardia, and sexual dysfunction. Vasodilators, yet another group of medications, have an affect on the smooth muscle tissue of arterioles, causing vasodilation and the reduction of systemic vascular resistance.

Calcium channel blockers, such as Calan, Cardizem, and Procardia, are also used in the treatment of high blood pressure. These medications cause vasodilation of peripheral arterioles by blocking the movement of extracellular calcium into the cells, resulting in decreased systemic vascular resistance. Side-effects from this medication can include headache, peripheral edema, and constipation.

About 75 percent of hypertensives have a mild case of the "disease," defined as systolic pressure between 140 and 150 or diastolic pressure between 90 and 100. For many of these patients, lifestyle changes primarily in regard to diet and exercise can lower blood pressure without the need for drugs. In fact, 30 percent of all hypertensives can probably manage their blood pressure with diet and exercise.

An additional 20 percent of so-called hypertensives do not really have high blood pressure. They suffer with what can be called "white-coat syndrome"—their blood pressure rises only under the stress of a visit to their doctors. Home monitoring will reveal this problem and prevent the unnecessary use of medications to control blood pressure.

Although hypertension often does not show any clinical manifestations, one of the telling complaints is headaches. Hypertension patients complain of headaches that often occur in the mornings and go away as the day progresses. The headaches are usually in the occipital area and may be nothing more than a complaint of stiffness or tightness in this region. Headache can be a sign of severe hypertension and from the Western viewpoint is thought to be due to changes in the cerebrospinal fluid. When the patient lies down, the fluid pressure increases, thus causing the headache. When they stand up, the cerebrospinal fluid pressure decreases and the headache goes away. Other possible signs can be dizziness, palpitations, blurry vision, and nosebleeds.

High blood pressure can be examined through the homeodynamic model. Constitutional factors, such as the health of the parents at conception and the quality of Jing that is passed to the fetus, are primary influences on the health of the

individual. Some families have a history of hypertension, and members of those families will have more of a propensity toward developing high blood pressure. Diet is naturally a factor. Excessive intake of hot-energy foods, such as alcohol and spicy foods, can create Internal Heat leading to Fire. This frequently affects the Liver, resulting in Ascendant Liver Yang or Fire, which can manifest as high blood pressure. Excessive intake of sodium can initiate hypertension in some patients. Sodium causes water retention and can affect the Spleen as well as the Kidney. By weakening the Spleen, excessive salt causes retention of Dampness which in turn obstructs the movement of Fluids, thus causing a Spleen and Kidney Yang Deficiency. Excessive sodium intake can also contribute to a Kidney Yin Deficiency. If the Kidney Yin is deficient it cannot nourish Liver Yin. Deficient Liver Yin results in hyperactivity of Liver Yang, which causes hypertension when it rises.

According to the homeodynamic model, long-standing chronic emotional states, such as anger, frustration, irritability, rage, and resentment, weaken the Liver. The buildup of negative emotions can produce stagnation and the subsequent rising of Yang energy, Heat, or Fire, all of which can rise into the head and chest. The distinction between Ascendant Liver Yang and Liver Fire Rising is that Ascendant Liver Yang is due to a combination of Deficiency and Excess patterns. Here the Liver Yin energy is deficient, either due to a Liver Blood Deficiency or a Kidney Yin or Yang Deficiency. The deficiency of Liver Yin results in an imbalance with the Liver Yang energy, which is now in excess.

Liver Fire Rising is a purely Excess

Heat condition and the symptoms manifest more Heat. The symptoms that are shared by both syndromes are negative emotions of anger and irritability, dizziness, headaches, tinnitus, and disturbed sleep or insomnia. In both cases the pulse will be wiry and the tongue will be red, with the sides more red than the rest of the tongue body. But in Liver Fire Rising we can also see symptoms of red eyes and face, a dry tongue, thirst, bitter taste in the mouth, constipation, and scanty and dark urine, all Heat signs. In severe cases there may be epistaxis. Ascendant Liver Yang and Liver Fire Rising can fuel Heart Fire to flare upward, resulting in palpitations and insomnia.

It should be noted that in some Ascendant Liver Yang cases the tongue may actually be pale if the underlying Liver Yin Deficiency is due to a Liver Blood Deficiency. If the underlying cause is Liver and Kidney Yin Deficiency, the tongue would appear red and peeled. Both Ascendant Liver Yang and Liver Fire Rising can result in hypertension and, in extreme cases, can also produce Wind Stroke through the creation of endogenous Liver Wind.

Another cause of hypertension is stress or overwork, either physical or mental. Occupational or family stress can deplete the Kidney Yin and Kidney Yang energies. In Five Element theory, the Kidney is the mother of the Liver; it supplies the Liver with Essence and Blood via its production of Marrow. Any depletion of Kidney energy will result in Liver Yin Deficiency, which then can catalyze Ascendant Liver Yang.

Deficient Kidney Yin can also cause Heart Yin Deficiency, precipitated by the Kidney's failure to nourish the Heart. On the other hand, Heart Yin Deficiency can lead to Kidney Yin Deficiency. When the Yin of the Heart is deficient, this results in Apparent Yang and the flaring up of Heart Fire. The symptoms produced are mental agitation, dizziness, tinnitus, insomnia, palpitations, and a rise in blood pressure.

The creation of Phlegm Fire can also cause hypertension when the Phlegm Fire rises up and blocks the Yang energies from reaching the head. This condition arises when a weak Spleen allows Dampness to develop which transforms into Phlegm from Heat, usually due to Liver Yang or Liver Fire. Phlegm Fire can cause high blood pressure and symptoms of agitation, dream-disturbed sleep, anxiety, and depression. Stagnation of Phlegm in the channels obstructs the flow of Qi and Blood and can cause a stroke.

Recommendations for treatment of hypertension include regular Amma therapy treatments, dietary change, herbal and vitamin supplementation, an exercise regimen of t'ai chi or hatha yoga, biofeedback, and in some cases counseling with a psychologist to help the patient deal with emotional problems and stress.

AMMA THERAPY TREATMENT

The Amma therapist will first review the patient's medical history and check any medications that the patient may be currently taking. The therapist should then consult the Physicians' Desk Reference to check the pharmacological actions, potential adverse reactions, and contraindications. Numerous patients are unaware not only of the side-effects of many of their medications, but they are also ignorant of the effects caused by the interactions of the medications with each other. Over the years we have seen many patients taking several medications simultaneously which together produce moderate to serious side-effects that are part of their current symptomology. It is for this reason that taking the time to investigate drug side-effects is of primary importance in creating a treatment strategy.

After reviewing the patient's medical history, the therapist will conduct a thorough assessment that will include all facets of the Four Traditional Methods. The therapist should inquire as to how long the patient has suffered with this problem, the length of time the patient has been on medication, and the patient's diet and exercise regimen. The therapist will also check the patient's tongue and pulse. The therapist will be interested in any family history of cardiovascular problems, and naturally will take the patient's blood pressure to get a baseline from which to work. It is helpful to instruct the patient to purchase his own blood pressure unit so that he can monitor his pressure at home in a more relaxing environment and get regular readings. It has been our experience that patients suffering from white-coat syndrome often wind up on medication unnecessarily. Patients who can monitor themselves have a decreased chance of misconstrued blood pressure readings.

The patient can use food forms to list in detail his daily intake of foods and drinks. These forms are an educational tool for the patient and also help the therapist to get a more realistic view of the patient's diet. Many patients think that they have a good diet until they complete a series of food forms, an exercise that forces them to face the realities of their dietary indiscretions. Keeping track of his diet by way of the food forms provides the patient with an opportunity to become knowledgeable of the hidden dangers in certain foods, such as sodium intake, of which he may have been previously unaware.

AMMA THERAPY ASSESSMENT

1. The Amma therapist should measure the patient's blood pressure. Measurement should be done before the treatment begins to see what the baseline numbers are.
2. Question the patient about his or her blood pressure history. For example, does the patient keep track of his/her own pressure readings? Seeing the consistency of readings is really the only way to determine the validity of a diagnosis of hypertension.
3. Question the patient about his diet. Does the diet consist of excessive salt intake, fried foods, and processed foods (which contain a lot of hidden sodium), or alcohol and hot and spicy foods, which can produce Internal Heat and Fire?
4. Ask the patient if he suffers from headaches that appear at the temples, behind the eyes, or on the lateral sides of the head. From a TCM perspective, such headaches point to Ascendant Liver Yang or Liver Fire Rising, two syndromes that can cause hypertension.

5. Question the patient as to whether he has the following symptoms, which are indicative of Liver Fire Rising: dizziness; tinnitus; hearing problems; dream-disturbed sleep or insomnia; dry mouth and throat; irritability or angry demeanor; red face or eyes; bitter taste; constipation; dark urine; epistaxis; hematemesis or hemoptysis.

6. Question the patient as to whether he has occipital or vertex headaches, insomnia, dizziness, numbness in the limbs, blurry vision, low back pain, ringing in the ears, night sweating, malar flush, five-palm heat, dry eyes, or constipation. Women may experience a loss of the period or scanty bleeding during periods. These are symptoms of a Liver and Kidney Yin Deficiency.

7. Question the patient as to whether she has the following symptoms, which are indicative of a Kidney and Heart Yin Deficiency: mental agitation, palpitations, insomnia, tinnitus, dizziness, hearing problems, low back pain, tidal fever or malar flush, night sweats, scanty dark urine.

8. Ask the patient if she is suffering from dizziness, insomnia, chest oppression, a feeling of heaviness in the head, disinterest in eating or drinking, food retention in the Middle Jiao, irritability, and a bitter taste in the mouth. These are symptoms of Phlegm Fire harrassing the Upper Jiao.

9. Look at the patient's tongue.
   + If the patient is suffering from Liver Fire Rising, the tongue will be red with the sides being more red; there will be a yellow coating and the tongue will be dry from the Fire.
   + If the patient is suffering from Ascendant Liver Yang, the tongue will also be red, and redder on the sides. However, if the upsurging Liver Yang is due to an underlying Liver Blood Deficiency, the tongue will be pale and dry.
   + If the patient has Phlegm Fire harrassing the Upper Jiao, her tongue will be red with a yellow slimy coating, and the tip may be very red with prickles.
   + If the patient has both a Liver and Kidney Yin Deficiency, the tongue will show as red and peeled, typical signs of Yin Deficiency.
   + If the patient has both Kidney and Heart Yin Deficiency, the tongue will be peeled and red, the tip will be redder, and there most likely will be a midline crack in the tongue that extends to the tip.

10. Observe the patient for exophthalmia, which is a sign of Ascendant Liver Yang. If the patient's eyes are red and dry, this would be a sign of Liver Fire Rising.

11. Observe the patient's emotional state. Anger, depression, anxiety, and irritability can all point to Liver Fire Rising, Ascendant Liver Yang, or Heart Fire.

12. Observe the patient's complexion. A red face, ruddy complexion, or red and/or purple blotches on the face indicate Heat and/or Blood Stagnation. Blood Stagnation is the Oriental corollary for atherosclerosis.

13. Observe the patient's rib cage.

Thoracic fullness is often seen in patients suffering from hypertension, due to stress blocking the flow of Qi and Blood in the chest.

14. Take the patient's pulses.
    + In cases of Liver Fire Rising, the pulse will be rapid, forceful, and wiry.
    + In cases of Ascendant Liver Yang, the pulse will also be wiry. However if the Ascendant Liver Yang is due to an underlying Liver Blood Deficiency, the pulse will be hesitant and thin.
    + In cases of Phlegm Fire harrassing the Heart, the pulse will be rapid and slippery.
    + In cases of Kidney and Heart Yin Deficiency the pulse will be rapid, overblown, and sometimes floating.

15. The Amma therapist should be aware when taking the pulses of the patient with high blood pressure that medication can often affect the pulse, causing it to become irregular or very slow. It is important to note this so that the therapist does not mistake the slow pulse for an Interior Cold condition or mistake the irregular pulse for a Blood Deficiency. If other signs and symptoms do not confirm or support this conclusion, medication must be suspected.

16. Palpate the patient's body tissue for fluid retention. In particular, palpate the ankles and feet for pitting edema. The clearest signs of fluid retention are to be found in the ankles and feet. When edema is present it can signify a Kidney imbalance or be resultant from the side-effects of such medications as Cardizem or Procardia.

ADDITIONAL TECHNIQUES

1. Begin the treatment by cupping the palms over both sides of the head and gently holding the area for approximately one minute. During the course of this treatment the therapist can return to using circular digital pressure at the temples, around the ears, and on the sides of the head.

2. Thumb stroke on GV20, laterally to the ears. Then apply alternate thumb stroking on GV20. The direction is inferior toward the occiput.

3. For very tight necks, traction the neck with both hands, the index fingers pressing up into GB12 and the fourth fingers pressing up into GB20. The therapist should keep the patient's chin tucked.

4. Use the appropriate additional techniques described in the Treatment for Stiff Neck and Shoulder Pain (chapter 16) and in the Treatment for Headaches (chapter 22).

5. Using the thumb and index finger to grasp Ht9 and SI1 simultaneously, manipulate both points to help reduce blood pressure. Repeat on the fifth digit of the opposite hand.

POINT LOCATION AND ACTION

1. Extra point (yin tang)

Location: Located on the midline between the medial ends of the two eyebrows.

Use the pad of the third finger to press this point. Relax the hand and rest the second and fourth fingers on Bl2.

Action: This point calms the Spirit, dispels Wind, and clears Heat. It is very effective in the treatment of hypertension.

2. GV20

Location: On the midline of the head halfway between the frontal hairline and the vertex of the external occipital protuberance, or 7 tsun from the posterior hairline and 5 tsun behind the anterior hairline.

Pressure is with the third finger or the thumb directly toward the feet. Hold the point for 20–30 seconds before slowly circling and releasing.

Action: GV20 calms the Spirit, clears the brain, subdues Liver Yang and Wind, and helps spread Liver Qi. It helps the Yang energies ascend to the head to clear the mind.

Comment: This is an Intersecting point of the Six Yang channels, either directly or through their other branches with the Governing Vessel.

3. GB20

Location: In a depression between the SCM and the upper portion of the trapezius.

This point can be accessed bilaterally, whether the patient is in the supine or prone position, by pressing the third finger up toward the occiput. If the third finger is not strong enough by itself, it may be combined with the second finger. Use the pads of the two fingers together to hook up under the occiput.

Action: GB20 subdues Interior Wind, Liver Yang, or Fire Rising. It is used to treat dizziness, stiffness in the neck, and headaches, which often accompany hypertension.

Comment: This is an Intersecting point of the Gall Bladder and San Jiao channels.

4. GB21

Location: Midway between GV14 and the acromion, on the highest point of the shoulder.

This point is pressed bilaterally from the supine or prone position, using the thumbs. The force is slightly medial and down toward the feet.

Action: GB21 relaxes the sinews and treats neck, shoulder, and back pain.

Comment: This is an Intersecting point of the Gall Bladder and San Jiao channels.

5. Lu1

Location: On the lateral aspect of the chest, in the intercostal space between the first and second ribs, 6 tsun lateral to the midline of the chest.

Using the pad of the index finger, third finger, or thumb, press down and direct the pressure toward the center of the chest.

Action: Lu1 regulates the Lung, catalyzes the descending function of the Lung, opens up the chest, and calms the patient. It treats tightness and pain in the chest and shoulders.

Comment: This point is the Mu point for the Lung. It is also an Intersecting point of the Lung and Spleen channels.

6. Sp20

Location: In the second intercostal space directly below Lu1, 6 tsun lateral to the Conception Vessel.

Using the pad of the index finger, third finger, or thumb, press down and direct the pressure toward the table.

Action: This point relaxes and opens up the chest and calms the patient.

7. CV17

Location: Midway between the nipples at the center of the sternum.

Pressure is activated with the pad of the middle finger gently pressing directly toward the table.

Action: CV17 releases stagnant emotional energy trapped in the chest and tonifies the Qi of the Upper Burner. This point helps breathing by opening up the chest, and releases emotional stress, tension, and pain in the chest.

Comment: This is the Mu point for the Heart Envelope and Upper Burner, and Influential point of the Qi. It is also an Intersecting point for the Spleen, Kidney, Small Intestine, San Jiao, and Heart Envelope channels.

8. CV12

Location: Midway between the end of the sternum and the umbilicus, or 4 tsun above the umbilicus on the anterior midline of the body.

The point is activated with the thumb or third finger. Rest one hand gently above CV12, palm down, to help stabilize the point pressure of the thumb or third finger of the opposite hand. Ask the patient to inhale, and to exhale slowly. As the patient exhales, apply pressure directly toward the table until a slight pulsation is felt. Hold the point for 15–30 seconds and then slowly release. As you release your pressure, begin circling your finger.

Action: CV12 harmonizes the Middle Burner, reverses the flow of Rebellious Qi, and strengthens the Spleen. This point is also helpful for bringing the emotional energy down from the chest toward the feet, and opening up the chest. It also treats cardiac pain.

Comment: This is the Mu point for the Stomach as well as for the Middle Burner. It is an Intersecting point of the Small Intestine, San Jiao, and Stomach channels. It is also the Influential point of the Yang Organs.

9. Ht3

Location: Between the medial end of the transverse cubital crease and the medial epicondyle of the humerus, with the elbow bent.

Grasp the elbow with your hand that is closest to the patient's body. Using the pad of your thumb, press laterally directly toward the joint space of the medial epicondyle of the humerus. Hold the point for approximately 15 seconds or longer, depending on the emotional condition of the patient.

Action: Ht3 calms the Shen and therefore the emotions. It helps clear Heat or Fire from the Heart and regulates the flow of Blood and Qi; it also treats chest pain.

Comment: This is the Sea and Water point of the Heart Channel.

10. TS-FA2

Location: One finger space below Ht3, on the medial side of the tendon.

Using the pad of the thumb, press into the tendon.

Action: This point calms the Spirit, treats pain in the heart area of the chest, and treats dizziness.

11. Co4

Location: In the center of the flesh between the first and second metacarpal bones, closer to the second metacarpal bone.

Grasp the patient's thumb so that the second and third fingers fall on the palmar aspect of the patient's hand. Gently push up on the palmar aspect of the web that lies between the thumb and index finger. Using the thumb of the opposite hand, place its lateral side on the radial edge of the second metacarpal bone, then roll the lateral edge of the thumb into the depression on the second metacarpal bone. Pressure is toward the second metacarpal bone.

Action: This point treats the face and head. It subdues Interior Wind from the head, and calms the mind in combination with Liv2. It is used as a distal point for treating the head and face, particularly for frontal headaches that accompany hypertension.

Comment: This is the Organ point of the Colon.

12. Co11

Location: In the depression at the lateral end of the transverse cubital crease; midway between Lu5 and the lateral epicondyle of the humerus, when the elbow is half-flexed.

Bend the patient's elbow and place your thumb on the point. Gently open the arm and press. The force is straight into the joint.

Action: Co11 benefits the sinews and joints and therefore can be used in relaxing and opening the circulation in the blood vessels and channels of the neck and shoulders. It clears Interior Heat, and is used for hypertension originating from Liver Fire Rising.

Comment: This is the Sea and Earth point of the Colon Channel.

13. TS-HA1

Location: On the palmar surface

between Ht8 and HE8 (P8).

Hold the patient's hand, placing the pad of the thumb on the point. Pressure is directly into the palm. Upon releasing, thumb stroke between the fourth and fifth metacarpals toward the fingertips.

Action: This point clears Heart Fire, subdues Wind, calms the Spirit, and reduces blood pressure.

14. St36

Location: 3 tsun below St35, 1 tsun lateral to the anterior crest of the tibia. (St35 is at the lateral foramen of the patella.)

Stand alongside the patient facing the patient's knee. Place the pad of the thumb of the hand closest to the patient's head on the point. Gently hold the foot with the other hand and tilt the leg toward your body as you press toward the tibia. This will direct more pressure into the point. This point may be held for 15–30 seconds. Circle as you release your pressure.

Action: This point tonifies the body. It regulates and tonifies the Stomach, Spleen, Lung, Kidney, and Colon, and regulates both Wei Qi and Nutrient Qi, thereby strengthening the resistance of the body against disease.

Comment: This is the Sea and Earth point of the Stomach Channel.

15. St40

Location: 8 tsun below St35 and 2 tsun lateral to the anterior crest of the tibia.

Pressure is with the pad of the thumb toward the tibia.

Action: This point calms the Spirit and transforms Phlegm and Dampness in all parts of the body.

Comment: This is the Luo point of the Stomach Channel.

16. Liv5

Location: 5 tsun proximal to the vertex of the medial malleolus, in a depression on the medial aspect of the tibia.

Pressure is applied with the pad of the thumb directly into the depression.

Action: Liv5 regulates the smooth flow of Liver Qi and helps to remove obstructions from the channel.

Comment: This is the Luo point of the Liver Channel.

17. Sp6

Location: 3 tsun proximal to the vertex of the medial malleolus, just posterior to the tibial border.

Stand at the foot of the table. Grasp the patient's leg with your hand and place the pad of the thumb on the point. Gently press toward the tibia until you feel a sulcus in the bone. Hold the point for 15–30 seconds and then slowly release, circling as you lighten your pressure. This point can be pressed bilaterally.

Action: Sp6 tonifies the Spleen, Liver, and Kidney. It is an important point for promoting the smooth flow of Liver Qi to help calm the Shen. It nourishes Blood and Yin and treats the symptoms of Kidney Yin Deficiency.

Comment: This point is the Intersecting point of the three Yin channels of the leg.

18. Sp4

Location: Approximately 1 tsun proximal to Sp3, in the depression distal and inferior to the base of the first metatarsal bone at the border of the red and white skin. This point may be pressed bilaterally.

Standing at the foot of the table, grasp the dorsum of the patient's foot with your hand so that the thumbs naturally fall below the arch of the foot. Pressure is with the thumb toward the metatarsal bone.

Action: Sp4 tonifies the Stomach and Spleen. As the Confluent point of the Penetrating Vessel, Sp4 influences the circulation of Qi and Blood in the chest.

Comment: This is the Luo point (Connecting Point) for the Spleen and is also a Confluent Point of the Penetrating Vessel.

19. Liv2

Location: 0.5 tsun proximal to the margin of the web between the first and second toes.

Grasp the patient's toe with your hand and press into the lateral joint space with your thumb. Angle your thumb to fit into the joint space. This point may be more tender than others and should be pressed gently at first and then with increasing pressure. Hold for 15–30 seconds and then slowly release, circling as you lighten your pressure.

Action: Liv2 helps to sedate Rising Liver Fire and Wind, releases stress, and calms the Spirit. It treats headaches due to Excess Liver Fire or Wind, dizziness, and insomnia.

Comment: Liv2 can be used in combination with Co4 to sedate the Liver Qi. This is the Spring and Fire point of the Liver Channel.

20. Liv3

Location: In the depression distal to the junction of the first and second metatarsal bones.

Pressure is applied with the pad of the thumb and directed toward the first metatarsal.

Action: This point tonifies the Liver; regulates the flow of Liver Qi and Blood;

subdues Liver Yang and Wind; clears Liver Fire; redirects Rebellious Liver Qi downward; and treats headaches, dizziness, and insomnia.

Comment: This is the Organ, Stream, and Earth point of the Liver Channel.

21. Ht7

Location: On the transverse crease of the palmar surface of the wrist, between the pisiform bone and the ulna, in the depression on the radial side of the tendon of the flexor carpi ulnaris.

Place the thumb pad between the pisiform bone and the end of the ulna. Hook with the thumb pad and pull toward the pisiform bone.

Action: Ht7 calms the mind and Spirit, clears Fire from the Heart, and treats anxiety and insomnia.

Comment: This is the Organ, Stream, and Earth point of the Heart Channel.

22. Ki6

Location: On the medial aspect of the foot, 1 tsun distal to the lower border of the medial malleolus.

Pressure is with the pad of the thumb into the point.

Action: Ki6 calms the Spirit, treats Kidney Yin Deficiency, and helps to open and relax the chest.

23. Ki2

Location: In the depression distal to the lower border of the tuberosity of the navicular bone.

Pressure is with the thumb or third finger into the depression.

Action: This point clears Apparent Yang from the Kidney; it also treats agitation, irritability, and uneasiness.

Comment: This is the Spring and Fire point of the Kidney Channel.

24. Bl14

Location: 1.5 tsun lateral to the lower border of the spinous process of the fourth thoracic vertebra.

Pressure is applied bilaterally, with the pad of the thumb or the third finger directed toward the table.

Action: Bl14 harmonizes the Heart and treats heart conditions, including hypertension.

Comment: This is the Yu point (Associated point) of the Heart Envelope.

25. Bl15

Location: 1.5 tsun lateral to the lower border of the spinous process of the fifth thoracic vertebra.

Pressure is with the pad of the thumb or the third finger, directed toward the table. Pressure is applied bilaterally.

Action: Bl15 calms the Shen. It treats mental agitation due to Heart Fire and also treats chest pain due to Blood Stasis.

Comment: This is the Yu point (Associated point) of the Heart.

26. Bl18

Location: 1.5 tsun lateral to the lower border of the spinous process of the ninth thoracic vertebra.

Pressure is applied bilaterally with the thumbs, straight down toward the table.

Action: This point regulates and tonifies the Liver. It treats Liver Qi Stagnation and subdues Liver Yang and Liver Fire.

Comment: This is the Yu point (Associated point) of the Liver.

APPENDIX

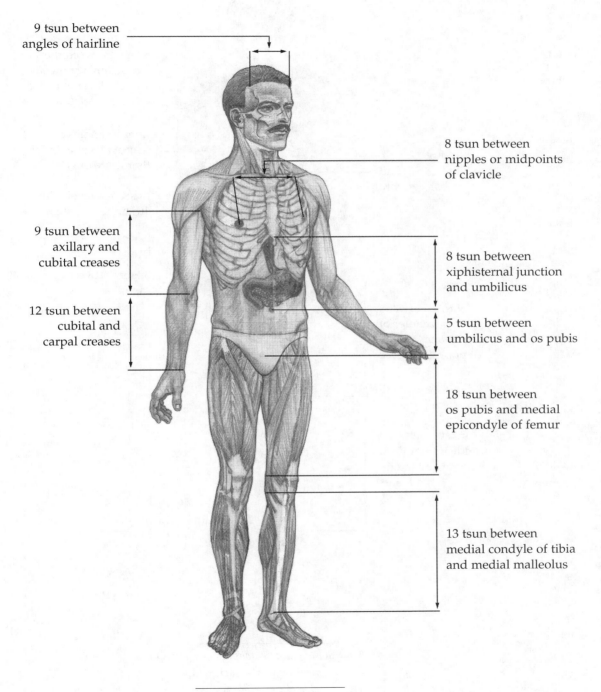

9 tsun between
angles of hairline

8 tsun between
nipples or midpoints
of clavicle

9 tsun between
axillary and
cubital creases

8 tsun between
xiphisternal junction
and umbilicus

12 tsun between
cubital and
carpal creases

5 tsun between
umbilicus and os pubis

18 tsun between
os pubis and medial
epicondyle of femur

13 tsun between
medial condyle of tibia
and medial malleolus

*Traditional Chinese acupuncture units of
measurement—front view*

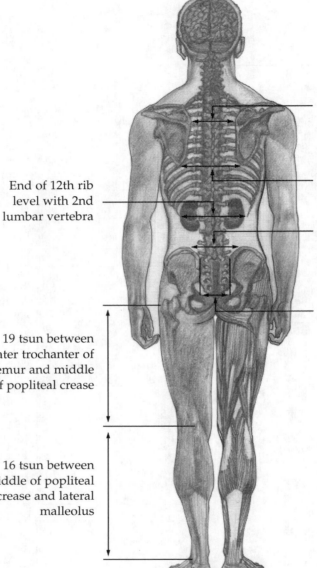

6 tsun between the
two scapula spine at
scapula level with 3rd
thoracic vertebra

Inferior angle of
scapula level with 7th
thoracic vertebra

End of 12th rib
level with 2nd
lumbar vertebra

Iliac crest level with
4th lumbar vertebra

3 tsun between
sacroiliac joints

19 tsun between
greater trochanter of
femur and middle
of popliteal crease

16 tsun between
middle of popliteal
crease and lateral
malleolus

Traditional Chinese acupuncture units of
measurement—back view

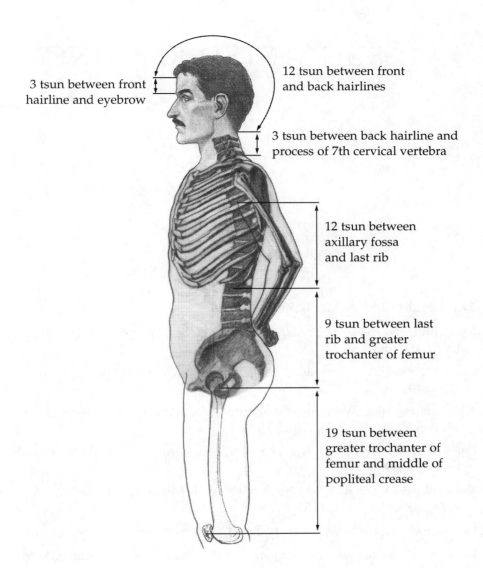

3 tsun between front
hairline and eyebrow

12 tsun between front
and back hairlines

3 tsun between back hairline and
process of 7th cervical vertebra

12 tsun between
axillary fossa
and last rib

9 tsun between last
rib and greater
trochanter of femur

19 tsun between
greater trochanter of
femur and middle of
popliteal crease

*Traditional Chinese acupuncture units of
measurement—side view*

SUGGESTED READING

Traditional Chinese Medicine

Chen, Jirui, and Nissi Wang, eds. *Acupuncture Case Histories from China*. Seattle, Wash.: Eastland, 1988.

Cheng, Xinnong, ed. *Chinese Acupuncture and Moxibustion*. Beijing: Foreign Languages Press, 1997.

Ellis, Andrew, Nigel Wiseman, and Ken Boss. *Fundamentals of Chinese Acupuncture*, Rev. ed. Brookline, Mass.: Paradigm, 1991.

Ellis, Andrew, Nigel Wiseman, and Ken Boss. *Grasping the Wind*. Brookline, Mass.: Paradigm, 1989.

Kaptchuk, Ted J. *The Web That Has No Weaver: Understanding Chinese Medicine*. Chicago, Ill.: Congdon & Weed, 1983.

Lade, Arnie. *Acupuncture Points: Images & Functions*. Seattle, Wash.: Eastland, 1989.

Li, Xuemei, and Jingyi Zhao. *Acupuncture Patterns & Practice*. Seattle, Wash.: Eastland, 1993.

Low, Royston. *The Secondary Vessels of Acupuncture: A Detailed Account of Their Energies, Meridians and Control Points*. Wellingborough, Great Britain: Thorsons, 1983.

Maciocia, Giovanni. *Foundations of Chinese Medicine: A Comprehensive Text for Acupuncturists and Herbalists*. Edinburgh, Scotland: Churchill Livingstone, 1989.

Mann, Felix. *Acupuncture: The Ancient Chinese Art of Healing and How It Works Scientifically*. New York: Random House, 1962.

O'Connor, John, and Dan Bensky, trans. and eds. *Acupuncture: A Comprehensive Text*. Seattle, Wash.: Eastland, 1993.

Porket, Manfred, Christian Ullmann, and Mark Howson, trans. *Chinese Medicine*. New York: Henry Holt, 1988.

Ross, Jeremy. *Zang Fu: The Organ Systems of Traditional Chinese Medicine*. 2nd ed. Edinburgh, Scotland: Churchill Livingstone, 1985.

Sohn, Robert C. *Tao and T'ai Chi Kung.* Rochester, Vt.: Destiny, 1989.

Uncshuld, Paul U., trans. *Nan-Ching: The Classic of Difficult Issues.* Berkeley, Calif.: University of California Press, 1986.

Veith, Ilza, trans. *Huang Ti Nei Ching Su Wen* (The Yellow Emperor's Classic of Internal Medicine). New ed. Berkeley, Calif.: University of California Press, 1949.

Wiseman, Nigel, trans. *Zhong Yi Xue Ji Chu.* (Fundamentals of Chinese Medicine) Rev. ed. Brookline, Mass.: Paradigm, 1995.

Zmiewski, Paul, and Richard Feit. *Acumoxa Therapy: A Reference and Study Guide.* Brookline, Mass.: Paradigm, 1989.

Zmiewski, Paul, and Richard Feit. *Acumoxa Therapy: A Reference and Study Guide II: The Treatment of Disease.* Brookline, Mass.: Paradigm, 1990.

Western Medicine

Anderson, James E. *Grant's Atlas of Anatomy.* 7th ed. Baltimore, Md.: Williams & Wilkins, 1978.

Cailliet, Rene. *Low Back Pain Syndrome.* 5th ed. Philadelphia, Pa.: F. A. Davis, 1995.

Cailliet, Rene. *Neck and Arm Pain.* 3rd ed. Philadelphia, Pa.: F. A. Davis, 1991.

Cailliet, Rene. *Shoulder Pain.* 3rd ed. Philadelphia, Pa.: F. A. Davis, 1991.

Cailliet, Rene. *Understanding Your Backache: A Guide to Prevention, Treatment, and Relief.* Philadelphia, Pa.: F. A. Davis, 1984.

Cox, James M. *Low Back Pain: Mechanism, Diagnosis, and Treatment.* 5th ed. Baltimore, Md.: Williams & Wilkins, 1990.

Cox, James M. *Low Back Pain: Mechanism, Diagnosis, and Treatment.* 5th ed. Baltimore, Md.: Williams & Wilkins, 1990.

Eisenberg, David M., et al. "Unconventional Medicine in the United States: Prevalence, Costs, and Patterns of Use." *New England Journal of Medicine,* 28 January 1993, 246–252.

Lappe, Marc. *Evolutionary Medicine: Rethinking the Origins of Disease.* San Francisco, Calif.: Sierra Club, 1994.

Levy, S. M. "Interventions in Behavioral Medicine." *Cancer* 50 (1982): 1928–35.

Lewis, Sharon Mantik, and Idolia Cox Collier. *Medical-Surgical Nursing: Assessment and Management of Clinical Problems.* 3rd ed. Saint Louis, Mo.: Mosby, 1992.

Lubec, G., et al. "Amino Acid Isomerisation and Microwave Exposure." *Lancet,* 9 December 1989, 1392–93.

Mendelsohn, Robert S. *Confessions of a Medical Heretic.* Chicago, Ill.: Contemporary Books, 1979.

Mendelsohn, Robert S. *How to Raise a Healthy Child . . . In Spite of Your Doctor.* New York: Ballantine, 1984.

Upledger, John E. *Craniosacral Therapy II: Beyond the Dura.* Seattle, Wash.: Eastland, 1987.

Upledger, John E., and Jon D. Vredevoogd. *Craniosacral Therapy.* Seattle, Wash.: Eastland, 1983.

Warfel, John H. *The Extremities: Muscle and Motor Points.* 5th ed. Philadelphia, Pa.: Lea & Febiger, 1985.

Warfel, John H. *The Head, Neck, and Trunk.* 5th ed. Philadelphia, Pa.: Lea & Febiger, 1985.

Wyngaarden, James B., Lloyd H. Smith, and Claude Bennett. *Cecil Textbook of Medicine.* 19th ed. Philadelphia, Pa.: W. B. Saunders, 1992.

Nutrition

Braverman, Eric, and Carl Pfeiffer. *The Healing Nutrients Within: Facts, Findings and New Research on Amino Acids.* New Canaan, Conn.: Keats, 1987.

Colbin, Annemarie. *Food and Healing.* New York: Ballantine, 1986.

Dufty, William. *Sugar Blues.* New York: Warner, 1975.

Matesz, Don. "The Sweet Taste of Qi." *Qi: The Journal of Traditional Eastern Health* 2 (1992): 22–29.

McDougall, John A., and Mary A. McDougall. *The McDougall Plan.* Piscataway, N.J.: New Century, 1983.

Oski, Frank. *Don't Drink Your Milk.* Syracuse, N.Y.: Molica, 1983.

Pfeiffer, Carl. *Mental and Elemental Nutrients.* New Canaan, Conn.: Keats, 1975.

Pitchford, Paul. *Healing with Whole Foods: Oriental Traditions and Modern Nutrition.* Berkeley, Calif.: North Atlantic, 1993.

Whitney, Eleanor Noss, and Sharon Rady Rolfes. *Understanding Nutrition.* 6th ed. New York: West Publishing, 1993.

Wholistic Psychology

Church, Dawson, and Alan Sherr. *Heart of the Healer.* New York: Aslan, 1987.

Dossey, B. M., and C. E. Guzzetta. "Implications for Bio-Psycho-Social-Spiritual Concerns in Cardiovascular Nursing." *Journal of Cardiovascular Nursing* 8 (1994): 72–88.

Hammer, Leon. *Dragon Rises, Red Bird Flies: Psychology, Energy & Chinese Medicine.* Barrytown, N.Y.: Station Hill, 1990.

Millenson, J. R. *Mind Matters: Psychological Medicine in Holistic Practice.* Seatle, Wash.: Eastland, 1995.

Morrison, R. "Interrelationship of the Mind, Body and Emotions in the Cancer Fight." *Radiologic Technology,* 62 (1990): 28–31.

Pelletier, Kenneth R. *Mind As Healer—Mind As Slayer: A Holistic Approach to Preventing Stress Disorders.* New York: Dell, 1977.

Sheldon, William, and S. S. Stevens. *The Varieties of Temperament: A Psychology of Constitutional Differences.* New York: Hafner, 1970.

BIBLIOGRAPHY

Anderson, James E. *Grant's Atlas of Anatomy,* 7th ed. Baltimore, Md.: Williams & Wilkins, 1978.

Braverman, Eric, and Carl Pfeiffer. *The Healing Nutrients Within: Facts, Findings and New Research on Amino Acids.* New Canaan, Conn.: Keats, 1987.

Cailliet, Rene. *Low Back Pain Syndrome.* 5th ed. Philadelphia, Pa.: F. A. Davis, 1995.

———. *Neck and Arm Pain.* 3rd ed. Philadelphia, Pa.: F. A. Davis, 1991.

———. *Shoulder Pain.* 3rd ed. Philadelphia, Pa.: F. A. Davis, 1991.

———. *Understanding Your Backache: A Guide to Prevention, Treatment, and Relief.* Philadelphia, Pa.: F. A. Davis, 1984.

Cantekin, E. I., T. W. McGuire, and T. L. Griffith. "Antimicrobial Therapy for Otitis Media with Effusion (Secretory Otitis Media)." *Journal of the American Medical Association* 266 (1991): 3309–17.

Cheng, Xinnong, ed. *Chinese Acupuncture and Moxibustion.* Beijing: Foreign Languages Press, 1997.

Church, Dawson, and Alan Sherr. *Heart of the Healer.* New York: Aslan, 1987.

Colbin, Annemarie. *Food and Healing.* New York: Ballantine, 1986.

Cox, James M. *Low Back Pain: Mechanism, Diagnosis, and Treatment.* 5th ed. Baltimore, Md.: Williams & Wilkins, 1990.

Dossey, B. M., and C. E. Guzzetta. "Implications for Bio-Psycho-Social-Spiritual Concerns in Cardiovascular Nursing." *Journal of Cardiovascular Nursing* 8 (1994): 72–88.

Dufty, William. *Sugar Blues.* New York: Warner, 1975.

Eisenberg, David M., et al. "Unconventional Medicine in the United States: Prevalence, Costs, and Patterns of Use." *New England Journal of Medicine,* 28 January 1993, 246–252.

Ellis, Andrew, Nigel Wiseman, and Ken Boss. *Fundamentals of Chinese Acupuncture.* Rev ed. Brookline, Mass.: Paradigm, 1991.

Lade, Arnie. *Acupuncture Points: Images & Functions.* Seattle, Wash.: Eastland, 1989.

Lappe, Marc. *Evolutionary Medicine: Rethinking the Origins of Disease.* San Francisco, Calif.: Sierra Club, 1994.

Levy, S. M. "Interventions in Behavioral Medicine." *Cancer* 50 (1982): 1928–35.

Lewis, Sharon Mantik, and Idolia Cox Collier. *Medical-Surgical Nursing: Assessment and Management of Clinical Problems.* 3rd ed. Saint Louis, Mo.: Mosby, 1992.

Low, Royston. *The Secondary Vessels of Acupuncture: A Detailed Account of Their Energies, Meridians and Control Points.* Wellingborough, Great Britain: Thorsons, 1983.

Lubec, G., et al. "Amino Acid Isomerisation and Microwave Exposure." *Lancet,* 9 December 1989, 1392–93.

Maciocia, Giovanni. *Foundations of Chinese Medicine: A Comprehensive Text for Acupuncturists and Herbalists.* Edinburgh, Scotland: Churchill Livingstone, 1989.

Matesz, Don. "The Sweet Taste of Qi." *Qi: The Journal of Traditional Eastern Health* 2 (1992): 22–29.

McDougall, John A., and Mary A. McDougall. *The McDougall Plan.* Piscataway, N.J.: New Century, 1983.

Mendelsohn, Robert S. *How to Raise a Healthy Child . . . In Spite of Your Doctor.* New York: Ballantine, 1984.

Morrison, R. "Interrelationship of the Mind, Body and Emotions in the Cancer Fight." *Radiologic Technology* 62 (1990): 28–31.

O'Connor, John, and Dan Bensky, trans. and eds. *Acupuncture: A Comprehensive Text.* Seattle, Wash.: Eastland, 1993.

Oski, Frank. *Don't Drink Your Milk.* Syracuse, N.Y.: Molica, 1983.

Pfeiffer, Carl. *Mental and Elemental Nutrients.* New Canaan, Conn.: Keats, 1975.

Pitchford, Paul. *Healing with Whole Foods: Oriental Traditions and Modern Nutrition.* Berkeley, Calif.: North Atlantic, 1993.

Porket, Manfred and Christian Ullmann, and Mark Howson, trans. *Chinese Medicine.* New York: Henry Holt, 1988.

Sheldon, William, and S. S. Stevens. *The Varieties of Temperament: A Psychology of Constitutional Differences.* New York: Hafner, 1970.

Sohn, Robert C. *Tao and T'ai Chi Kung.* Rochester, Vt.: Destiny, 1989.

Uncshuld, Paul U., trans. *Nan-Ching: The Classic of Difficult Issues.* Berkeley, Calif.: University of California Press, 1986.

Upledger, John E. *Craniosacral Therapy II: Beyond the Dura.* Seattle, Wash.: Eastland, 1987.

Upledger, John E., and Jon D. Vredevoogd. *Craniosacral Therapy.* Seattle, Wash.: Eastland, 1983.

Veith, Ilza, trans. *Huang Ti Nei Ching Su Wen* (The Yellow Emperor's Classic of Internal Medicine). New ed. Berkeley, Calif.: University of California Press, 1949.

Warfel, John H. *The Extremities: Muscle and Motor Points.* 5th ed. Philadelphia, Pa.: Lea & Febiger, 1985.

———. *The Head, Neck, and Trunk.* 5th ed. Philadelphia, Pa.: Lea & Febiger, 1985.

Whitney, Eleanor Noss, and Sharon Rady Rolfes. *Understanding Nutrition.* 6th ed. New York: West Publishing, 1993.

Wiseman, Nigel, trans. *Zhong Yi Xue Ji Chu* (Fundamentals of Chinese Medicine). Rev. ed. Brookline, Mass.: Paradigm, 1995.

Wyngaarden, James B., Lloyd H. Smith, and Claude Bennett. *Cecil Textbook of Medicine.* 19th ed. Philadelphia, Pa.: W. B. Saunders, 1992.

INDEX

for Spleen, 323, 338, 352
for Stomach, 324, 338, 352
Yuan Qi, 316
Yuan points, 64, 254
Zang Organs, 60, 154–155
Zang-Fu, 132, 134, 153

Zhang Xiang Xue Shou, 58
Zhen Qi. *See* True Qi.
Zheng Qi. *See* Upright Qi.
Zhi, 121–122
Zhong Qi. *See* Center Qi.
Zong Qi. *See* Pectoral Qi.